Male Infertility

Karthik Gunasekaran • N Pandiyan
Editors

Male Infertility

A Clinical Approach

Springer

Editors
Karthik Gunasekaran
Metromale Clinic,
Gunasekaran Hospital Pvt Ltd
Chennai
India

N Pandiyan
Department of Andrology and Reproductive Medicine
Chettinad Hospital and Research Institute
Chennai
India

ISBN 978-81-322-3602-3 ISBN 978-81-322-3604-7 (eBook)
DOI 10.1007/978-81-322-3604-7

Library of Congress Control Number: 2016953337

Printed on acid-free paper

This Springer imprint is published by Springer Nature
The registered company is Springer (India) Pvt. Ltd.
The registered company address is 7th Floor, Vijaya Building, 17 Barakhamba Road, New Delhi 110 001, India

Preface

Infertility in men is an important cause of barren marriage. Male infertility is on the rise and the world wide prevalence of male infertility now stands at 7 %, an incidence even more than diabetes mellitus. Yet sadly, we, the medical community at large, have chosen to ignore this problem. Until a few decades ago, this area was wide open with almost all medical practitioners handling the field. Besides urologists, gynecologists, and embryologists who are probably the rightful inheritors of the field, specialists in venereology, dermatology, endocrinology, and internal medicine were also practicing male infertility with very little or formal training in the field. Universities offering training in this branch of reproductive medicine were also few.

The advent of assisted reproductive technologies and intracytoplasmic sperm injection (ICSI) made a paradigm change in the management of male infertility. However, an increase in failed ICSI procedures and declining male fertility have made physicians dwell deep into the realm of male infertility. Many hitherto unproven therapies have fallen into disrepute. Many conditions untreatable few decades ago have become treatable now with the introduction of ICSI and sperm retrieval techniques. There is an urgent need for good understanding of the principles and practice of male infertility. This book hopes to fulfill this need.

The chapters in this book have been hand-picked to provide the gynecologists, urologists, endocrinologists, and fertility specialists in-depth information about male infertility and aim to serve as a reference point with detailed descriptions and practical analysis by leading practitioners in the field of men's health.

We would like to thank our teachers, our patients, the andrology fellows, our contributing authors, and all other research staff, without whom this book would not have been possible. We specially acknowledge the great contribution rendered by Dr. C. Siddharth, Embryologist and Andrologist, in the initial phase of the project.

We value your feedback; this will help us improve the future editions of the book.

Chennai, India — Karthik Gunasekaran
Chennai, India — N. Pandiyan

Acknowledgments

The Editors gratefully acknowledge the help rendered by many people to make this book a reality.

Dr. Shah Dupesh Khan, Chief Consultant in Andrology and Men's Health, Women's Center, Chennai, has been a source of continuous, constant, and great support in getting this book to the present shape. Besides contributing chapters in time, he also helped immensely in the numerous correspondences with the authors and in editing this book.

Authors from various parts of the world contributed chapters, mostly on time, despite their numerous professional commitments, thus helping the timely release of this book.

Our publisher, Springer and its dynamic executives: Ms. Eti has been instrumental for the launch of this book; Mr. Kumar and Mr. Mahesh gently but constantly prodded us and helped in completion of this book by their continuous reminders to all of us.

Chennai, India — Karthik Gunasekaran
Chennai, India — N. Pandiyan

Contents

About the Editors

Karthik Gunasekaran graduated from Madras Medical College in General Surgery with a gold medal in Urology. Interest in Pelvic Floor Dysfunction made him pursue a Fellowship in Urogynecology from the Cleveland Clinic Foundation, USA. On his return, he founded the Indian Urogynecological society, the first society for Urogynecology and Pelvic Floor Dysfunction in India. An avidly sought after speaker and surgical demonstrator, he pioneered the use of mesh in pelvic floor surgery in India.

Men's health, a field which spawned his interest, was yet a nascent area in medicine in India, and Dr. Karthik began his training with Prof. Pandiyan at the Chettinad Hospital and Research Institute in Chennai. Preceptorships in male infertility at the Turek Clinic in the United States under Dr. Paul Turek and sexual health in San Diego Sexual Medicine under Prof. Irwin Goldstein followed. A certification in sexual health training was obtained when Dr. Karthik completed his FECSM from Oxford University, UK. He is of the firm belief that men's health is taking a back seat in India, especially in fertility and sexual health. He founded the Metromale Clinic, a first of its kind all male clinic for male fertility and sexual health in Chennai. His weekly live talk show, Dr. X, on the Sun Network, is critically acclaimed and has over a million hits on YouTube. He currently serves as Director of Metromale Clinic and is also the Managing Director of Gunasekaran Hospitals Pvt Ltd in Chennai.

He lives in Chennai with his wife Manu and children Sara and Arav.

Prof. Dr. N. Pandiyan currently is the Head of the Department and Chief Consultant in Andrology and Reproductive medicine, Dept. of Andrology and Reproductive medicine, Chettinad Super Specialty Hospital, Kelambakkam, Chennai, and the Chief Editor of Chettinad Health City Medical Journal. He has had a long and distinguished academic and professional career. He won many gold medals and prizes, during his undergraduate and postgraduate medical courses. He was awarded first rank in the University of Madras for excellence in Post Graduate Diploma and Degree in Obstetrics and Gynaecology. He scored first rank at All India level in MNAMS examination. He was the only Scholar from India in Gynaecology for the prestigious Commonwealth scholarship programme in 1985, which earned him Fellowship in Male and Female infertility at University of Nottingham, UK, for

2 years. Upon his return to India, he established the first joint Infertility Clinic in Government General Hospital, Chennai, in 1987, earning the unique distinction of pioneering the beginning of Andrology and Reproductive Medicine, the new sub-specialty of Obstetrics and Gynaecology, in the country.

Dr. Pandiyan was also responsible for setting up of Infertility Centres in many private institutions and trained numerous aspiring gynaecologists from all over India. On the academic side, he held many prestigious posts as Head of Departments in Chennai and Brunei Darussalam; Examiner for many local, national, and international level examinations; invited speaker for many national and international conferences; serving on the expert committees of ICMR and Department of Science and Technology; one among the doyens in this specialty to formulate National Guidelines for the practice of ART; and author of several publications and books related to human reproduction. The Tamil Nadu Dr. MGR Medical University recognized his yeoman services in this field and awarded him with "Life time achievement award". He is still continuing his academic mission of training young medical graduates in all aspects of human reproduction, motivating research and innovative thinking in this sub-specialty.

Anatomy and Development of the Male Reproductive System

1

Sneha Guruprasad Kalthur and Guruprasad Kalthur

The male reproductive system includes the gonads, external genitalia, reproductive tracts, and accessory sex glands (Fig. 1.1). It has two major functions: production of male gametes known as spermatozoa and delivery of the male gametes into the female reproductive tract (Table 1.1).

Penis It is the male organ of copulation which comprises of an attached portion called root (that lies within the perineum) and a free, pendulous part called body which is completely covered by a thin, dark colored skin. At the neck of the penis, the skin is folded upon itself to form the prepuce (foreskin) which covers the glans to a varying extent and that can be retracted back and forth. The root consists of three masses of erectile tissue, which includes two crura and a bulb, while the body is composed of three masses of erectile tissue (two corpora cavernosum and one corpus spongiosum). The shape of the penis in a flaccid state is cylindrical, and during erection, it resembles a triangular prism with rounded angle. Erection of the penis is a neurovascular phenomenon independent of muscular compression. Factors responsible for the erection are the rapid inflow of blood from the helicine arteries which fill the spaces of corpora cavernosa leading to distention of the erectile tissue. The distended corpora cavernosa retards the outflow of blood by compressing the veins (Woodhouse and Kellett 1984).

S.G. Kalthur (✉)
Department of Anatomy, Kasturba Medical College, Manipal University,
Manipal, Karnataka 576104, India
e-mail: sneha.guruprasad@manipal.edu

G. Kalthur
Division of Clinical Embryology, Department of Obstetrics and Gynecology,
Kasturba Medical College, Manipal University, Manipal, Karnataka 576104, India

K. Gunasekaran, N. Pandiyan (eds.), *Male Infertility*,
DOI 10.1007/978-81-322-3604-7_1

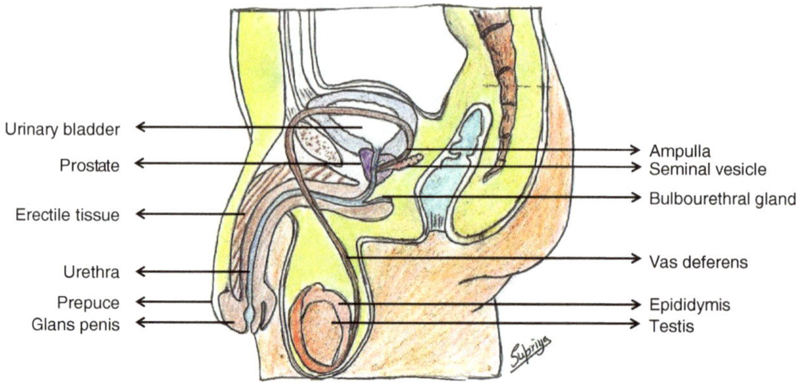

Fig. 1.1 Parts of male reproductive system

Table 1.1 Outlines the components of the male reproductive system

Components of the male reproductive system	
External genital organ	Penis
Gonads	A pair of testicles
Reproductive tracts	Epididymis, vas deferens, ejaculatory duct, penile part of urethra
Accessory sex glands	Prostate, seminal vesicle, and bulbourethral glands

Scrotum It is a cutaneous fibromuscular sac containing the testes and the lower part of the spermatic cords (Fig. 1.2). The layers of this sac from outside to inside include the skin, dartos muscle, external spermatic, and cremasteric and internal spermatic fasciae. The scrotum is divided into right and left halves by a cutaneous raphe. The scrotal skin is thin and pigmented and bears scattered hairs. In addition, it has numerous sweat glands and sebaceous glands whose secretion has a characteristic odor. The external appearance of the scrotum varies according to the temperature and age of the male. It is smooth, elongated, and flaccid in elderly men and under warm conditions, whereas it is short, corrugated, and closely applied to the testes in cold conditions and also in the younger age groups. The movement of the testes away from and close to the body depending on the temperature is possible due to the contraction and relaxation of the dartos muscle (Waites 2012).

Testes Testes are the primary reproductive organs or male gonads. They are responsible for sperm production (gametogenesis) and testosterone production (steroidogenesis) in the male. During the fetal period of life, these organs are located high in the abdominal cavity. However, before birth, they descend downward to the inguinal canal into a sac known as the scrotum. An adult man has a pair of testis which measures about 4–5 cm in length, 3 cm in width, and 2.5 cm in thickness, weighing around 10–15 g each. Each testis lies obliquely within the scrotum with a convex anterior aspect and nearly straight posterior aspect which is attached to the spermatic cord. The testis is covered by three layers, which are, from outside to inside,

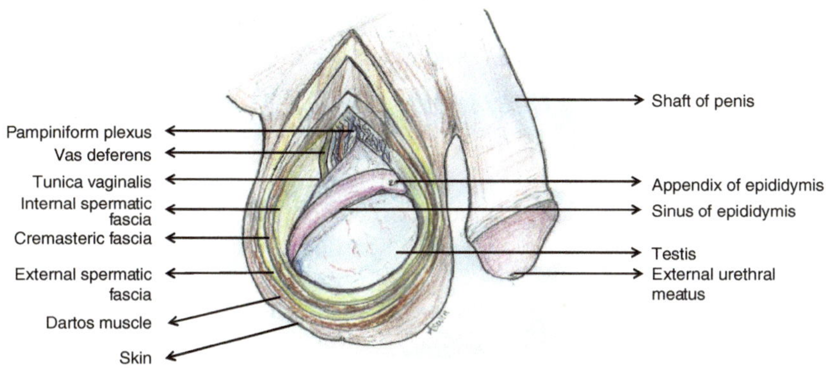

Fig. 1.2 Scrotum and its contents

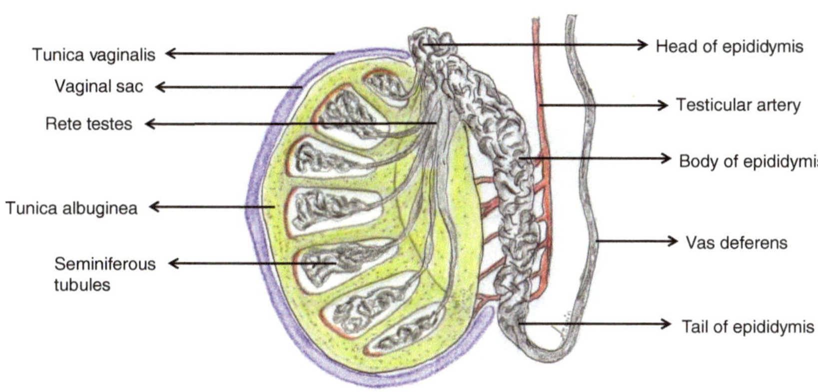

Fig. 1.3 Cross section of testis and epididymis

the tunica vaginalis, a thick fibrous layer of tunica albuginea, and tunica vasculosa. The testis invaginates the tunica vaginalis from behind, and hence the layer covering closely to testis becomes the visceral layer, while the other is called the parietal layer. Both the layers are (Fig. 1.3) separated from one another by a space filled with serous fluid which acts as a lubricant and allows the movement of the testis within the scrotum. The testicular capsule is made up of collagenous and hard tunica albuginea which covers the testis all round and is thickened in the posterior aspect to form the mediastinum testis. A thin layer of connective tissue with blood vessels is present below this layer. The blood vessels, lymphatics, and the genital ducts enter or leave the testis at mediastinum (Johnson 2012).

Septa from the mediastinum of the testis extend internally in a fanlike fashion to divide it into approximately 250 lobules. The largest and longest lobules are found in the center of the testis with each lobule having one to four convoluted seminiferous tubules. The free ends of the seminiferous tubules open into channels known as rete testis within the mediastinum. The connective tissue between the seminiferous tubules contains the Leydig cells and several layers of contractile peritubular myoid cells (Standring 2015).

Seminiferous Tubules Each testis contains around 400–600 seminiferous tubules measuring 70–80 cm in length and 0.12–0.3 mm in diameter. Each tubule is surrounded by a basal lamina which has stratified epithelium consisting of spermatogenic stem cell and the support cells called Sertoli cells (Tubules 1992).

(a) *Sertoli cells:* They are the epithelial support cells present in the seminiferous tubules. Structurally, Sertoli cells are tall, simple columnar cells, which extend from the basement membrane to the lumen of the seminiferous tubule (Fig. 1.4). They are connected to each other by tight junctions to form the blood-testis barrier that divides the tubule into basal (close to the basal lamina) and adluminal (toward the lumen) compartment. The blood-testis barrier isolates the spermatogenic cells and the mature spermatozoa from blood. Differentiating spermatozoa nestle in pockets, in the peripheral cytoplasm of these cells. Sertoli cells produce the testicular fluid and androgen binding protein which binds to and concentrates testosterone. They also help to translocate the differentiating spermatogenic cells to the lumen and phagocytose the degenerating germ cells. They also remove the surplus cytoplasm remaining after the process of spermiogenesis (Grisworld 1998).

(b) *Leydig cells:* These cells are present in the interstitial connective tissue of the testis. They have round nuclei and a polygonal cell body found individually or in clusters. There are two types of Leydig cells: fetal type and adult type. The fetal type starts appearing from the 8th week of intrauterine development and is replaced by the adult type by the third week of neonatal life. Leydig cells secrete testosterone and thus play a significant role in spermatogenesis (Saez 1994).

(c) *Spermatogonia*: They are the stem cells from which spermatozoa are produced. Spermatogonial cells are located on the basal lamina of the seminiferous tubules. Based on their nuclear dimension and chromatin structure, they are classified into dark A type (Ad), pale A type (Ap), and type B cells. The spermatogonial cell population is maintained by mitotically dividing Ad cells which are under the control of androgens. Ap cells also divide mitotically and are the precursors of type B cells that enter the spermatogenic cycle (Rooij and Russell 2000).

(d) *Spermatocytes*: Primary spermatocytes are diploid but have duplicated sister chromatids. Therefore, the DNA content of these cells is 4 N. Primary spermatocytes are large cells with large round nuclei in which the nuclear chromatin is condensed into dark, threadlike coiled chromatids at different stages in the process of crossing over. These cells give rise to secondary spermatocytes with haploid chromosome and DNA content of 2 N (Rooij and Russell 2000).

(e) *Spermatids*: The secondary spermatocytes rapidly undergo second meiotic division to form haploid spermatids. One primary spermatocyte gives rise to four

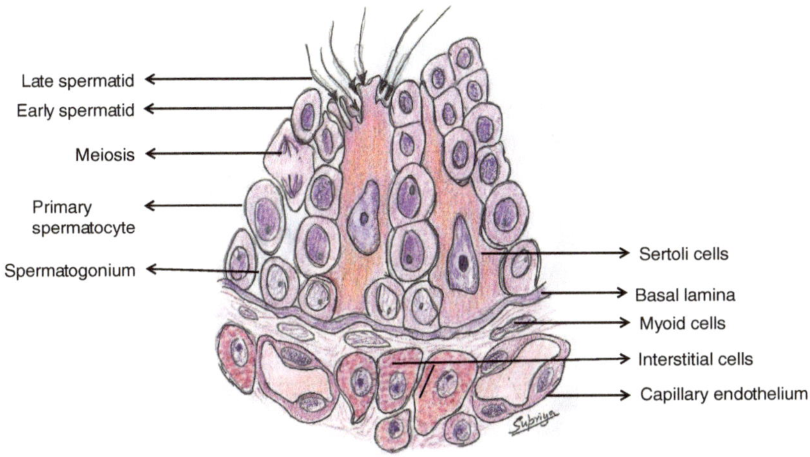

Fig. 1.4 Histology of seminiferous tubule

spermatids. However, few may degenerate during the process of further maturation. Spermatids undergo a series of cytoplasmic and nuclear changes in a process known as *spermiogenesis*. Finally, the functionally mature spermatozoa will be released from the wall of the seminiferous tubule into the lumen by a process called *spermiation* (Rooij and Russell 2000).

Epididymis The efferent ductules perforate the tunica albuginea at the mediastinum and leave the testis to form the epididymis. It can be divided into three parts: a globular head or caput, body, and tail or cauda region. In the head region, the ductules form conical lobules which open into the single duct of epididymis through lobular ducts measuring 15–20 cm in length. The lobular ducts coil and form the body and tail of epididymis. The coils are held together by fibrous connective tissue. The epithelial lining of the epididymal duct contains mainly principal and basal cells and few apical and clear cells. The principal cells are tall columnar cells with apical microvillus termed as stereo cilia. The cells help in reabsorbing the fluid generated from the testicular secretions (Bedford 1978).

Spermatic Cord It is a collection of vessels (testicular artery, testicular veins, testicular lymph vessels, cremasteric artery, and artery of vas deferens), nerves (autonomic nerves and genital branch of the genitofemoral nerve), remnants of the processus vaginalis, and vas deferens which suspends the testis in the scrotum. The left cord is slightly longer than the right, and therefore left testis is at a lower level than the right (Moore et al. 2013).

Vas Deferens It is a cordlike structure which can be palpated between the finger and thumb in the upper part of the scrotum. It is a thick-walled muscular duct measuring approximately 45 cm in length that helps in transporting the spermatozoa from the epididymis to the urethra. It is tortuous in its initial part but becomes straight as it ascends upward (Moore et al. 2013).

Male Urethra It is about 20 cm in length and extends from the neck of the bladder to the external meatus of the glans penis. It can be divided into three parts: prostatic urethra, membranous urethra, and penile urethra. Prostatic urethra is around 3 cm in length which passes through the prostate from base to the apex. It is the widest and the most dilatable portion of the urethra. The membranous urethra on the other hand is the least dilatable portion of urethra measuring about 1.25 cm in length and lies between the urogenital diaphragm, surrounded by the sphincter urethra muscle fibers. The penile urethra is about 15.75 cm in length and is enclosed in the bulb and corpus spongiosum of the penis (Standring 2015).

Seminal Vesicles These are a pair of accessory sex glands located between the bladder and rectum. It is a pyramidal, contorted tube measuring 5 cm in length with the base directed upward lying on the posterior surface of the bladder. The upper ends of the glands are widely separated and their lower ends are close together. On the medial side of the each vesicle, the terminal part of the vas deferens is present. Each seminal vesicle narrows down and joins with the vas deferens of the same side to form the ejaculatory duct (Standring 2015).

The walls of the seminal vesicle contract during ejaculation and expel their secretions into the ejaculatory duct. This helps in washing the spermatozoa out of the urethra. It produces an alkaline secretion which contributes to approximately 70 % of the ejaculate. It is rich in substances which help in nourishing the spermatozoa.

Prostate Gland It is a fibromuscular glandular organ shaped like an inverted cone which surrounds the prostatic urethra. It is approximately 3 cm long and lies in between the neck of the bladder above and the urogenital diaphragm below. The prostate has numerous glands which are embedded in connective tissue and smooth muscles. The ducts of the prostate gland open into the prostatic urethra. The posterior wall of the penile urethra has a longitudinal ridge called urethral crest on either side of which the prostatic sinus are present. The prostatic glands open into these grooves. On the summit of the urethral crest, the prostatic utricle is present, which is an analog of the uterus and vagina in females. On the edge of the mouth of the utricle, openings of the two ejaculatory ducts are present. The prostate gland produces a thin milky fluid which is rich in citric acid and acid phosphatase. Approximately 30 % of the seminal plasma is from the prostatic secretion which is added to the seminal fluid at the time of ejaculation. The smooth muscles of the prostate gland contract to squeeze the prostate and empty their secretion into prostatic urethra (Standring 2015).

Ejaculatory Ducts It is around 2 cm in length which is formed on either side by the union of duct of the seminal vesicle with the ampulla of the vas deferens. The

Table 1.2 Neurovasculature of male reproductive system

Region	Blood supply	Nerve supply
Penis	Internal pudendal artery (deep and dorsal artery of penis, artery of bulb)	S2, 3, 4
Scrotum	Femoral artery (external pudendal), internal pudendal artery (scrotal)	Anterior 1/3rd – L1 Posterior 2/3rd – S3
Testis	Testicular artery	T10, 11
Epididymis	Testicular artery	T 10, 11
Vas deferens	Artery of vas deferens	Pelvic plexus
Seminal vesicle and ejaculatory duct	Internal pudendal artery (inferior vesical and middle rectal)	Pelvic plexus
Prostate	Internal pudendal artery	Prostatic plexus
Bulbourethral glands	Internal pudendal artery (artery to bulb)	Pelvic plexus

two ejaculatory ducts pierce the posterior surface of the prostate and open into the prostatic part of the urethra (McNeal 1981).

Bulbourethral Glands Also known as Cowper's glands are a pair of small, round, and lobulated masses of 1 cm diameter which lies lateral to the membranous urethra above the perineal membrane and the penile bulb. The excretory ducts pass obliquely and penetrate the perineal membrane. It opens by a small orifice on the floor of the bulbar urethra. The secretions are poured into the urethra as a result of erotic stimulation.

Ejaculation It is the process by which the spermatozoa mixed with the seminal fluid are ejected from the penile urethra. During sexual excitement, the external urethral meatus of the glans penis become moist due to secretions of the bulbourethral gland. At the time of orgasm, friction on the glans penis and also the simultaneous stimulation of sympathetic nerve fibers supplying the smooth muscles of duct of the epididymis, vas deferens, seminal vesicles, and prostate gland take place; as a result, the smooth muscle contracts, and the spermatozoa along with secretions from seminal vesicle and prostate gland are discharged into prostatic urethra. Rhythmic contractions of the bulbospongiosus muscle compress the urethra as a result of which the semen is ejected antegrade from the penile urethra. During this process, the reflux of semen into the bladder is prevented by contraction of the sphincter of the bladder (Giuliano and Clément 2005) (Table 1.2).

1.1 Development of Male Reproductive System

The genetic sex of an embryo is determined at the time of fertilization by the sperm that fertilizes the oocyte. However, the distinct morphological characteristics of male and female gonads do not appear until about week 7 of development. The

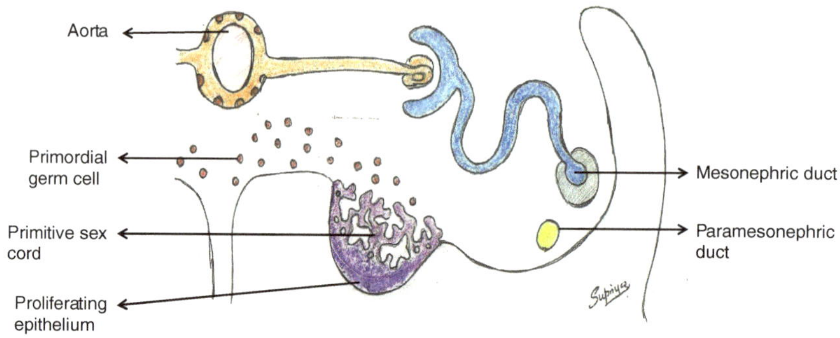

Fig. 1.5 Transverse section through lumbar region showing indifferent gonad with primitive sex cord

early genital system is called as indifferent stage of development due to the similarity in the development of gonads of both sexes. Therefore, in the early stage of development, all human embryos are potentially bisexual (Rao and Burnett 2013). The gonads develop from three sources: coelomic epithelium (mesothelium), intermediate mesoderm (mesenchyme), and primordial germ cells (Fig. 1.5).

1.2 Stages of Development of the Bipotential Gonad

The primordial germ cells are large, spherical primitive sex cells of about 25–30 mm, with a granular cytoplasm and are rich in lipids. The human primordial germ cells are discernible at about day 21 of embryonic life and are seen among the endodermal cells in the wall of the yolk sac near the origin of the allantois. Thus, they are at first, at some distance away from their eventual definitive location in the genital or gonadal ridge. During the 5th week, the primordial germ cells migrate, probably by an amoeboid movement, along the dorsal mesentery of the hindgut (Fig. 1.6) and reach the 10th thoracic level region of the developing embryo, the future gonadal ridge. During their migration, they proliferate by mitosis and are approximately 30,000 in number by the time they reach the genital ridge. Even though the mechanism of migration is not clearly understood, several factors such as SCF (stem cell factor) and its receptor C-kit (a tyrosine kinase receptor) are proven to be crucial for their migration and survival. The coelomic epithelium which lines the anterior internal side of the mesonephric (Wolffian) body thickens to form the genital or gonadal ridge. The Intermediate mesoderm (mesenchyme) forms the stromal cells which later become Leydig cells in the testis and thecal cells in the ovary. By week 6, the primordial germ cells invade the genital ridges and are incorporated into the primary sex cords (Fig. 1.7a, b), which proliferate and grow from the coelomic epithelium into the underlying mesenchyme to form the primary sex cords. At this stage, the "indifferent gonad" consists of an outer cortex and an inner medulla. In embryos with an "XX" chromosomal constitution, the cortex forms an ovary, and the medulla regresses; in one with an XY chromosome complex, the medulla differentiates into a testis, and the cortex regresses (Rao and Burnett 2013).

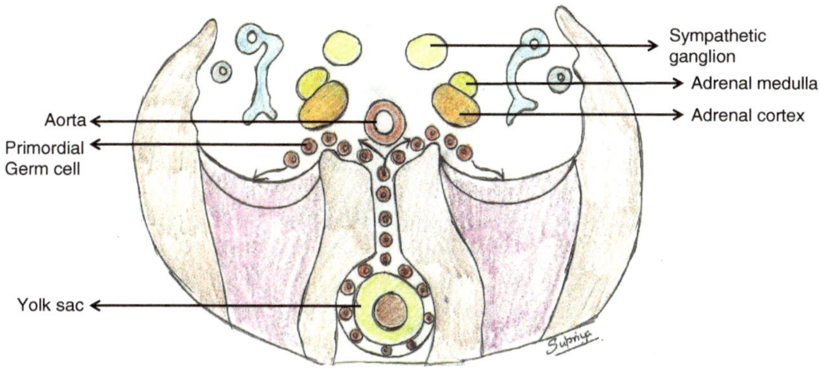

Fig. 1.6 Transverse section through lumbar region showing migration of primordial germ cell through dorsal wall of yolk sac

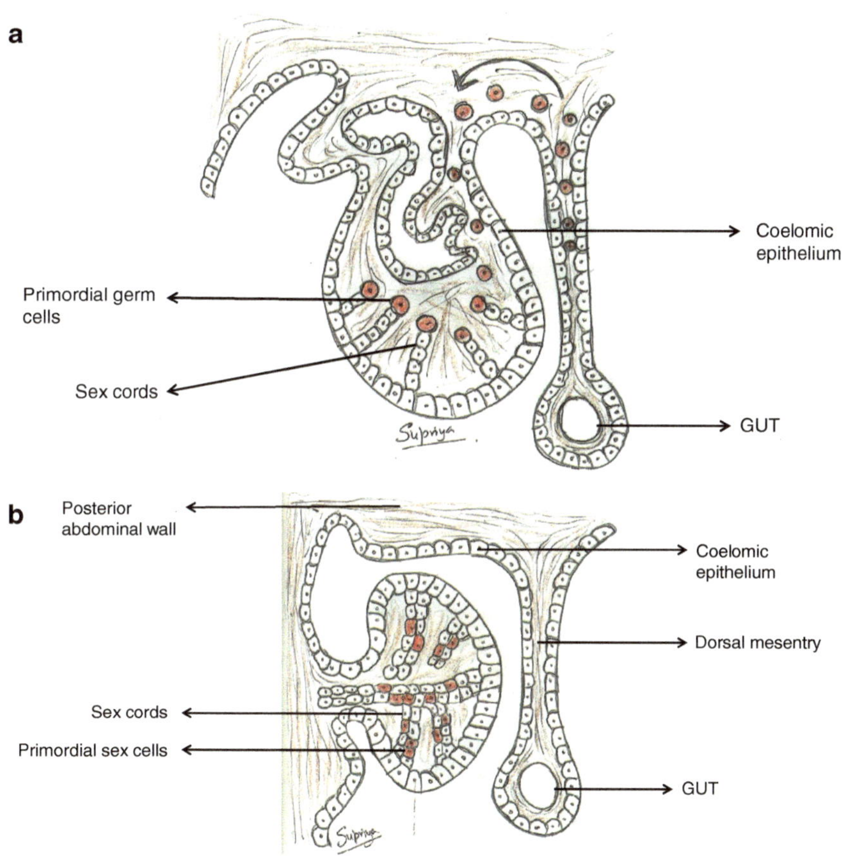

Fig. 1.7 (**a**) Transverse section through lumbar region showing migration of primordial germ cell through dorsal wall of yolk sac and formation of sex cords from coelomic epithelium. (**b**) Transverse section through lumbar region showing proliferation of primitive sex cords and incorporation of primordial germ cell in sex cord

1.3 Testicular Differentiation

The male gonad develops into the testis during week 7 of development which is driven by the "XY" genetic constitution of the embryo. The primary sex cords proliferating from the coelomic epithelium condense and extend into the medulla of the gonad. In the medulla, the cords branch, their deep ends anastomose, and they form the rete testis. These events are regulated by "SRY" gene (termed as sex-determining region) on the short arm of "Y" chromosome present on the somatic cells – Sertoli cells. The expression of SRY gene upregulates the SOX-9 gene (Morais et al. 1996) and anti-Mullerian hormone (AMH). Under the influence of SRY protein, the surrounding mesenchymal cells differentiate in to Leydig cells which secrete testosterone (Fig. 1.8).

The prominent sex cords become the seminiferous or testicular cords which soon lose their connections with the coelomic epithelium because of the development of a thick fibrous capsule, the tunica albuginea which is interposed early, between the coelomic epithelium and the rest of the gland. Development of the tunica albuginea is a characteristic and diagnostic feature of testicular development. The seminiferous or testicular cords develop into the seminiferous tubules, whose deep portions narrow to form the tubuli recti, which converge on the rete

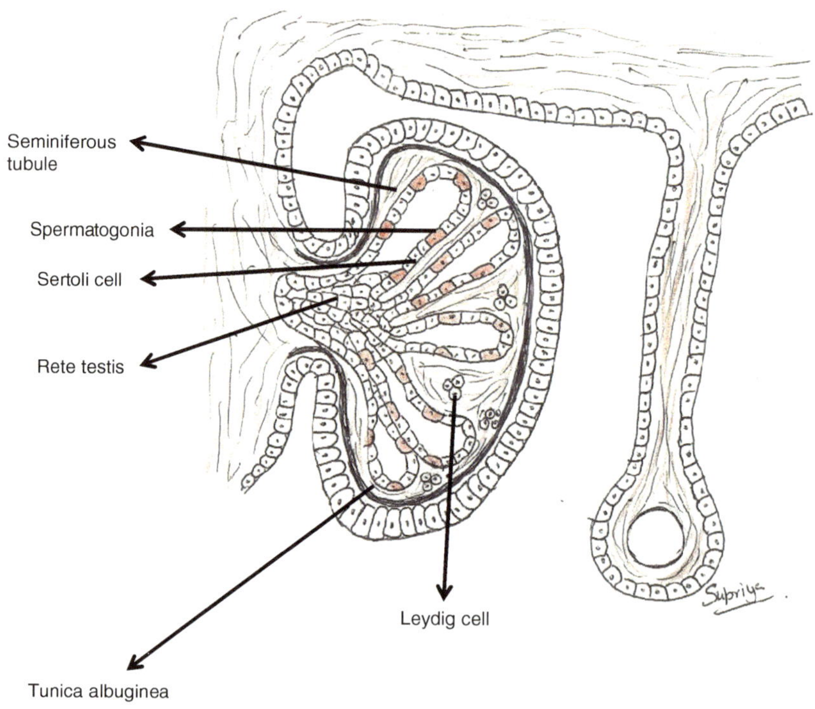

Fig. 1.8 Transverse section through lumbar region showing canalization of seminiferous tubule and formation of Leydig cell

testis. By 4th month the testicular cords become horseshoe shaped to form the seminiferous tubule and are solid until puberty. The seminiferous tubules become separated by mesenchyme which gives rise to the interstitial cells of Leydig. The walls of the seminiferous tubules, as a result of their cellular duality of origin, are composed of two types of cells: supporting or sustentacular cells of Sertoli, derived from the coelomic epithelium, and the spermatogonia, derived from the primordial germ cells (Hanley et al. 2000).

1.4 Descent of Testis

Toward the end of the second month, the urogenital mesentery attaches the testis and mesonephros to the posterior abdominal wall. With degeneration of the mesonephros, the attachment serves as a mesentery for the gonad. The testis is connected to the scrotal swelling by caudal genital ligament and a fibrous cord called the "gubernaculum testis." The continuous shortening of the gubernaculum pulls the testis from the upper part of the abdomen to the scrotum along with the peritoneal sac "processus vaginalis" which gets later obliterated at birth and forms a covering of testis known as the tunica vaginalis. Normally, the testes reach iliac fossa by the 3rd month of intrauterine (IU) life, inguinal canal by the 7th month of IU life, superficial inguinal ring by the 8th month of IU life, and scrotum by the 9th month of IU life. The process is influenced by hormones, including androgens and Mullerian inhibitory substance (Hutson et al. 1997). During descent, blood supply to the testis from the aorta is retained, and testicular vessels extend from their original lumbar position to the testis in the scrotum (Fig. 1.9).

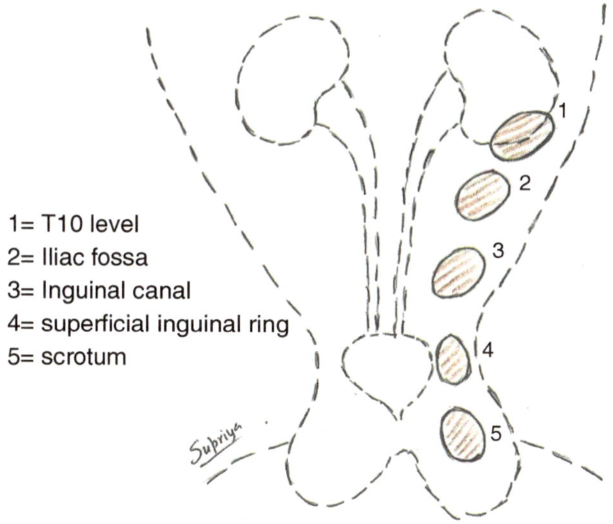

Fig. 1.9 Descent of testis during intrauterine life

1.5 Development of Genital Tracts

The genital tracts have the same appearance in both male and female embryos until week 7 of development, consisting of the two paramesonephric or Mullerian ducts and two mesonephric or Wolffian ducts (Fig. 1.10). Under the influence of testosterone and AMH, the Mullerian duct system starts regressing, while the Wolffian duct system persists. The persistent mesonephric tubules, after regression of the mesonephric (Wolffian) body, participate in the formation of the excretory tracts of the testis, forming the vasa efferentia or efferent ductules. The efferent ductules open into the adjacent mesonephric duct which becomes the ductus epididymidis (epididymis), vas deferens, and ejaculatory duct. The cranial most part of mesonephric duct forms the appendix of epididymis (Standring 2015) (Fig. 1.11).

1.6 Development of Male Genital Glands

The three accessory glands – seminal vesicle, prostate, and bulbourethral gland – all develop near the junction between the mesonephric ducts and pelvic urethra. At the 10th week of development, from mesonephric duct near the attachment of pelvic urethra, a glandular sprout arises giving rise to seminal vesicle. The portion of vas deferens (mesonephric duct) between the seminal vesicle and urethra gives rise to ejaculatory duct. Multiple endodermal outgrowths arising from the prostatic part of

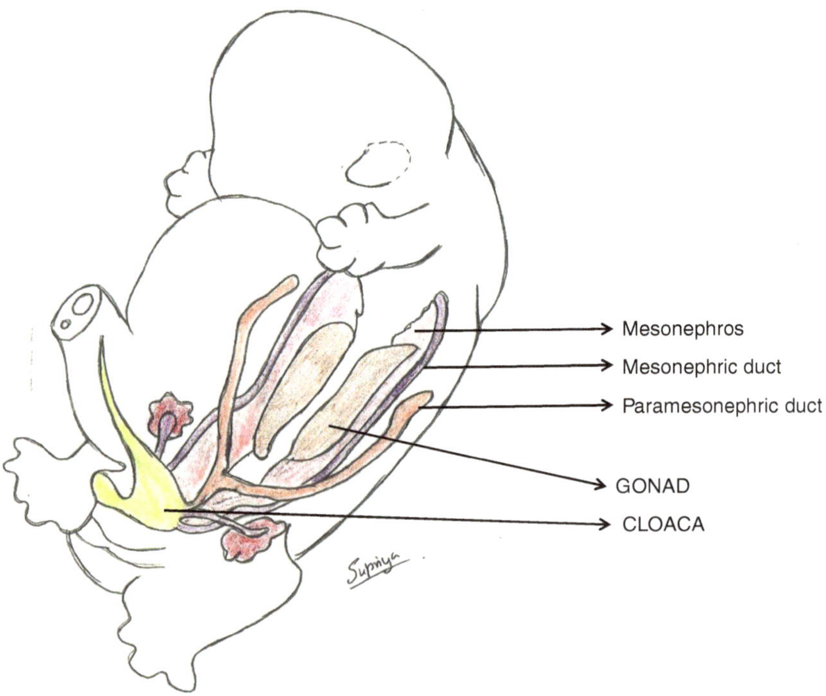

Fig. 1.10 Genital ducts in the 6th week in both sexes

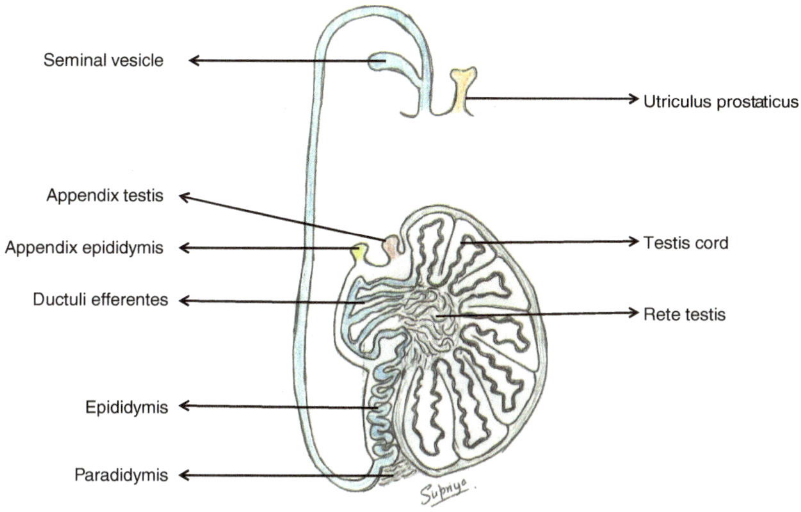

Fig. 1.11 Fate of genital ducts in male in 4th month of IUL

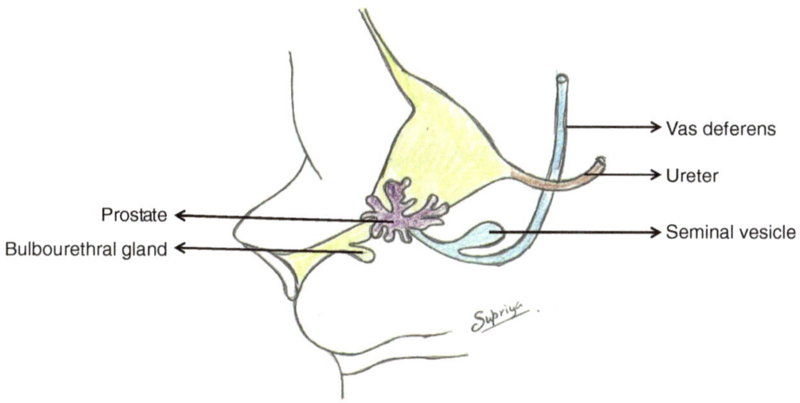

Fig. 1.12 Development of seminal vesicle, prostate, bulbourethral gland during 10–12 week of intrauterine life

urethra differentiate into prostatic glandular epithelium to form the prostate gland (Macleod et al. 2010). Bulbourethral glands (Cowper's) develop from paired outgrowths from the spongy part of urethra, and the mesenchyme differentiates into the stroma and smooth muscle (Fig. 1.12).

1.7 Development of External Genitalia

The cloacal membrane is surrounded by cloacal fold which meets anteriorly to form genital tubercle. The cloacal membrane is divided by the urorectal septum into urogenital and anal membrane. Likewise, the cloacal fold is divided into genital

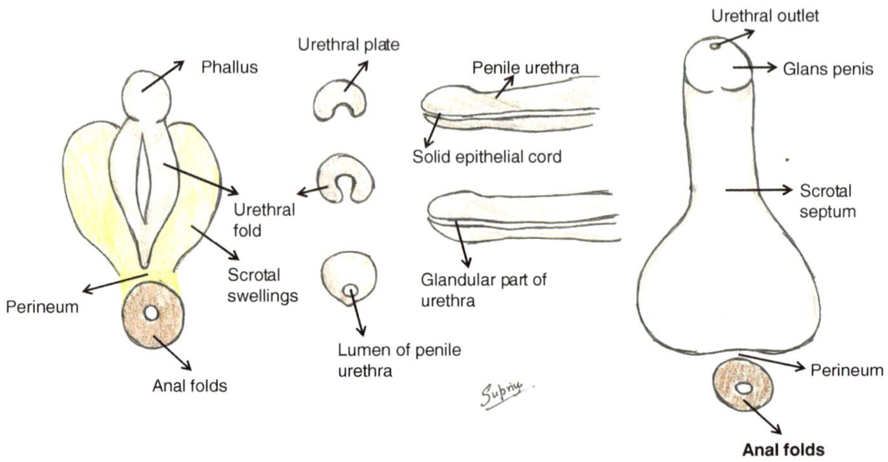

Fig. 1.13 Development of external genitalia in male

Table 1.3 Embryonic origin of the parts of male reproductive system

Embryonic structure	Adult male structure
Bipotential gonad	Testes
Primordial germ cell	Sperm
Somatic support cell	Sertoli cells
Stromal cells	Leydig cells
Cranial part of mesonephric duct	Appendix of epididymis
Mesonephric duct	Epididymis, vas deference, seminal vesicle, ejaculatory duct
Mullerian duct	Appendix of testes, prostatic utricle
Urogenital sinus	Prostate gland, bulbourethral gland
Genital tubercle	Penis
Urogenital folds and urethral plate	Penile urethra/ventral penis
Labioscrotal folds	Scrotum

(urethral) and anal folds. A genital swelling is formed just lateral to the urethral fold. The genital tubercle, the genital fold, and the genital swelling are at an indifferent stage because the male and female genitalia cannot be differentiated at this stage. Elongation of the genital tubercle begins in the 10th week during which genital tubercle enlarges to form the phallus (penis) and urethral folds close over the urethral plate forming the penile urethra. A solid cord of ectoderm is formed in the glans which becomes canalized to form the glandular urethra. The genital swellings form the scrotum. All these changes are mediated by dihydrotestosterone (DHT) (Macleod et al. 2010) (Fig. 1.13, Table 1.3).

Conclusion

The development of the male reproductive system is a very complex process well organized in time and space. A problem with any one of the key developmental steps may affect a man's future fertility and/or capacity to father a conception. Further research into the developmental anatomy of the male reproductive system is warranted as much is yet to be discovered.

References

Bedford JM. Anatomical evidence for the epididymis as the prime mover in the evolution of the scrotum. Am J Anatomy. 1978;152(4):483–507.

Giuliano F, Clément P. Physiology of ejaculation: emphasis on serotonergic control. Eur Urol. 2005;48(3):408–17.

Griswold MD. The central role of Sertoli cells in spermatogenesis. 1998.

Hanley NA, Hagan DM, Clement-Jones M, Ball SG, Strachan T, Salas-Cortes L, McElreavey K, Lindsay S, Robson S, Bullen P, Ostrer H. SRY, SOX9, and DAX1 expression patterns during human sex determination and gonadal development. Mech Dev. 2000;91(1):403–7.

Hutson JM, Hasthorpe S, Heyns CF. Anatomical and functional aspects of testicular descent and cryptorchidism 1. Endocr Rev. 1997;18(2):259–80.

Johnson AD, editor. The testis: biochemistry. Oxford: Elsevier; 2012.

Macleod DJ, Sharpe RM, Welsh M, Fisken M, Scott HM, Hutchison GR, Drake AJ, Van Den Driesche S. Androgen action in the masculinization programming window and development of male reproductive organs. Int J Androl. 2010;33(2):279–87.

McNeal JE. The zonal anatomy of the prostate. Prostate. 1981;2(1):35–49.

Moore KL, Dalley AF, Agur AM. Clinically oriented anatomy. Philadelphia: Lippincott Williams & Wilkins; 2013.

Morais DS, Hacker A, Harley V, Goodfellow P, Swain A, Lovell-Badge R. Sox9 expression during gonadal development implies a conserved role for the gene in testis differentiation in mammals and birds. Nat Genet. 1996;14(1):62–8.

Rao PK, Burnett AL. Development of the male reproductive system. In: Clinical urologic endocrinology. London: Springer; 2013. p. 11–24.

Rooij DG, Russell LD. All you wanted to know about spermatogonia but were afraid to ask. J Androl. 2000;21(6):776–98.

Saez JM. Leydig cells: endocrine, paracrine, and autocrine regulation. Endocr Rev. 1994;15(5):574–626.

Standring S, editor. Gray's anatomy: the anatomical basis of clinical practice. London: Elsevier Health Sciences; 2015.

Tubules AR. Testosterone and spermatogenesis. J Androl. 1992;13(2):172–84.

Waites GM. Temperature regulation and the testis. Testis. 2012;1:241–79.

Woodhouse CR, Kellett MJ. Anatomy of the penis and its deformities in exstrophy and epispadias. J Urol. 1984;132(6):1122–4.

Physiology and Endocrinology of Spermatogenesis

2

R. Bharath

2.1 Introduction

Spermatogenesis is the process by which the primordial germ cells, called the spermatogonial stem cells, transform into highly specialized mature spermatozoa. This is a complex process which takes place in the male gonad (Testis) and involves several steps. Spermatogenesis is controlled by several endocrine and paracrine/autocrine testicular factors (Mahmoud and Eitan 2004). Most of the current knowledge on the exact sequence of mammalian spermatogenesis and its regulation emerge from studies on rodent models. Though the basic sequence of spermatogenesis remains the same among mammals, the number and type of cells, their relationship with each other, and the duration of different stages vary greatly among the species (Kerr and De Kretser 2010). Differences in the life expectancy and offspring number play a major role in the differences seen in spermatogenesis among different species, i.e., primates and rodents (Ehmcke et al. 2006).

2.2 Testis

Testis, the male gonad, subserves two important functions in an adult male: (1) production of male sex hormones, specifically testosterone, and (2) production of the male gamete, the spermatozoa. Gametogenesis or spermatogenesis occurs in the seminiferous tubules which occupies the bulk of the testicular volume. These

R. Bharath, MD, DNB (Endo)
Arka Center for Hormonal Health Pvt. Ltd.,
G-67, (Old no.125), First Avenue, Anna Nagar East, Chennai 600102, India
e-mail: bharathramji78@gmail.com

K. Gunasekaran, N. Pandiyan (eds.), *Male Infertility*,
DOI 10.1007/978-81-322-3604-7_2

tubules are separated by intertubular space which contains Leydig cells, blood vessels, nerves, and lymphatics.

2.3 Stages of Spermatogenesis

The basic steps of spermatogenesis include (1) generation of daughter cells which can transfer the genetic material to the next generation through the process of reproduction and (2) maintenance of a self-renewable germ cell line for sustaining the abovementioned process (Joachim et al. 2007). In order to fulfill both the aims, the germ cells undergo two types of cell division: mitosis and meiosis. The entire process occurs in a specialized compartment of testis called "seminiferous tubules." The spermatogenic process is divided into four important steps:

1. The proliferation and differentiation of spermatogonia into spermatocytes
2. Meiotic division of spermatocytes to spermatids
3. Spermiogenesis – the process of transformation of round spermatids to elongated spermatozoa
4. Spermiation – release of spermatozoa into the lumen of seminiferous tubules

2.3.1 Seminiferous Tubules

Seminiferous tubules constitute around 60 % of the testicular volume indicating their importance in determining the testicular size. There is an ethnic difference in the testicular weights with Hispanic men having greater testicular weight compared to White and Chinese men. This difference is due to the contribution of seminiferous tubules to the testicular volume. The tubule length varies between 450 and 600 m in different ethnic groups. The tubules are divided into basal and luminal compartments and are supported by layers of myofibroblasts. Seminiferous epithelium contains two types of cells: (1) Sertoli cells (SC) and (2) germ cells (GC) (Kerr and De Kretser 2010).

2.3.2 Sertoli Cells

Sertoli cells are somatic cells present in the seminiferous tubules and they constitute 25 % of the tubular cell population. SC increase in number till approximately 15 years of age beyond which their numbers remain constant. They are the supporting cells for the proliferating germ cell population. Each SC supports a defined number of germ cells (Griseold 1995). SC not only provides structural support to germ cells but also give nutritional and immunological support to them. They are the most important paracrine mechanism of spermatogenic control. Structurally, Sertoli cells are tall columnar cells extending from the basement membrane of seminiferous epithelium. Along with several proteins, they form a physiological barrier for the germ cells called the "blood-testis barrier" (BTB) (discussed below). SC have receptors for gonadotropins (FSH and LH) and testosterone. The important functions of SC include:

1. Providing nutrition to germ cells
2. Maintenance of integrity of seminiferous epithelium
3. Secretion two important hormones – anti-Mullerian hormone (AMH) and inhibin.
4. Production of various factors like androgen-binding protein, plasminogen activator, lactate, transport and functional proteins like transferrin and ceruloplasmin, growth factors, etc.
5. Facilitating spermiation

2.3.3 Blood-Testis Barrier

As mentioned above, the BTB is formed by SC and also by several component proteins like actin filaments, actin-binding proteins, and cisternae of endoplasmic reticulum. Structurally BTB divides seminiferous tubule into basal compartment and ad-luminal compartment. Functionally, it divides the pre-leptotene/leptotene spermatocyte from postmeiotic germ cells. The main purpose of the BTB include (1) maintenance of immunological barrier for developing germ cells to prevent autoimmune orchitis and (2) providing a suitable intratubular milieu for effective germ cell development as against a blood milieu in the intertubular space. While the tight junctions of BTB prevent the exposure of postmeiotic germ cell antigens to the immune system, the gap junctions facilitate the migration of pre-leptotene/leptotene spermatocytes to the ad-luminal compartment and also provide suitable hormonal milieu for gem cell development. The BTB is a dynamic barrier because of the constant restructuring process it undergoes in order to facilitate germ cell migration (Yan et al. 2008).

2.3.4 Spermatogenic Stages

As mentioned above, the spermatogenic cycle is a complex process by which the spermatogonia differentiates into mature spermatozoa. Spermatogonia are derived from primordial germ cells which migrate into the testis during fetal life. They transform into gonocytes which are capable of multiplication by the process of mitosis. After a period of multiplication, they migrate to the basement membrane of the seminiferous epithelium and are called spermatogonia (de Kretser et al. 1998). Based on the morphology, different types of spermatogonia can be identified in the seminiferous tubules. They are pale type A spermatogonia (Ap) containing pale staining nuclei, dark type A spermatogonia (Ad) containing deeply staining, homogenous nuclei, and type B spermatogonia.

Type A spermatogonia form the pool of self-renewable stem cells whereas type B spermatogonia enter into the process of meiosis and are the precursors of spermatocytes. Spermatogonia undergo repeated mitotic divisions to produce daughter cells but these divisions are incomplete. Hence, the cells are interconnected to one another through cytoplasmic bridges. The connection persists throughout the subsequent stages of spermatogenesis until the mature spermatids are released into the lumen of seminiferous tubules. This helps in synchronization of germ cell maturation (Kierszenbaum 2002).

2.3.4.1 Spermatocytes

Type B spermatogonia attach to the basal compartment of the seminiferous epithelium and undergo the process of meiosis to form the primary spermatocyte. Meiosis starts with DNA synthesis of type B spermatogonia which results in the duplication of the chromosomes. Thus, each chromosome contain two chromatids and hence the DNA content of primary spermatocyte is tetraploid (4C). Meiosis is subdivided into (1) prophase, (2) metaphase, (3) anaphase, and finally (4) telophase. Two successive meiotic divisions occur which result in the synthesis of four spermatids from each primary spermatocyte. Prophase is a lengthy process which takes around 1–3 weeks and is further subdivided into (1) leptotene, (2) zygotene, (3) pachytene, (4) diplotene, and finally (5) diakinesis. Leptotene stage of the prophase starts in the basal compartment and further steps are continued after the spermatocytes cross the blood-testis barrier to reach the ad-luminal compartment. The primary spermatocyte undergoes first meiotic division to form secondary spermatocyte which in turn becomes round spermatid through the second meiotic division.

2.3.4.2 Spermiogenesis

The round spermatids become elongated spermatozoa which attains motility. This is accomplished through the following events:

1. Acrosome formation
2. Nuclear condensation
3. Reduction of cytoplasm
4. Formation of tail
5. Reorganization of cellular organelles.

The detailed discussions of steps of spermatogenesis are seen elsewhere.

2.4 Neuroendocrine Regulation of Spermatogenesis

The complex process of spermatogenesis is regulated by two major mechanisms:

1. Extrinsic or neurohormonal regulation
2. Intrinsic or autocrine/paracrine regulation

2.4.1 Extrinsic Regulation

Neuroendocrine regulation of the testis is often termed as "hypothalamo-pituitary-testicular axis." This axis is mainly controlled by the gonadotrophin-releasing hormone (GnRH).

2.4.1.1 Gonadotrophin-Releasing Hormone

GnRH is a decapeptide which is secreted and released from the hypothalamic neurons. It is the major regulator of secretion of follicle-stimulating hormone (FSH) and luteinizing hormone (LH) from the gonadotrophs of the anterior pituitary. GnRH is secreted in pulsatile manner and each pulse of GnRH is accompanied by a simultaneous pulsatile secretion of LH. The pulses of GnRH are controlled by "GnRH pulse generator" which is under the influence of several neurotransmitters, the most important among them called as "kisspeptin."

2.4.1.2 Kisspeptin

Kisspeptin is a hypothalamic neuropeptide coded by the KiSS1 gene. Kisspeptin is a neuromodulator that acts upstream of GnRH. It is controlled by sex steroid feedback mechanism and is also responsive to metabolic signals. Kisspeptin is recognized as a crucial regulator of onset of puberty, gonadotrophin secretion, and fertility. It acts on the GPR-54 receptor located on the GnRH neurons and increases the GnRH pulsatility and consequently LH secretion. Activation of kisspeptin neurons triggers the onset of puberty in male and female by stimulating the "GnRH pulse generator." However, there is an anatomical and functional dimorphism in kisspeptin neuronal system between male and female, which explains the greater role of kisspeptin in different stages of menstrual cycle in female. Genetic mutations in KiSS1 gene are associated with hypothalamic form of hypogonadism in men (Skorupskaite and George 2014).

2.4.1.3 Gonadotrophins (LH and FSH)

LH and FSH belong the family of glycoprotein hormones with two subunits, the α subunit which is common for both and the β subunit which is unique and offers specificity. They are secreted by the gonadotrophs which constitute 7–10% of the cells in the anterior pituitary gland. Gonadotrophins are secreted in pulsatile manner in response to GnRH secretion. Their secretion increases during neonatal period which helps in the gonadal development. After a few months of the neonatal gonadotrophin surge, their secretion reaches a nadir level until the onset of puberty. In adults, LH and FSH secretion remain stable in male but markedly vary in female depending on the reproductive cycle. The plasma half-life of FSH (120–240 min) is longer than that of LH (30–90 min). This difference is attributed to the higher sialic acid content in FSH compared to LH (Matsumoto and Bremner 2011).

2.4.1.4 FSH

The most important function of FSH in male is the stimulation of spermatogenesis. FSH acts through the FSH receptor present in the Sertoli cells of testis. FSH receptor is a G-protein-coupled receptor with an extracellular hormone-binding domain (which binds to FSH), a seven helical transmembrane domain, and an intracellular domain. Binding of FSH to its receptor causes structural alteration in the seven membrane-spanning domains. This in turn stimulates the G proteins coupled with the receptor to activate adenylate cyclase which increases the intracellular cAMP levels. Apart from this mechanism, binding of FSH to FSH receptor triggers several intracellular pathways like protein kinase A (PKA) pathway, MAP kinase pathway, calcium pathway, and the phosphatidylinositol 3-kinase (PI3-K) pathway. Through these multipronged approach, FSH stimulates several transcription factors which are involved in germ cell proliferation, provides metabolic support to germ cells, helps in the transportation of glucose (which is converted to lactate to provide energy), and facilitates transferrin secretion which is vital for maintaining spermatogenesis (Walker and Cheng 2005). Secretion of FSH is regulated by two paracrine factors, activin and follistatin secreted from the pituitary and also inhibin B secreted from the Sertoli cells of testis (see later). These factors belong to the TGF-β family and their combined action determines the effective secretion of FSH. Men with inactivating mutations of FSH-β gene and FSH receptor are generally infertile with azoospermia or oligospermia, respectively (Matsumoto and Bremner 2011).

2.4.1.5 LH

The main function of LH in males is through its action on the Leydig cells of testis which produce testosterone, the most important male hormone. Leydig cells express receptors for LH on their surface and LH binds to these receptors. The downstream pathway is mediated through cAMP-dependent activation of PKA (similar to FSH action). In Leydig cells, this pathway leads to the production of proteins that regulate steroidogenesis and testosterone biosynthesis. Though Sertoli cells and germ cells do not have receptors for LH, spermatogenesis is indirectly regulated by LH through increasing the intratesticular testosterone concentration. Men with inactivating mutations of LH-β gene or LH receptor lack pubertal development with arrested spermatogenesis or azoospermia and infertility. This explains the role of intratesticular testosterone concentration in normal spermatogenic process (Matsumoto and Bremner 2011).

In short though FSH and LH (by increasing the intratesticular testosterone) help in spermatogenesis, their actions differ according to the stage of spermatogenesis. While FSH has greater effect on the maturation of spermatogonia, early meiosis, and conversion of spermatogonia to pachytene spermatocytes, LH has its predominant effect on the completion of meiosis and on spermiation. Both have similar effect on spermiogenesis (Matsumoto and Bremner 2011).

2.4.1.6 Other Factors of Extrinsic Regulation

Another neuromodulator which plays a major role in gonadotrophin secretion is leptin which is produced from peripheral adipose tissue. Leptin receptors are expressed in GnRH-secreting neurons through which it positively regulates the gonadal axis. Leptin accelerates GnRH pulsatility and in turn stimulate gonadotrophins secretion. Environmental stress, through the secretion of corticotrophin-releasing hormone (CRH) and glucocorticoid, negatively regulates hypothalamo-pituitary-gonadal axis.

2.4.2 Intrinsic Regulation

The two important cells in human testis which are involved in the autocrine/paracrine regulation of spermatogenesis are (1) Leydig cells and (2) Sertoli cells.

2.4.2.1 Leydig Cells

Leydig cells constitute 10–20 % of the intertubular cell population. They are derived from the mesenchymal fibroblasts present in the intertubular space. They are the major source of testosterone synthesis from cholesterol which acts as the substrate. The steps in the steroidogenic pathway and their control are beyond the scope of this chapter. Testosterone, once synthesized from Leydig cells, diffuses into the systemic circulation. The concentration of intratesticular testosterone is several times greater than its systemic concentration. Especially, higher levels of testosterone are found near the basement membrane of the seminiferous tubules indicating its role in spermatogenesis (Kerr and De Kretser 2010).

2.4.2.2 Testosterone

Testosterone is the predominant male hormone secreted from the Leydig cells of testis. It is synthesized from cholesterol, which acts as its substrate, through the steriodogenic pathway, under the control of LH. After synthesis, it is secreted into the circulation, where it is either bound to albumin (54–68 %) and sex hormone-binding globulin (SHBG) (30–44 %) or present in unbound or (free) form (0.5–3 %). The biological actions of testosterone, including its effect on male sexual differentiation and maturation, development of secondary sexual characters, epiphysis growth, and metabolic actions, are mediated by the free form. Intratesticular testosterone concentration is 100–200-fold higher than its serum concentration. As androgen receptors are present in Sertoli cells, testosterone and consequently LH mediate their effect on spermatogenesis (discussed above) through Sertoli cells. Administration of LH as human chorionic gonadotropin (HCG) alone in hypogonadal men maintains spermatogenesis once it is initiated by the combination of FSH and HCG treatment. However, administration of testosterone in hypogonadal men suppresses sperm production by reducing the endogenous LH. This explains the role of LH (HCG) in increasing the intratesticular testosterone and thereby maintaining spermatogenesis. Exogenous testosterone administration in turn suppresses LH secretion by acting at the level of hypothalamus and pituitary. This completes the feedback inhibition loop of hypothalamo-pituitary-testicular axis. Testosterone is aromatized to estradiol by the enzyme aromatase. Like testosterone, intratesticular level of estradiol is 100-fold higher than the serum level. Recent studies have thrown light on the importance of higher levels of estradiol in testis and its role in spermatogenesis (Matsumoto and Bremner 2011).

2.4.2.3 Estrogen

Estradiol (E2) is the most abundant and active form of estrogen in both male and female. E2 is derived in male by the peripheral aromatization of testosterone by the enzyme called aromatase. Aromatase enzyme is expressed widely in adipose tissue, testis, and brain. Estrogen exerts its genomic action through two major receptors – estrogen receptor 1 (ER1) and estrogen receptor 2 (ER2) which are located in the nucleus. The non-genomic actions of estrogen are mediated through nonclassical membrane-bound G-protein-coupled receptors called as GPR30/GPER. Recent studies have shown the presence of estrogen receptors (ER1, ER2, and GPR30/GPER) in human testicular Sertoli cells and germ cells (Lambard et al. 2004; Carreau et al. 2010). Also, GPER is found in hypothalamus. Through mouse models, it has been proven than estrogen plays a significant role in spermatogenesis. Estrogen modulates germ cell proliferation, differentiation, survival, and apoptosis. Estrogen also acts at the hypothalamic level to regulate the gonadotrophin secretion. Most of these actions are mediated through ER2 and GPER. The functional and clinical significance of these findings needs further detailed studies.

2.4.2.4 Inhibin B

Inhibins are glycoproteins belonging to TGF-β family of proteins. They are composed of α- subunit which is connected to either a β_A or β_B subunit to form inhibin A or inhibin B, respectively. Inhibin B is the predominant inhibin present in male. It is produced by the Sertoli cells in response to FSH stimulation. Inhibin B in turn controls FSH through negative feedback mechanism. Inhibin B is the marker of Sertoli cell function. It is present in childhood and levels rise during puberty to reach the adult range by mid puberty. In contrast to the prepubertal inhibin level which is exclusively indicative of Sertoli cell function, inhibin B production in adult men is dependent on the presence of certain germ cells in the seminiferous tubules, most likely involving the pachytene spermatocytes and early spermatids. While, prepubertal boys with cryptorchidism will have normal inhibin B levels (indicating intact Sertoli cells) when compared to those with congenital or acquired anorchia, adult men with early spermatogenic failure and Sertoli cell-only syndrome will have low inhibin B levels when compared to normal adult men or men with late spermatogenic failure. The physiology of inhibin B levels in adult men helps us to understand the role of germ cells in the control of Sertoli cell function (Andersson and Skakkebaek 2001) (Fig. 2.1).

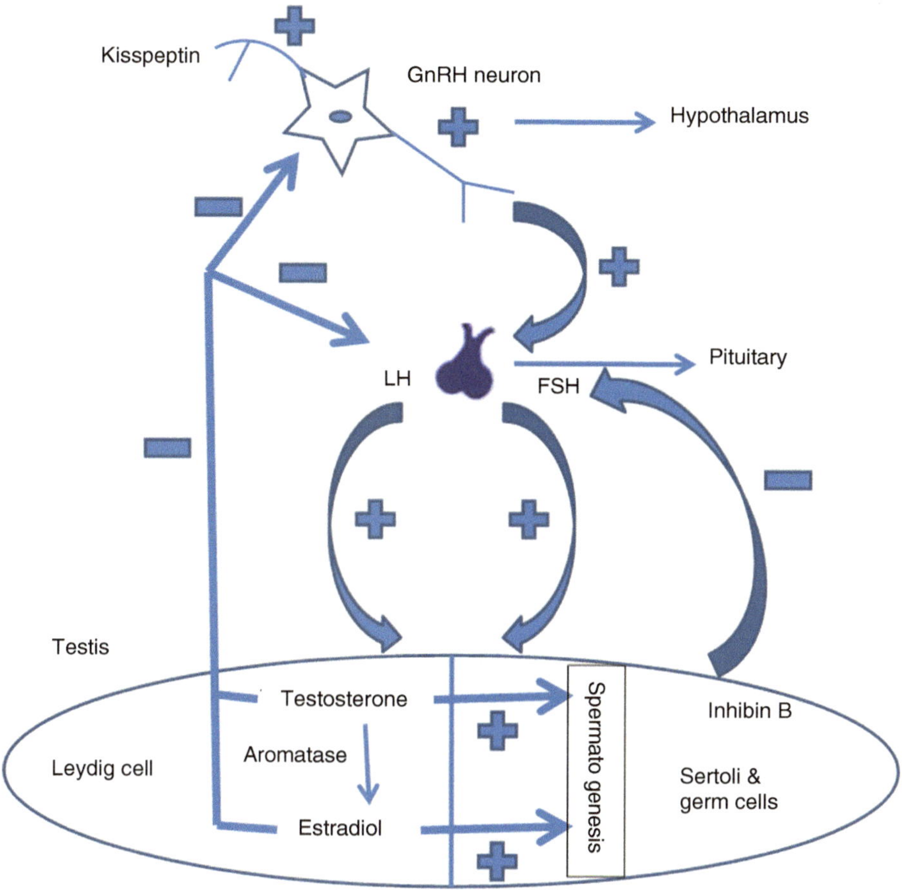

Fig. 2.1 *Hypothalamo-pituitary-testicular axis (graphical representation). GnRH* gonadotropin-releasing hormone, *LH* luteinizing hormone, *FSH* follicle-stimulating hormone, – feedback inhibition, + stimulation

Conclusion

The process of spermatogenesis involves a complex interplay of several endocrine, paracrine, and autocrine factors. Endocrine regulation of spermatogenesis is finely controlled by the kisspeptin, gonadotropin-releasing hormone, the gonadotropins, and the testicular steroidogenic pathway. A thorough knowledge of the physiology is the key to successful management of patients suffering from disorders of spermatogenesis.

References

Andersson AM, Skakkebaek NE. Serum inhibin B levels during male childhood and puberty. Mol Cell Endocrinol. 2001;180(1–2):103–7.
Carreau S, Wolczynski S, et al. Aromatase, oestrogens and human male reproduction. Philos Trans R Soc Lond B Biol Sci. 2010;365(1546):1571–9.
de Kretser DM, Loveland KL, et al. Spermatogenesis. Hum Reprod. 1998;13 Suppl 1:1–8.
Ehmcke J, Wistuba J, Schlatt S. Spermatogonia, physiology, pathology and clinical relevance. Hum Reprod Update. 2006;12:275–82.
Griseold MD. Interaction between germ cells and sertoli cells in the testis. Biol Reprod. 1995; 52:211–6.
Joachim W, Jan-Bernd S, Marc L. Mammalian spermatogenesis. Funct Dev Embryol. 2007;1: 99–117.
Kerr JB, De Kretser D. Functional morphology of the testis. In: Jameson JL, De Groot LJ, editors. Endocrinology. 6th ed. Philadelphia: Saunders Elsevier; 2010. p. 2440–68.
Kierszenbaum AL. Genomic imprinting and epigenetic reprogramming: unearthing the garden of forking paths. Mol Reprod Dev. 2002;63:269–72.
Lambard S, Galeraud-Denis I, et al. Human immature germ cells and ejaculated spermatozoa contain aromatase and oestrogen receptors. J Mol Endocrinol. 2004;32(1):279–89.
Mahmoud H, Eitan L. Regulation of spermatogenesis by paracrine/autocrine testicular factors. Asian J Androl. 2004;6:259–68.
Matsumoto AM, Bremner WJ. Testicular disorders. In: Melmed S, Polonsky KS, editors. Williams textbook of endocrinology. 12th ed. Philadelphia: Saunders Elsevier; 2011. p. 688–777.
Skorupskaite K, George JT. The kisspeptin-GnRH pathway in human reproductive health and disease. Hum Reprod Update. 2014;20(4):485–500.
Walker WH, Cheng J. FSH and testosterone signaling in Sertoli cells. Reproduction. 2005;130: 15–28.
Yan HH, Mruk DD, et al. Blood-testis barrier dynamics are regulated by testosterone and cytokines via their differential effects on the kinetics of protein endocytosis and recycling in Sertoli cells. FASEB J. 2008;22:1945–59.

3 Ultrastructure of Human Spermatozoa

Priya Kannan

3.1 Introduction

The sperm is a complex cell with a specialized function and structure compared to other cells of the body. Sperm cells are transcriptionally and translationally inactive; its DNA is tightly condensed in an almost crystalline state, packaged by protamines, and is produced in large numbers. Its objective is to deliver the intact haploid genome to the oocyte at the site of fertilization. The sperm must conserve the DNA, transport it to the site of fertilization, recognize the egg and start the process of fertilization. The human sperm migrates from the site of deposition – vagina, through the cervix into the uterus and then to the site of fertilization – ampullary region of the fallopian tube. During the travel, it completes its process of functional maturation – a process termed as *capacitation*.

To accomplish these processes, the sperm has a highly specialized structure. The structure of the sperm was first described in 1677 by Antonie van Leeuwenhoek. Advances in microscopy and the optics have immensely improved our knowledge on the description made by van Leeuwenhoek. While light microscopy can show major abnormalities in the sperm, it cannot reveal information about the submolecular structures. Electron microscopy and transmission electron microscopy have provided the much-needed details on the ultrastructure of sperm. The human spermatozoon can be grossly divided into two regions – the head and the flagellum (the tail).

P. Kannan, MBBS, MMed., MCE
Academy of Clinical Embryologists, Bangalore, India

Medical Genetics, The Tamil Nadu Dr. MGR Medical University, Chennai, India

Garbba Rakshambigai Fertility Centre,
4, 6th Cross Street, United India Colony, Kodambakkam, Chennai, India
e-mail: kaypriya2000@gmail.com

K. Gunasekaran, N. Pandiyan (eds.), *Male Infertility*,
DOI 10.1007/978-81-322-3604-7_3

3.1.1 Flagellum

The spermatozoa are typically 'stripped-down' cells with a long flagellum to propel them. It is devoid of organelles such as endoplasmic reticulum or ribosomes (Alberts et al. 2002). The tail or the flagellar region of the sperm is designed for motility of the sperm. The flagellar structure that serves as the 'tail' of the sperm is complex in higher vertebrates such as humans. The tail of the sperm can be divided into four regions (Fawcett 1975) with distinct anatomy related to their function:

- The short connecting piece
- The midpiece
- The principal piece
- The terminal piece

The structure of flagellum has:

1. The axoneme which runs throughout the length of the flagellum
2. The outer dense fibres (ODFs) which surround the axoneme in the midpiece and principal piece
3. The mitochondrial sheath (MS), which is located in the midpiece
4. The fibrous sheath (FS) which is located in the principal piece

Understanding the proteins which make up each of these flagellar structures and how these proteins interact to produce the normal flagellar beat would throw light on understanding the molecular genetics behind the reduced sperm motility in infertile animals, and humans.

3.2 Axoneme

Axoneme of the axial filament stretches across the full length of the flagellum and constitutes the motor apparatus of the sperm tail. The organization of the axoneme is similar to that of cilia and flagella of all eukaryotic cells. It has two central microtubules surrounded by nine evenly spaced microtubular doublets – the classic 9+2 pattern. The nine peripheral doublets are numbered in a clockwise direction from 1 to 9. The first doublet is situated on a place perpendicular to that of the two central microtubules. Each doublet consists of an A subunit with a complete microtubule of 26 nm in diameter and a B subunit which is an incomplete microtubule (C shaped in cross section) that is attached to the A subunit. Tubulin is the structural component of the microtubules (Farrell 1982; Curry and Watson 1995). The A tubule is made of 13 protofilaments that are aligned side by side. The B tubule is made from 10 protofilaments. Extending from A microfilament to B microfilament are 'arms' which play a crucial role in flagellar movement. The principal component of the arms is dynein (Porter and Johnson 1989; Holzbaur and Vallee 1994; Milisav 1998). Activation of the axonemal dynein ATPase results in sliding of adjacent outer doublet microtubules and it has been proposed that these sliding results in flagellar bending (Tash and Means 1982). The doublets are connected by the protein nexin (Clermont et al. 1990). The central microtubules are interconnected by linkages and are surrounded by a pair of spiral fibres that are attached to the microtubules. The spiral fibres form the central sheath from which radial spokes go out to the A subunit of the doublet (Pederson 1970).

3.3 Connecting Piece

The connecting piece connects the flagellum and the sperm head. It is about 0.5 μ in length and consists of:

1. Capitulum
2. Segmented columns

The capitulum is a dome-shaped fibrous structure. Proteinaceous filaments run between the capitulum and the caudal surface of the nucleus. The capitulum is the site of the centrioles. It is positioned at right angles to the axis of the flagellum. Only the proximal centriole is seen in a mature spermatozoon as the distal centriole disintegrates during spermiogenesis. The centriole plays a major role in the formation of the axoneme during spermiogenesis and also a major part in fertilization and the events following fertilization. The structure of the centriole is the same as that of an axoneme but without the central pair of microtubules and has peripheral triplet in place of doublets.

The segmented columns fuse proximally into major and minor columns and attach to the capitulum. The columns attach to the outer dense fibre in the midpiece distally.

3.4 Centrosome

As early as 1887, it was postulated by Theodor Boveri that the oocyte has all elements required for embryonic development except the active division centre (Baltzer 1967). In a somatic diploid cell, the mitotic spindle is the key to the distribution of the genomic material. The spindle is derived from the centrosome. The centrosome and centriole are a part of the MTOC (microtubule-organizing centre). The centrosome consists of two centrioles and the pericentriolar material (PCM). The centriole is a pair of cylinders arranged perpendicularly, whereas the aster and the spindle fibres are derived from PCM (Palermo et al. 1994). The centriole displays the distinct 9+0 pattern of nine triplet microtubules. This differs from the axoneme by the absence of the central pair of microtubule. Earlier reports suggested that mammalian gametes lack centrioles. It was proven beyond doubt that centrioles are indeed part of the mitotic division in humans (Sathananthan et al. 1991) and in other species too (Guen and Crozet 1989). Sathananthan et al. described in detail the anatomy of centrioles in human reproduction. They showed that the human oocyte does not possess any centriole and the sperm has two centrioles – proximal and distal. The proximal centriole is located in the connecting piece, next to the basal plate of the sperm head. It has a pinwheel structure of nine microtubules surrounded by electron dense material referred to as the 'black box'. The distal centriole is located perpendicular to the proximal and is aligned with the flagellum that forms the axoneme during spermiogenesis (Sathananthan et al. 1991; 1996).

The two major functions of the centrosome are (1) nucleation of microtubule and (2) mitotic spindle formation (Schatten 1994; Bornens et al. 1990). In all mammalian species, except the mice, the sperm centrosome nucleates the aster. This brings about the apposition of the female and male pronuclei. It has been demonstrated that injection of the tail alone can induce aster formation (Van Blerkom and Davis 1995). After the fusion of the gametes, the tail of the sperm is incorporated into the ooplasm. The centriole duplicates during the pronuclear stage. Centrioles have been detected up to the stage of blastocyst (Sathananthan et al. 1996). In humans, only the male gamete has an active centrosome and is the structure responsible for the first mitotic division (Palermo et al. 1994).

3.5 Outer Dense Fibre

The axoneme of the sperm is surrounded by the outer dense fibre. Each of the peripheral microtubule doublets has an outer dense fibre. They are individual fibres that are teardrop shaped, with an outer rounded edge that tapers towards the axoneme. Cranially, these fibres fuse with the connecting piece. These are suggested to facilitate sperm movement, mediated by protein phosphorylation, and serve as protector of the sperm during its passage in the male and female tracts (Tash and Means 1983). It is also suggested to act as the stiffening rods within the sperm tail.

3.6 Midpiece

The midpiece of the flagellum is about 3.5 μm in length and runs from the distal end of the connecting piece to the annulus. It is an electron dense circumferential band marking the junction between the midpiece and principal piece. A recent report by Guan and colleagues in BMC Developmental Biology 2009 described the development of the annulus, in the formation of the mature spermatozoon. Its function has not clearly been established, but it may constitute a diffusion barrier between the two compartments and/or facilitate mitochondria migration and alignment along the axoneme.

The midpiece has a mitochondrial sheath with a species-specific number of mitochondria. The mitochondria are arranged in a helical pattern around the axoneme. The human spermatozoon has a helix composed of 11–15 gyres. The mitochondrial structure in the sperm is the same as that in other cell types but has greater stability.

It is resistant to osmotic changes which might help resist stretching and compression of the mitochondria during flagellar beat. It is the site of energy production of spermatozoa and its position allows ready supply of ATP to the axoneme. The flagella activity requires energy which is obtained in the form of ATP. The ATP is supplied by the mitochondria and is hydrolyzed by ATPase in the dynein arms in the presence of magnesium.

3.7 Principal Piece

This is the longest flagellum extending from the annulus to the proximal end of the terminal piece. It is approximately 55 μm in length. It has a fibrous sheath which is the cytoskeletal structure surrounding the axoneme and the outer dense fibres. The sheath consists of two columns that is circumferentially connected by a series of closely packed filaments called ribs. In the human sperm, the ribs are 10–20 nm apart and 50 nm thick. The function of the fibrous sheath appears to be similar to that of outer dense fibres – to act as stiffening rods and provide rigid support to the flagellum and determining its planar beat (Lindemann et al. 1992). It has been seen that sperms with disorganized fibrous sheath have disrupted motility indicating its importance in motility of the sperm.

3.8 Terminal Piece

Beyond the fibrous sheath is the terminal piece of the flagellum, which is about 3 μm in length. The microtubules of the axoneme terminate in this region. The dynein arms disappear first and the A subunit takes a hollow appearance. The central pair of the microtubules terminates, after which two of the peripheral outer doublets move to the centre. The doublets separate and the open B tubule disappear. The pattern that remains is a single central tubule surrounded by a circle of single microtubule covered by plasma membrane.

3.8.1 Flagellum: Role in Infertility

The connection between male infertility and ciliopathy was first disclosed by the observation of a common ultrastruc-tural abnormality in sperm flagella and epithelial cilia in patients with Kartagener syndrome (Camner et al., 1975).

Defects in the axonemal structure of the sperm causes defects in motility, and often leads to male subfertility. These affect fertilisation. Male infertility is linked with symptoms or diseases such as Kartagener syndrome or cystic fibrosis. These result in a deficiency in the components of cilia and flagella, they are called "immotile cilia syndrome" or "primary ciliary dyskinesia," or more recently, "ciliopathy," which includes deficiencies in primary and sensory cilia.

A recent study by Mitchell et al in 2012, had assessed the morphology of the sperm flagellum by light microscopy and compared it to axonemal deficiencies. The study included 41 patients with known axonemal abnormalities. They could correlate flagellar abnormalities to axonemal deficiencies such as correlations between missing outer dynein arms and abnormal, short or coiled flagellum. There found a negative correlation between misassembly and spermatozoa of irregular flagella. They concluded that light microscopy analysis of flagellar abnormalities may help to identify correct diagnosis and sperm abnormalities.

The green alga Chlamydomonas has been used to generate many useful mutants for studying cilia and flagella, including mutants for the outer and inner dynein arms and other substructures (Kamiya, 2002). In animals, sperm from marine invertebrates have contributed to our understanding of the molecular architecture of flagella and the mechanism of their motility.

In humans, most such cells are multiciliated are seen in nasal and trachea epithelia , the lachrymal sac, brain ventricles (ependymal cilia), male efferent ducts and female oviducts (Fallopian tubes). The structures of the axonemes in motile multicilia have a 9 + 2 micro- tubule lattice with dynein arms, apparently the same as those in sperm flagella, although there are several reports showing minor differences in their components. The cilia is found in many parts of the male reproductive system. They are seen in epididymis, vas deferens as well. Atleast 20n genes have been identified thaqt result in ciliopathy (Inaba and Mizuno, 2016).

Knockout mice are powerful models for studying ciliopathy. However, in most cases, loss of axonemal dyneins results in embryonic lethality. This is not compatible with the symptoms of human ciliopathy, in which patients are alive and show fertility, making it possible to carry out family studies.

3.8.1.1 Centrosome

Since centrosome is critical, for the event of fertilization, the study of centrosome is relevant especially in the scenario of failed fertilization and other such clinical scenarios. There were studies by Sathananthan where he reported that incidence of centriolar abnormalities were more in immotile and non-progressively motile spermatozoa (Sathananthan et al. 1996).

Structural defects in the flagellum that have been noted are changes in the composition or number of axonemal microtubules, impairment of dynein arms. The absence of dynein arms is one of the frequent causes of sperm immobility. Disorganization of the mitochondrial sheaths or absence can impair sperm motility. A lack of ATP can also lead to sperm degeneration (Kupker et al. 1998).

3.8.1.2 Head

The function of the head of the sperm is well defined – it is to conserve the paternal DNA and deliver it to the oocyte at the time of fertilization. To achieve this, the following are indispensible:

1. The DNA should be held in a stable form.
2. The sperm should penetrate the oocyte surface.
3. Capability of membrane fusion.

The basic structure of head of the sperm is common to all mammalian species, but there can be differences in shape and size of the nucleus and the acrosome. The head of the human spermatozoa is called pleomorphic. The sperm head is about 4.5 μm in length and it is about 3.5 μm at its widest part and is slightly flattened.

3.9 Acrosome

The acrosome, which is derived from the Golgi apparatus, is a membrane-bound vesicle forming a cap-like covering on the cranial part of the nucleus. In humans, the acrosome is relatively small and covers about two third of the nucleus. This results from the topographic development over the Sertoli cell cytoplasm in the late stages of spermiogenesis, by contracting the nucleus to result in its unique shape. The acrosome has two membranes – the outer and the inner. The inner membrane is right below the plasma membrane and continues as the inner acrosome membrane which lies above the nuclear envelope. The membranes are parallel to each other and the space in between them is filled with acrosomal matrix (Huang and Yanagimachi 1985). The matrix has hydrolytic enzymes such as hyaluronidase and acrosin, a proteinase in inactive zymogen form – proacrosin and a second zymogen called sperminogen (Siegel et al. 1987). Other enzymes that are present in acrosomal matrix are acid phosphatase, phospholipases, N-acetylglucosaminidase and collagenase.

Eutherian sperms have an equatorial region which is situated at the posterior border of the acrosomal cap. The acrosomal membranes in the equatorial segment are electron dense. There is no acrosomal matrix in this segment. It is the site of accumulation of vimentin (Virtanen et al. 1984). It is hence a stable membrane structure which plays the role of stabilizing this critical region during in acrosome reaction and zona penetration. It is at the border between the anterior acrosome and the equatorial segment; thus, when the acrosome fuses with the plasma membrane, the integrity of the sperm cell is maintained.

There have been many theories of penetration of the sperm, such as enzymatic or mechanical or both. The very narrow, sharply defined penetration slit made by the sperm in the zona does not conform to the purely enzymatic penetration. Evidence has also suggested that by thrust force alone, the sperm cannot penetrate the zone. Hence, the use of both mechanisms has been proposed (Green 1988).

3.10 Perinuclear Material

The perinuclear material is situated between the acrosome and the nucleus. It is a thin layer stabilized by disulphide bonds. It acts like cement between the acrosome and nucleus. Posterior to the acrosome, the perinuclear material forms the acrosome sheath. This structure is composed of two distinct regions separated by a shallow grove. The anterior region has an electron dense material parallel to the plasma membrane, which has a series of rounded projections extending towards the plasma membrane (Pedersen 1972b). The posterior region of the sheath has granular material with oblique cord-like structures (Koehler 1972).

3.11 Nucleus

The nucleus of the sperm has a haploid set of chromosome. It is the result of the process of spermiogenesis, the specialized process that changes the round spermatids into a mature sperm with its distinct shape. The size of the nucleus is decreased in the process by chemical and architectural modifications. The DNA in the sperm is complexed with protamines which lead to chromatin condensation. The DNA remains inactive and does not replicate until the protamines disintegrate after the entry into the oocyte (Johnson and Lalancette 2010). The protamine, which allows packaging of the sperm chromatin, neutralizes the charges of the phosphate ester backbone in the DNA. There are disulphide bonds between free thiols which give the nucleus its highly stable keratinoid nature.

Nucleus shape is species specific and is determined by the sperm genotype. Human sperms exhibit a variety of nuclear shapes. The heterogeneity in nuclear shape may be due to the difference in chromatin condensation. The posterior ring is a circumferential junction between the plasma membrane and nuclear envelope with a series of striations (Pedersen 1972b). It is a diving point between the flagellum and head. The implantation fossa of the sperm tail is situated at the base of the nucleus.

The nucleus of the sperm is extremely well packaged. The genome is repackaged into a crystalline state. During the condensation process, there is elimination of RNA, replacement of somatic histones by protamines and formation of chromatin-stabilizing disulphide bonds (Balhorn et al. 1984). Though most histones are replaced by protamines, there are some areas where the somatic-like structure is retained. In some cases, these regions are differentially marked by modified histones in a manner reminiscent of the epigenetic states observed in somatic or stem cells (Hammoud et al. 2009). This may influence the order in which genes are repackaged into a nucleosomal bound state and/or expressed following fertilization (Rousseaux et al. 2008). Recent research has led to believe that there could be more to sperm than just delivering the paternal DNA. The role of the three main structural genetic elements of the sperm nucleus, chromatin, RNA, and the nuclear matrix beyond the sperm nucleus, has been suggested by researchers which may have an impact on embryonic development.

3.12 Cytoplasmic Droplet

It is the residual cytoplasm from the process of spermiogenesis. It forms a collar shaped covering of the midpiece of the flagellum. It usually has redundant organelles such as ribosomes and mitochondria.

3.13 Plasma Membrane

The plasma membrane forms the outer boundary of all cells. It maintains the cell integrity and functions as a dynamic interface between the cell and its environment. The plasma membrane of the sperm has regional specialization with specific physical, chemical and immunological parameters. It also undergoes reorganization during its transport in the female reproductive tract during the process of capacitation.

There are five domains in the plasma membrane of the sperm, depending on the part of the sperm it is associated with. The head of the sperm has three domains covering the acrosome, equatorial region and the post acrosomal region. The flagellum has two domains covering the principal piece and the midpiece. The domains are different in their affinity for plant lectins, difference in the distribution of glycocalyx, membrane fluidity, lipid composition, intra-membranous particle distribution, binding pattern for monoclonal antibodies and membranous surface charge (Koehler 1981; Friend 1982; Villaroya and Scholler 1986 and Yanagimachi et al. 1972). The specialization allows for more efficient performance of tasks which culminates in fertilization.

3.14 Midpiece Region

The plasma membrane overlying the mitochondria contains chains of particles that follow the mitochondrial helix. In the interstices, the particles are absent and hence the plasma membrane is closely applied to the mitochondrial sheath (Philips 1970). These particles were first discovered in guinea pig by Friend and Fawcett in 1974. The main function of the plasma membrane over the mitochondrial sheath is to permit substances that are of significance in metabolism during capacitation.

3.15 Principal Piece Region

The axonemal complex is attached to the plasma membrane through a 'zipper', which is a longitudinal double row of staggered intra-membranous particles that overlay the dense outer fibre number 1 (Friend and Fawcett 1974). The particles of the zipper attach to the ribs of the fibrous sheath. They may have a role in controlling the axonemal functions such as the change in the flagellar beat during capacitation. The membrane of the midpiece is separated from the principal piece by the annulus.

3.16 Anterior Acrosomal Region

The plasma membrane covering the anterior acrosome has a major role in fertilization. It recognizes and binds to the zona pellucida and fuses with the outer acrosomal membrane during cortical exocytosis, during acrosome reaction. The presence of glycocalyx is high in this region of plasma membrane. The membrane in this region exhibits fusogenic properties, which facilitates the processes in the initiation of the acrosome reaction. At the end of the acrosome reaction, the inner acrosomal membrane becomes the limiting membrane of the anterior region of the head.

3.17 Equatorial Region

This is the site of fusion of the plasma membrane with the oocyte. The plasma membrane in this region is stable. Physiological changes occur in the plasma membrane in this region around the time of acrosome reaction, without much of structural changes, as sperm oocyte fusion cannot happen without the acrosome reaction.

3.18 Post-acrosomal Region

In humans, this part consists of indistinct striations posteriorly and an anterior domain consisting of an irregular smooth ridge around the base of the acrosome (Pedersen 1972a, b).

3.18.1 Head: Role in Infertility

Pathology of acrosome has been most commonly implicated in causing subfertility in males. This could include partial or complete lack of acrosome or disorganization of the acrosome membrane. This will result in the alteration in the shape of the sperm head commonly called the round sperm head. This could also implicate a failure in the late stages of spermiogenesis. This will cause inability of the sperm to elicit an acrosome reaction, hence being unable to penetrate the zona pellucida. When all the sperms in the semen sample have a round head, it is termed globozoospermia. When there is separation of the flagellum from the head, the resulting structure is called the pin head (Zaneveld and Polakowski 1977).

The latest abnormality that has come as another armamentarium in the hands of reproductive specialists is the sperm DNA fragmentation. This is an abnormality when there are incomplete chromatin condensations displaying single-stranded DNA rather than double-stranded DNA (Johnson et al. 2011). This has been implicated in IVF failures, poor embryonic development and hence male subfertility.

Conclusion

A spermatozoon is a highly specialized cell. The importance of sperm has been never more highlighted than in the present age of advanced reproductive medicine. Though the morphological criteria have been recommended by WHO, the understanding of ultrastructure of sperm will contribute to the diagnosis and treatment conditions which contribute to subfertility.

As for correlation between ultrastructure of sperm and fertilization capacity in IVF, Alebit et al. in 1992 concluded that sperm alterations in tail do not affect the fertilizing capacity, whereas decondensation of nuclear chromatin regardless of acromosal defect was mentioned as one of the major reasons for IVF failure by Chitale and Rathur as early as 1995. In the era of ICSI, there have been no conclusive studies correlating the severity of sperm defects to success in ICSI. Yet again, the sperm remains as elusive as ever!

References

Alberts B, Johnson A, Lewis J, et al. Molecular biology of the cell. 4th ed. New York: Garland Science; 2002.

Balhorn R, Weston S, Thomas C, Wyrobek A. DNA packaging in mouse spermatids. Synthesis of protamine variants and four transition proteins. Exp Cell Res. 1984;150:298–308. doi:10.1016/0014-4827(84)90572-X.

Baltzer F. Theodor Boveri; Life and Work of a Great Biologist, 1862–1915. Univ of California Press; 1967.

Barratt CL, Kay V, Oxenham SK. The human spermatozoon – a stripped down but refined machine. J Biol. 2009;8(7):63.

Boivin J, Bunting L, Collins JA, Nygren KG. International estimates of infertility prevalence and treatment-seeking: potential need and demand for infertility medical care. Hum Reprod. 2007;22:1506–12. doi:10.1093/humrep/dem046.

Bornens M, Bailly E, Gosti F, Keryer G. The centrosome: recent advances on structure and functions. Prog Mol Subcell Biol. 1990;11:86–114.

Camner P, Mossberg B, Afzelius BA. Evidence of congenitally nonfunctioning cilia in the tracheobronchial tract in two sub-jects. Am Rev Respir Dis. 1975;112:807–9.

Clermont Y, Oko R, Hermo L. Immunocytochemical localization of proteins utilized in the formation of outer dense fibers and fibrous sheath in rat spermatids: an electron microscope study. Anat Rec. 1990;227:447–57.

Curry MR, Watson PF. Sperm structure and function. In: Gemetes- the spermatozoon. New York: Press Syndicate of the University of Cambridge; 1995. p. 45–70.

Farrell KW. Purification and reassembly of tubulin from outer doublet microtubules. Methods Cell Biol. 1982;24:61–78.

Fawcett DW. The mammalian spermatozoon. Dev Biol. 1975;44:394–436. Guan J, Kinoshita M, Yuan L. Spatiotemporal association of DNAJB13 with the annulus during mouse sperm flagellum development. BMC Dev Biol. 2009;9:23.

Friend DS. Plasma membrane diversity in a highly polarized cell. J Cell Biol. 1982;93:243–9.

Friend DS, Fawcett DW. Membrane differentiation in freeze-fracture mammalian sperm. J Cell Biol. 1974;63:641–64.

Green DPL. Sperm thrusts and the problem of penetration. Biol Rev Camb Philos Soc. 1988;63:70–105.

Guan J, Kinoshita M, Yuan L. Spatiotemporal association of DNAJB13 with the annulus during mouse sperm flagellum development. BMC Dev Biol. 2009;9:23. doi:10.1186/1471-213X-9-23.

Guen LE, Crozet N. Microtubule and centrosome distribution during sheep fertilization. Eur J Cell Biol. 1989;48:239–49.

Hammoud SS, Nix DA, Zhang H, Purwar J, Carrell DT, Cairns BR. Distinctive chromatin in human sperm packages genes for embryo development. Nature. 2009;460:473–8. doi:10.1038/nature08162.

Holzbaur EL, Vallee RB. DYNEINS: molecular structure and cellular function. Annu Rev Cell Dev Biol. 1994;10:339–72.

Huang TTF, Yanagimachi R. Inner acrosomal membrane of mammalian spermatozoa: its properties and its possible function in fertilization. Am J Anat. 1985;174:249–68.
Johnson GD, Lalancette C. The sperm nucleus: chromatin, RNA, and the nuclear matrix. Reproduction. 2010;141(1):21–36. doi:10.1530/REP-10-0322.
Johnson GD, Lalancette C, Linnemann AK, ´de´ric Leduc F, Boissonneault G, Krawetz SA. The sperm nucleus: chromatin, RNA, and the nuclear matrix. Reproduction. 2011;141:21–36.
Kamiya R. Functional diversity of axonemal dyneins as studied in Chlamydomonas mutants. Int Rev Cytol. 2002;219:115–55.
Kazuo Inaba, Katsutoshi Mizuno. Sperm dysfunction and ciliopathy. Reproductive Medicine and Biology 2016;15:77–94.
Koehler JK. Human sperm head ultrastructure: freeze etching study. J Ultrastruct Res. 1972;39: 520–39.
Koehler JK. Lectins as probes of the spermatozoon surface. Arch Androl. 1981;6:197–217.
Kupker W, Schulze W, Diedrich K. Ultrastructure of gametes and intracytoplasmic sperm injection: the significance of sperm morphology. Hum Reprod. 1998;13 Suppl 1:99–106.
Lindemann CB, Orlando A, Kanous KS. The flagellar beat of rat sperm is organized by the interaction of two functionally distinct populations of dynein bridges with a stable central axonemal partition. J Cell Sci. 1992;102:249–60.
Milisav I. Dynein and dynein-related genes. Cell Motil Cytoskeleton. 1998;39:261–72.
Mitchell V, Sigala J, Ballot C, Jumeau F, Barbotin AL, Duhamel A, Rives N, Rigot JM, Escalier D. and Peers MC. Light microscopy morphological characteristics of the sperm flagellum may be related to axonemal abnormalities. Andrologia. 2015;47:214–220. doi: 10.1111/and.12249
Palermo G, Munne S, Cohel J. The human zygote inherits its mitotic potential from male gamete. Hum Reprod. 1994;9:1220–5.
Pedersen H. Further observations on the fins structure of the human spermatozoa. Z Zelforsch. 1972a;123:305–15.
Pedersen H. The postacrosomal region of the spermatozoa of man and Macacaarctoides. J Ultrastruct Res. 1972b;40:366–77.
Pederson H. Observations on the axial filament of the human spermatozoa. J Ultrastuct Res. 1970; 33:451–62.
Porter ME, Johnson KE. Differential localization of two isoforms of the regulatory subunit RII alpha of cAMP-dependent protein kinase in human sperm: biochemical and cytochemical study. Annu Rev Cell Dev Biol. 1989;5:119–51.
Rousseaux S, Reynoird N, Escoffier E, Thevenon J, Caron C, Khochbin S. Epigenetic reprogramming of the male genome during gametogenesis and in the zygote. Reprod Biomed Online. 2008;16:492–503. doi:10.1016/S1472-6483(10)60456-7.
Sathananthan AH, Kola I, Osborna J, Trounson A. Centrioles in the beginning of human development. Proc Natl Acad Sci U S A. 1991;88:4806–10.
Sathananthan AH, Ratnam SS, Ng SC, Tarin JJ, et al. The sperm centriole: its inheritance, replication and perpetuation in early human embryos. Hum Reprod. 1996;11:345–56.
Schatten G. The centrosome and its mode of inheritance: the reduction of the centrosome during gametogenesis and its restoration during fertilization. Dev Biol. 1994;165:299–335.
Siegel MS, Bechtold DS, Willard JC, Poakoski KL. Partial characterization and purification of human sperminogen. Biol Reprod. 1987;36:1063–8.
Tash JS, Means AR. Regulation of protein phosphorylation and motility of sperm by cyclic adenosine monophosphate and calcium. Biol Reprod. 1982;26:745–63.
Tash JS, Means AR. Cyclic adenosine 3′5′ monophosphate, calcium and protein phosphorylation in flagellar motility. Biol Reprod. 1983;28:75–104.
Van Blerkom J, Davis P. Evolution of the sperm aster microinjection of isolated human sperm centrosomes into meiotically mature human oocytes. Hum Reprod. 1995;10: 2179–82. Virtanen I, Bradley RA, Paasivuo R, Lehto VP. Distinct cytoskeletal domains revealed in sperm cells. J Cell Biol. 1984;99:1983–91.
Villaroya S, Scholler R. Regional heterogeneity of human spermatozoa detected with monoclonal antibodies. J Reprod Fertil. 1986;76:435–47.

Virtanen I, Bradley RA, Paasivuo R, Lehto V-P. Distinct cytoskeletal domains revealed in sperm cells. J Cell Biol. 1984;99:1983–91.
Yanagimachi R, Noda YD, Fujimoto M, Nicholson G. The distribution of negative surface charges on mammalian spermatozoa. Am J Anat. 1972;135:497–520.
Zaneveld LJD, Polakowski KL. Collection and physical examination of the ejaculate. In: Hafez ESE, editor. Techniques of human andrology. Amsterdam: Elsevier-North Holland; 1977. p. 147–72.

4 A Clinical Approach to Male Infertility

N. Pandiyan and Shah Dupesh Khan

4.1 Introduction

Infertility has become a public health problem afflicting an estimated one in ten couples globally (Boivin et al. 2007). Approximately 48.5 million couples engaging in unprotected intercourse suffer from involuntary childlessness (Martinez et al. 2006). Male infertility alone contributes to approximately 60 % of the problem and has become a major health concern, the incidence of male infertility ranging from 2.5 to 12 % across different regions around the world (Agarwal et al. 2015). The actual incidence may be even higher, due to a general lack of data and underreporting in certain patriarchal cultures and groups where men refuse to be clinically evaluated. Sadly, despite these hard-hitting facts, clinical andrology remains a subject of neglect. The infertility specialist is frequently a gynecologist, with little or no understanding in assessing an infertile male. Frequently, the diagnosis of male infertility is based on a single laboratory value of the semen analysis, which ultimately decides the course of treatment for the infertile male. Thus, it is not the patient who is being treated, but the sperm which has become the cellular patient. The semen picture, in a majority, will not give any clues to the actual underlying pathology (Cummins and Jequier 1994).

N. Pandiyan, MD, DGO, MNAMS (✉)
Department of Reproductive Medicine, Chettinad Hospital and Research Institute, Chettinad University, Rajiv Gandhi Salai, Kelambakkam, Chennai, TN 603103, India
e-mail: pandiyan1@yahoo.com

S.D. Khan, MBBS, DCE, FASM, (PhD)
Andrology and Sexual Medicine, The Women's Center, Center of Excellence for Mens Health, Burkit Road, T-Nagar, Chennai, TN 600017, India

Fortis Healthcare, Fortis Malar Hospitals, Adyar, Chennai, TN 600020, India

K. Gunasekaran, N. Pandiyan (eds.), *Male Infertility*,
DOI 10.1007/978-81-322-3604-7_4

Table 4.1 Outlines the major causes of male infertility

Causes of male infertility (WHO)
Idiopathic
Isolated abnormalities of semen and sperm parameters
Varicocele
Immunological infertility
Genital tract infection
Primary testicular failure
Kallmann's syndrome
Klinefelter's syndrome
Cryptorchidism
Obstruction
Ejaculatory dysfunction
Erectile dysfunction
Genetic causes: Y-chromosome microdeletion

The exact etiopathological mechanism through which varicocele and antisperm antibodies contribute to male infertility remains to be elucidated

4.2 Goal and Indications for Evaluation of the Infertile Male

Male infertility can be attributed to a variety of conditions; however, most of the time an exact cause is not found, but if found, not all can be treated and/or corrected. An abnormal semen picture may be the only finding; in these cases, the cause of infertility is termed *idiopathic*. The aim of male infertility evaluation is to identify and treat potentially correctable causes. The identification of genetic disorder during male infertility workup would help in counseling the couple about the potential risks involved to the offspring and also help guide the couple to alternate treatment strategies. Potential serious conditions like testicular cancer and pituitary tumors may also present with infertility and/or sexual dysfunction as the only primary symptom during an assessment (Honig et al. 1994).

In a large WHO study involving over 8500 couples from 25 countries, a standardized classification system for categorizing the various causes of male infertility was published. This study clearly showed that the single most common etiology of male infertility belonged to the *idiopathic abnormalities of the semen* category (25 %), followed by varicocele (Comhaire 1987). Nevertheless, with our recent understanding of genetic causes, this study is in need of a review. The various causes of male infertility are summarized in Table 4.1. Varicocele is however a debatable cause of male infertility.

4.3 The Relevance of Clinical History Taking

Numerous medical conditions/pathologies can afflict male fertility both directly and indirectly. An in-depth history taking should comprehensively assess the patients (a) past fertility, (b) past investigations and treatments for infertility,

(c) presence of associated systemic diseases and/or treatments for the same, (d) current and past medication history, (e) past and recent history of surgeries with particular emphasis to surgeries performed in the inguinal/pelvic/testicular region, (f) chemotherapies and/or radiotherapy, (g) the occupational exposure to potential toxins/chemicals, (h) personal lifestyle factors like smoking and alcohol consumption and/or drug abuse, (i) family history of infertility and other congenital defects, and finally (j) sexual history. An in-depth sexual history is very important in the workup of an infertile male since the coital frequency/week is significantly associated with the chance of conception (Macleod and Gold 1953). A chance of conception significantly increases when coital frequency approaches ≥3 time/week as compared to ≤2 times/week. History about the patient's libido, erection, and ejaculation should also be elucidated as a pathology affecting any of these areas could reduce the number of successful sexual contacts leading to infertility. An outline of the various components in a male infertility clinical history taking is given in Table 4.2. An important point of noteworthy mention is that numerous medical drugs can potentially impair the male's fertility. Their mechanism of action could be by either affecting spermatogenesis, sperm motility, or sperm fertilizing capacity. Commonly used antibiotics, proton pump inhibitors, antihypertensive medications, calcium channel blockers, statins, beta-blockers, and psychotropic medications can all potentially impair male fertility and/or sexual function leading to difficulties with achieving a conception (Pandiyan 2007). A clinical history should thoroughly elucidate as to whether the patient *is or was* on any medication for any comorbid illness.

4.4 Clinical Examination of an Infertile Male

Clinical examination of an infertile male forms an important initial tool in the assessment of male infertility. A general examination is as important as a genital exam. The patient's height, weight, and BMI (body mass index) along with blood pressure should be documented before the systemic and local examination. The degree of androgenization can be assessed by looking for a male pattern of hair distribution and by questioning the patient on the frequency of shaving (to assess facial hair growth). An assessment of the distribution of body hair should also be made. Sparse hair distribution combined with gynecomastia and eunuchoidal body proportions is suggestive of Klinefelter's syndrome which can be clinically picked by watchful observation of the patient's phenotype. An assessment of the patient's cardiovascular and respiratory system is also to be made routine. Here, the presence of bronchiectasis combined with situs inversus is suggestive of dyskinetic cilia syndrome where the semen picture would also show varying degrees of immotile spermatozoa (Schidlow 1994). Careful inspection of the abdomen and inguinal region may show up scars that may potentially indicate past hernia surgery and/or orchidopexy that the patient might have forgotten to mention during the clinical history taking. Pediatric hernia surgeries carry a potential risk of iatrogenic injury to the vas deferens (Sheynkin et al. 1998). Genital examination should include details of the penile anatomy. The penis is examined and the position of the external urethral

Table 4.2 Highlights the various components that have to be assessed in the examination of an infertile male

Components of history taking in the assessment of an infertile male
1. Fertility history
Duration of marriage and infertility
Past conception with present and/or previous partner
Duration of infertility
Previous fertility investigations and treatments
2. Medical history
Past/present history of diabetes, hypertension, respiratory tract disease, and liver disease
Past/present history of neurological diseases and treatments
Past/present history of high fever
Past/present history of medication and duration of use
Past/present history of urinary tract infections/sexually transmitted disease
3. Surgical history
Past history of vasectomy, testicular surgeries like varicocelectomy and hydrocelectomy
Past history of inguinal hernia surgery, sympathectomy, prostatectomy
Past history of bladder neck operations
Any other history of urethral strictures
Past history of penile surgeries for hypospadias/epispadias
4. Developmental and childhood history
Past history of mumps/any other viral illness
Past history scrotal injury
Past history of testicular torsion
Past history of treatment for testicular maldescent and the age of treatment
Puberty and its onset, sexual development
5. Occupational and environmental history
Any history of exposure to heat, toxic factors, carcinogenic dyes, tannins, etc.
Any history of excess consumption of alcohol, smoking, and other drug abuse
Any history of exposure to high heat and exposure to sexually transmitted infections
6. Family history
Any family history of infertility, congenital birth defects
Any family history of cryptorchidism, metabolic syndrome, and other endocrine disorders
7. Sexual history
Frequency of intercourse
Libido
Erectile function
Ejaculation
Lubricant usage

meatus is noted. The presence of any hypospadias or epispadias should be documented. Phimosis should also be excluded. Palpation of the penile body may reveal hardened areas due to fibrous plaque formation within the cavernosal tissue that is suggestive of Peyronie's disease (Gelbard 1995). This is followed by examination of the testes, for its size and consistency. Testicular size is estimated to calculate volume; the testicular size has a moderate degree of correlation to sperm production (Johnson et al. 1980).

The mean average testicular volume of South Indian men is 6 cc (Dupesh and Pandiyan 2015). Estimation of testicular volume can be done using a Prader orchidometer, and these measurements correlate well with ultrasound measurements, although a good correlation >0.8 is obtained only with good clinical experience (Behre and Nashan 1989). A simpler method for estimating testicular size involves the use of a washable steel scale; in this method, the testis is stabilized firmly between the index and thumb, length (l) is measured in centimeters (cm) from the upper pole to the lower pole, and breadth (b) and height (h) along the midaxis are recorded. Volume is estimated by $l \times b \times h/2$ (length × breadth × height the product divided by two). This method gives an excellent correlation with ultrasound-based measurements and is routinely used in our clinic (Shah and Pandiyan 2015). From the clinical perspective, a small but firm testis along with elevated FSH is suggestive of hypergonadotropic hypogonadism, while small soft testis with low FSH is suggestive of hypogonadotropic hypogonadism (Pandiyan 1999). For male patients with low FSH and low LH, cranial imaging with *serum prolactin measurement* should be done to rule out pituitary pathology (De Kretser 1979). The presence of maldescended testis and anorchia should be documented and warrant further investigation. The epididymis should also be palpated. One should also look out for the classical Bayle's sign, where the epididymis is palpable and augmented and soft suggestive of an obstruction (Schoysman 1982). A normal epididymis is usually firm in consistency. Presence of nodularity is rare finding and could be due to a past history of tuberculous epididymo-orchitis.

The presence or absence of the vas deferens must be carefully examined on both sides. The vas deferens can be palpated with the patient in a supine position, within the vessels of the spermatic cord, as a firm threadlike structure that snaps between the examiner's fingers. The bilateral absence of vas deferens is suggestive of congenital bilateral absence of vas deferens (CBAVD) and is an extreme phenotypic variant of CFTR gene mutations (Costes et al. 1994). Unnecessary surgical exploration can be avoided in these cases. CBAVD is commonly associated with agenesis of the seminal vesicles, absence of sperm in the ejaculate with absent fructose in semen. In both unilateral and bilateral absence of vas deferens, an abdominal ultrasound for renal anomalies is warranted (McCallum et al. 2001). A varicocele is defined as distension of the venous pampiniform plexus in the spermatic cord, and assessment should be done only in the upright position. Grade 3 varicoceles are usually easily identified; however, to diagnose smaller grades accurately, Doppler studies are necessary.

4.5 Investigating an Infertile Male: A Prudent Approach

Semen analysis remains the cornerstone test in the workup of an infertile male. A conventional semen analysis gives information about the male's testicular germ cell function, secretory function of the male's accessory sex organs, and also about the patency of the male reproductive tract. It is very important to understand that semen parameters of concentration, motility, and morphology show a high degree of variance with time, place, and region both among individuals and also within the same individual. Semen analysis remains a controversial but *necessary test* and has numerous pitfalls: (a) it is a subjective test, with results varying between technical personnel and within the same personnel who are assessing the sample (Barroso et al. 1999); (b) semen parameters of both fertile and infertile men show considerable degree of overlap between parameters, and very low sperm counts have led to documented spontaneous pregnancies (Thomson et al. 1993); (c) none of current semen parameters, namely, sperm concentration, motility, and morphology, have good predictive power in estimating a couple's fertility potential (Ford 2010); and (d) it is important to understand that the relation between sperm concentration, sperm motility, and fertility is not a simple one. The role of the female partner and her fertility play a key role in deciding whether a conception would occur. It is now well known that a reproductive pathology in the female can reduce the fertility potential of a male presenting with a so-called "normal" spermiogram.

The clinical utility of semen analysis however cannot be overemphasized in extreme presentations like azoospermia, total asthenozoospermia, necrozoospermia, and globozoospermia. We still do not understand the molecular basis to male infertility; pathological changes resulting in subfertility rarely reflect onto a conventional semen analysis. The World Health Organization (WHO) has published over five editions so far reviewing diagnostic criteria and protocols for semen analysis in different times. It recently published the fifth edition of the Laboratory Manual for the Examination and Processing of Human Semen in 2010 (WHO manual, 5th edition. 2010). On an interesting note, while the first four editions were "consensus" based on expert opinions, the latest edition was published after a multicenter study. Numerous men who were previously diagnosed with oligozoospermia, asthenozoospermia, and teratozoospermia have now been included in the normal range as per the new manual's diagnostic cutoffs. Thus, many men might have been subjected to unwanted and unwarranted surgeries/therapies for infertility based on these criteria (Pandiyan 2012). Semen analysis thus remains a number game.

The aforementioned facts do not mean that a semen analysis is a redundant test, but it is important to take a deep look at the patient from a clinical perspective and listen to his story and only then can the right diagnosis be made from a clinical standpoint. Common instructions given to the male patient before a semen analysis are as follows: a] Patients are advised to abstain from sexual intercourse for a period ranging from 2 to 7 days before a semen analysis as per the WHO criteria. However, a retrospective analysis of our data from over 2130 patients clearly showed that all the three semen parameters, namely, concentration, motility, and morphology do not vary significantly as a result of ejaculatory abstinence. Any variation noted was still within the normal range (Shah and Pandiyan ISAR 2015).

In our clinic, we do not recommend patients to collect a sample after a specified period of ejaculatory abstinence. (a) Sample collection should be done in a sterile wide-mouthed container; any spillage should be reported immediately as this could potentially lead to a diagnosis of hypospermia. (b) Lubricant usage is not recommended during sample collection, and collection should be done in a private room adjacent to the andrology laboratory. Postcollection, the semen is allowed to liquefy for 20–30 min, after which a macroscopic estimation of semen volume, pH, liquefaction, and viscosity is done. This is then followed by a microscopic assessment of sperm concentration, motility, and morphology as per WHO 2010 guideline values. Reference values are given in Table 4.3.

4.6 Endocrine Workup of an Infertile Male

Serum FSH is usually the only endocrine test required for most patients with male infertility. If there is concomitant sexual dysfunction, then estimation of serum LH, prolactin, total testosterone, and free testosterone is required. Thyroid evaluation is not required in most men presenting with male infertility unless there is family history or elevated prolactin. Serum FSH is done in patients presenting with a sperm count <10 million/ml. Highly elevated values of FSH presenting along with azoospermia or severe oligozoospermia are suggestive of seminiferous tubular failure or an ongoing failure of the germinal epithelium. Elevated FSH and LH is suggestive of testicular failure, either acquired or possibly Klinefelter's syndrome. Very low FSH and LH could be due to a pituitary pathology or could be congenital (Kallmann's syndrome) and requires prompt intervention. Serum FSH within the normal range in azoospermic patients indicates an obstructive cause and needs further evaluation to assess the exact level/site of obstruction. A low ejaculate volume along with normal FSH and a semen picture showing azoospermia possibly indicates an obstruction at the level of the ejaculatory duct or vas deferens (Pandiyan 1999). Tables 4.4 and 4.5 and Fig. 4.1 give an algorithm for the basic workup of azoospermia.

Table 4.3 Reference values given are 5th centile and are used as lower cutoff limits of normality

Semen analysis parameters	WHO 2010 guideline values
Volume	1.5 ml
Sperm concentration/ml	15×10^6/ml
Total sperm count/ejaculate	39×10^6/ejaculate
Total motility	40 %
Progressive motility	32 %
Morphology	4 %
Vitality	58 %

Results should not be overinterpreted from a clinical standpoint

Table 4.4 Outlines the possible findings in patients suspected with nonobstructive azoospermia

Condition	FSH	Testes size	Semen volume	Feature
Hypogonadotropic Hypogonadism	Low or undetectable	Small and soft	Normal	Hyposmia or anosmia present
Seminiferous tubular failure	Elevated	Small, soft, and firm	Normal	–
Borderline azoospermia	Normal to mild elevation	Normal to slightly small	Normal	Biopsy shows hypospermatogenesis or maturation arrest

Reproduced with permission from Pandiyan (1999)

Table 4.5 Outlines the possible findings in patients suspected with obstructive azoospermia

Condition	FSH	Testes size	Semen volume	Feature
Ejaculatory duct obstruction	Normal	Normal	Very low	Absent
Vasal aplasia	Normal	Normal	Very low	Absent
Epididymal obstruction	Normal	Normal	Normal	Present
Vasal obstruction	Normal	Normal	Normal	Present
Intratesticular obstruction	Normal	Normal	Normal	Present

Reproduced with permission from Pandiyan (1999)

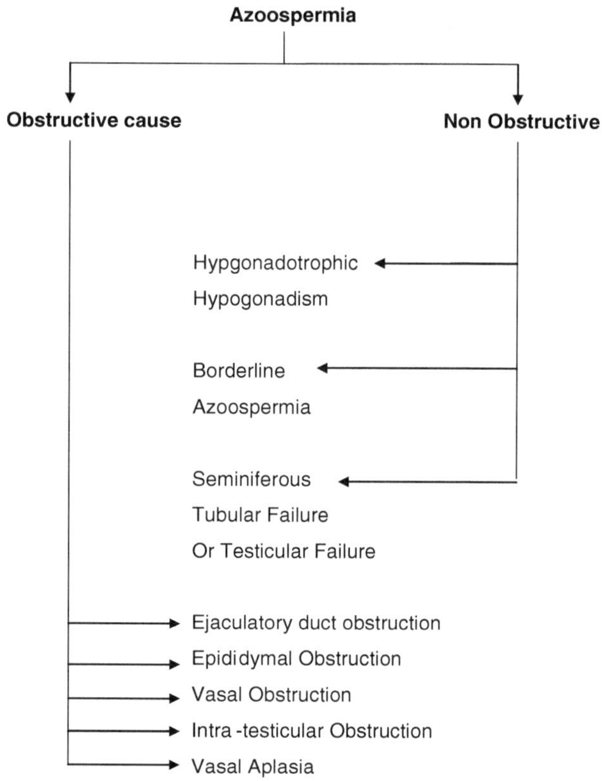

Fig. 4.1 Gives an outline of the differential diagnosis of azoospermia

If a nonobstructive cause is suspected, proceed as below to discern a possible etiology.

4.7 Genetics in Male Infertility

Genetic testing of the infertile male is done in select conditions. Genetic testing is done to assess the presence of Y-chromosome microdeletions that are commonly seen in 10–15 % of patients who are diagnosed with nonobstructive azoospermia (NOA) (McElreavey et al. 2000). Y-chromosome microdeletion is a known cause of spermatogenic failure. From the clinical standpoint, there are three types of deletions, namely, AZFa, AZFb, and AZFc. AZFa and AZFb have poor prognosis for sperm retrieval from the testis and are associated with Sertoli cell only or maturation arrest (McElreavey et al. 2000). The type of deletion affects the outcome of a testicular sperm extraction procedure done in these groups of patients. In AZFc deletion, there is a good chance of sperm retrieval from at least 50 % of patients presenting with these deletions; however, in AZFa and AZFb deletions, there is virtually *no chance* of finding sperm during retrieval (McElreavey and Krausz 1999). While a clear-cut relationship between the genotype and phenotype remains to be established, numerous studies have supported these observed trends. Y-chromosome microdeletion studies are not done routinely in many centers. We feel it may serve as an important prognostic test, as a prelude to predicting sperm retrieval for men presenting with NOA. Prior to ART, Y-chromosome microdeletion studies are vital to counsel couples regarding the possible chances of perpetuating male infertility to their male offsprings. Genetic testing of an infertile male is also indicated in patients where the clinical evaluation suggests Klinefelter's or Kallmann's syndrome and in patients with unilateral or bilateral absence of vas deferens, where a CFTR gene mutation would be expected.

4.8 Tests of Sperm Function, Qua Vadis

A number of sperm function tests have been utilized in the clinical setting in the past. Sperm function tests like acrosome reaction and induced acrosome reaction to calcium ionophore have demonstrated an increase in spontaneous acrosome reaction of sperm of infertile men compared to fertile controls (Fenichel et al. 1991). The clinical significance of these findings remains unknown. Other tests of specialized sperm function include sperm zona pellucida test and sperm penetration assays. Although a good degree of correlation is seen between these assays and the fertilizing ability of sperm in a conventional IVF cycle (Oehninger et al. 2000), these tests are again rarely used in a clinical setting, since male factor infertility is predominantly managed by ICSI worldwide. Tests, such as the postcoital test, have fallen out of favor, due to a lack of standardization in the test methodology, lack of definition as to what constitutes a normal test, and poor reproducibility (Griffith and Grimes 1990). Other newer tests, like the sperm creatinine kinase assay or assessment of markers of abortive apoptosis and hyaluronic acid binding assay, may help in sperm selection during ICSI (Huszar et al. 2007) but have no clinical utility in the evaluation of an infertile male.

A newer test that has recently caught the fancy of the clinical fraternity is the sperm DNA fragmentation assay. DNA integrity in the sperm is maintained by disulfide cross-linkages between proteins called protamines; this allows the compact packaging of the genetic material. After the spermiation process, the spermatozoa are transcriptionally inactive; thus, any damage occurring to the nuclear material cannot be potentially repaired in the sperm themselves. DNA damage in the sperm can occur during sperm transit in the male reproductive tract or due to endogenous endonuclease activity, heat exposure, reactive oxygen species, and/or potential gonadotoxin exposure (Lopes et al. 1998). Sperm DNA fragmentation has also been claimed to be associated with poor embryo quality, an increase in miscarriage rates, and also general poorer ICSI outcomes (Sakkas and Alvarez 2010). Commonly used tests to assess DNA fragmentation include conventional single-gel electrophoresis (COMET assay), terminal deoxy UTP nick end labeling (TUNEL), and lastly sperm chromatin structure assay (SCSA). From a clinical standpoint, we need to understand that although tests of DNA fragmentation may give some clinical information on the percentage of fragmentation of DNA, none of these tests actually give any information on the exact nucleotide sequences that are actually involved in fragmentation. Importantly, we are looking at a small subpool of spermatozoa for DNA fragmentation that may not be representative of the actual spermatozoa that reach the site of fertilization in vivo. Lastly, one must not forget that the oocyte in itself possesses a nucleotide excision repair (NER) mechanism, where potentially any fragmented nucleotide sequence in the sperm would be repaired (Ashwood and Edwards 1996). Considering the limited prognostic power of the DNA fragmentation test, we do not recommend these tests in the routine evaluation of an infertile male. Based on the current evidence and available literature, the ASRM practice committee guidelines also do not recommend routine DNA fragmentation analysis in the workup of an infertile couple (ASRM 2006, 2013). On a conclusive note, we would also like to point out that currently none of presently available sperm function tests have adequate sensitivity or specificity to predict IVF/ICSI treatment outcomes. The need to develop and validate ICSI-specific sperm function tests is the future.

4.9 Antioxidants in the Treatment of Male Infertility

Reactive oxygen species (ROS) have been blamed as a causative factor for numerous pathologies from head to foot. They have been implicated in the causative mechanism of stroke (Allen and Bayraktutan 2009) and also in diabetic foot (Cianci and Hunt 2007). However, it is not clear whether they are the cause or consequence of the pathology. ROS play an important physiological role in inducing apoptosis, which is an essential and indispensable cell function in all body tissues (Simon et al. 2000). Furthermore, antioxidant usage in cancer remains a conundrum (Seifried et al. 2003).

Not surprisingly, ROS have also been implicated in male infertility, and antioxidants to quench ROS have been prescribed rampantly around the globe (Ranjani et al. 2013). There are no large-scale high-quality randomized double-blind placebo-controlled trials to assess whether the antioxidants significantly contribute to improved semen parameters and improvement in pregnancy rates. A major confounding factor for any such study would be the inherent natural variability of semen, which has constantly been misinterpreted and misused to show clinical improvement with antioxidant usage. For the time being, till high-quality evidence is published, we do not recommend the routine usage of antioxidants in the management of idiopathic male infertility.

4.10 Treatable Conditions in Male Infertility

Most causes of obstructive azoospermia and some causes of aspermia are the only treatable conditions in male infertility from a clinical viewpoint. Obstructive azoospermia (OA) can be managed by surgical correction of the obstruction, exception being vasal aplasia where a surgical sperm retrieval can be performed. Patients with hypogonadotropic hypogonadism can be managed with gonadotropin therapy. For patients with retrograde ejaculation, a method of noninvasive sperm retrieval from the bladder can be done (Pandiyan et al. 1998). For all other conditions like severe oligozoospermia, asthenozoospermia, or a combination of semen parameter abnormalities, it would be wise to go with controlled ovarian hyperstimulation (COH) with IUI or ICSI and save time for the patient rather than try unproven empirical therapies. Depending on the women's age and duration of infertility, male patients with even 1 million/ml of motile sperm postwash could be given a cycle of IUI, although for patients where <1 million/ml of postwash recovery is obtained, it would be wise to go with ICSI.

A varicocele is invariably present in approximately 40 % of infertile males. Varicocelectomy in the management of male infertility remains *highly controversial*. We do not know the exact mechanism by which a varicocele contributes to impaired semen parameters or DNA fragmentation or just male infertility in general. *Indiscriminate varicocelectomy* in the management of the infertile male in the *era of ICSI* is not recommended, as assisted reproductive technology has shorter time to pregnancy rates and better results in general (Csokmay and DeCherney 2009).

4.11 Ethics of Treatment of Male Infertility

Prior to the advent of ICSI, all men with nonobstructive azoospermia due to seminiferous tubular dysfunction and most men with severe oligoasthenoteratozoospermia were untreatably infertile. Introduction of ICSI in 1992, Palermo and colleagues revolutionized the management of severe male infertility. However, it was soon recognized that a significant percentage of men, ranging from 15 to 35 %, with nonobstructive azoospermia and severe oligozoospermia (Foresta et al. 2001) may have Y-chromosome microdeletions. All these men would transmit these defects to all their offsprings, thereby perpetuating male infertility. Are we justified in doing this? This is a point to ponder.

CBAVD was an untreatable condition, until the introduction of ICSI and epididymal sperm aspiration (Pandiyan 1995). CBAVD is a genetic condition due to a defect in the CFTR gene; these patients may also transmit their defect to the offspring, raising the question, should we be treating these men at all? Men with balanced autosomal translocation may manifest NOA or severe oligozoospermia (Pandiyan and Jequier 1996). Treatment of these men with ICSI will lead to the birth of offspring with unbalanced translocation if the mother is also a carrier of balanced translocations.

Conclusions

With the advent of microassisted fertilization techniques, it would seem clinical andrology is but a redundant field. We would like to differ; microassisted fertilization techniques can never overcome the underlying pathology that leads to male infertility in the first place. At this juncture, we would like to stress that a man should not be judged by his semen alone and the sperm should not become the "cellular patient." The value of a good in-depth clinical evaluation must never be underestimated. Last of all, we would also like to advice caution with the utilization of microassisted technologies as it bypasses all natural selection process that is involved in sperm selection. Much research has to be done into this novel field of andrology before coming to a sound conclusion. The need of the hour we believe is *more clinical andrology and not less*.

References

Agarwal A, Mulgund A, Hamada A, Chyatte MR. A unique view on male infertility around the globe. Reprod Biol Endocrinol. 2015;13(1):37.

Allen CL, Bayraktutan U. Oxidative stress and its role in the pathogenesis of ischaemic stroke. Int J Stroke. 2009;4(6):461–70.

Ashwood-Smith MJ, Edwards RG. Genetics and human conception DNA repair by oocytes. Mol Hum Reprod. 1996;2(1):46–51.

Barroso G, Mercan R, Ozgur K, Morshedi M, Kolm P, Coetzee K, Kruger T, Oehninger S. Intra- and inter-laboratory variability in the assessment of sperm morphology by strict criteria: impact of semen preparation, staining techniques and manual versus computerized analysis. Hum Reprod. 1999;14(8):2036–40.

Behre HM, NASHAN D, Nieschlag E. Objective measurement of testicular volume by ultrasonography: evaluation of the technique and comparison with orchidometer estimates. Int J Androl. 1989;12(6):395–403.

Boivin J, Bunting L, Collins JA, Nygren KG. International estimates of infertility prevalence and treatment-seeking: potential need and demand for infertility medical care. Hum Reprod. 2007;22(6):1506–12.

Cianci P, Hunt TK. Adjunctive hyperbaric oxygen therapy in the treatment of the diabetic foot. In: Levin and O'Neal's the diabetic foot with CD-ROM. London: Elsevier Health Sciences; 2007. p. 339.

Comhaire F. Towards more objectivity in the management of male infertility. The need for a standardized approach. Int J Androl. 1987;7:1–53.

Costes B, Girodon E, Ghanem N, Flori E, Jardin A, Soufir JC, Goossens M. Frequent occurrence of the CFTR intron 8 (TG) n 5T allele in men with congenital bilateral absence of the vas deferens. Eur J Hum Genet: EJHG. 1994;3(5):285–93.

Csokmay JM, DeCherney AH. Discriminate use of varicocelectomy in light of advances in assisted reproductive technologies. In: Biennial review of infertility. Humana Press; 2009; pp. 249–57.

Cummins JM, Jequier AM. Treating male infertility needs more clinical andrology, not less. Hum Reprod. 1994;9(7):1214–9.
De Kretser DM. Endocrinology of male infertility. Br Med Bull. 1979;35(2):187–92.
Fenichel P, Donzeau M, Farahifar D, Basteris B, Ayraud N, Hsi BL. Dynamics of human sperm acrosome reaction: relation with in vitro fertilization. Fertil Steril. 1991;55(5):994–9.
Ford WC. Comments on the release of the 5th edition of the WHO laboratory manual for the examination and processing of human semen. Asian J Androl. 2010;12(1):59–63.
Foresta C, Moro E, Ferlin A. Y chromosome microdeletions and alterations of spermatogenesis. Endocr Rev. 2001;22:226–39.
Gelbard MK. Relaxing incisions in correction of penile deformity due to Peyronie's disease. J Urol. 1995;154(4):1457–60.
Griffith CS, Grimes DA. The validity of the postcoital test. Am J Obstet Gynecol. 1990;162(3): 615–20.
Honig SC, Lipshultz LI, Jarow J. Significant medical pathology uncovered by a comprehensive male infertility evaluation. Fertil Steril. 1994;62(5):1028–34.
Huszar G, Jakab A, Sakkas D, Ozenci CC, Cayli S, Delpiano E, Ozkavukcu S. Fertility testing and ICSI sperm selection by hyaluronic acid binding: clinical and genetic aspects. Reprod Biomed Online. 2007;14(5):650–63.
Johnson L, Petty CS, Neaves WB. The relationship of biopsy evaluations and testicular measurements to over-all daily sperm production in human testes. Fertil Steril. 1980;34(1):36–40.
Lopes S, Jurisicova A, Sun JG, Casper RF. Reactive oxygen species: potential cause for DNA fragmentation in human spermatozoa. Hum Reprod. 1998;13(4):896–900.
MacLeod J, Gold RZ. The male factor in fertility and infertility. VI semen. Quality and certain other factors in relation to ease of conception. Obstet Gynecol Surv. 1953;8(4):604–6.
Martinez G, Daniels K, Chandra A. Fertility of men and women aged 15–44 years in the United States: national survey of family growth. Natl Health Stat Report. 2006;2010(2012):1–28.
McCallum TJ, Milunsky JM, Munarriz R, Carson R, Sadeghi-Nejad H, Oates RD. Unilateral renal agenesis associated with congenital bilateral absence of the vas deferens: phenotypic findings and genetic considerations. Hum Reprod. 2001;16(2):282–8.
McElreavey K, Krausz C, Bishop CE. The human Y chromosome and male infertility. In: The genetic basis of male infertility. Berlin/Heidelberg:Springer; 2000. p. 211–32.
McElreavey K, Krausz C. Male infertility and the Y chromosome. Am J Hum Genet. 1999;64(4): 928–33.
Oehninger S, Franken DR, Sayed E, Barroso G, Kolm P. Sperm function assays and their predictive value for fertilization outcome in IVF therapy: a meta-analysis. Hum Reprod Update. 2000;6(2):160–8.
Pandiyan N, Pandiyan R, Muthiah S, Moorthy PS, Kanakaraj S. Sperm retrieval from the bladder-A simple non-invasive technique. Fertil Steril Int Ed. 1998;70:1187.
Pandiyan N. Medical drugs impairing fertility. In: Reproductive health and the environment. Netherlands: Springer; 2007. p. 187–205.
Pandiyan N. Semen analysis – a numbers game. CHCMJ. 2012;1(1):2–3.
Pandiyan N. Handbook of andrology. 1st ed. Chennai: T.R. Publication Pvt. Ltd; 1999.
Pandiyan N. Cryopreservation of epididymal spermatozoa. Curr Sci. 1995; 69(11):699–900.
Pandiyan N, Jequier AM. Genetics: mitotic chromosomal anomalies among 1210 infertile men. Hum Reprod. 1996;11(12):2604–8.
Practice Committee of the American Society for Reproductive Medicine. The clinical utility of sperm DNA integrity testing. Fertil Steril. 2006;86(5):S35–7.
Practice Committee of the American Society for Reproductive Medicine. The clinical utility of sperm DNA integrity testing: a guideline. Fertil Steril. 2013;99(3):673–7.
Ranjani S, Benziger A, Pandiyan N. Nutraceuticals in sperm abnormalities. Chettinad Health City. 2013;2(4):133–6.
Sakkas D, Alvarez JG. Sperm DNA fragmentation: mechanisms of origin, impact on reproductive outcome, and analysis. Fertil Steril. 2010;93(4):1027–36.
Schidlow DV. Primary ciliary dyskinesia (the immotile cilia syndrome). Ann Allergy. 1994;73(6): 457–68.

Schoysman R. Epididymal causes of male infertility: pathogenesis and management. Int J Androl. 1982;5(s5):120–34.

Seifried HE, McDonald SS, Anderson DE, Greenwald P, Milner JA. The antioxidant conundrum in cancer. Cancer Res. 2003;63(15):4295–8.

Dupesh S, Pandiyan N. Abstinence: does it make any sense? Paper presented at the Indian Society for Assisted Reproduction (ISAR). 2015. p. 10–12.

Sheynkin YR, Hendin BN, Schlegel PN, Goldstein M. Microsurgical repair of iatrogenic injury to the vas deferens. J Urol. 1998;159(1):139–41.

Simon HU, Haj-Yehia A, Levi-Schaffer F. Role of reactive oxygen species (ROS) in apoptosis induction. Apoptosis. 2000;5(5):415–8.

Thomson JA, Lincoln PJ, Mortimer P. Paternity by a seemingly infertile vasectomised man. BMJ. 1993;307(6899):299–300.

World Health Organization. WHO laboratory manual for the examination and processing of human semen. 5th ed. Geneva: World Health Organization; 2010.

5 Interpretation of Semen Analysis

Satya Srini Vasan

5.1 Introduction

Infertility is defined as the inability to conceive after one year of unprotected intercourse and affects globally about 15–20 % of couples. Of these, 30–40 % can be attributed to an identifiable male factor, 30–40 % to female factors, and the remaining 20 % to a combination of both male and female factors (Guttmacher 1956; Thonneau et al. 1991). Although many couples may present with an obvious and identifiable cause for the subfertility, there are cases with unexplained reasons for the delay in conception. Traditional semen analysis is the first test used to evaluate the male partner. This chapter discusses the basics of semen analysis and interpretation of the results in the light of the 2010 WHO Laboratory Manual for the Examination and Processing of Human Semen.

Evaluation of the man begins with a thorough history and physical examination and proceeds to laboratory examination. The initial screening evaluation of the male should include, at a minimum, a reproductive history and two semen analyses. If possible, the two semen analyses should be separated by a time period of at least 1 month. It is important to correlate history with the results of semen analysis because a person's medical history might affect the results of the semen analysis and, hence, fertility potential. Important considerations include past exposures to chemicals, heavy metals, pesticides, and extreme heat (specifically the workplace environment as well as recreational activities, such as frequency of hot tubs and use of a heated waterbed). Recreational drug use, as well as prescription medications, history of sexually transmitted infections, and other communicable diseases, genital infections, and genital injuries as well as fertility history are to be considered for evaluation (Sigman et al. 2009).

S.S. Vasan, DNB (Surgery, Urology)
Andrology, Manipal Ankur Andrology and Reproductive Services,
422, 20th Main, I Block, Rajajinagar, Bangalore 560010, India
e-mail: vasan@manipalankur.com

K. Gunasekaran, N. Pandiyan (eds.), *Male Infertility*,
DOI 10.1007/978-81-322-3604-7_5

5.2 Semen Analysis

Semen analysis is the most widely used test to predict male fertility potential. It provides information on the functional status of the seminiferous tubules, epididymis, and accessory sex glands, and its results are often taken as a surrogate measure of a man's ability to father a pregnancy. Although this test reveals useful information for the initial evaluation of the infertile male, it is not a test of fertility (Jequier 2010). It provides no insights into the functional potential of the spermatozoon to fertilize an ovum or to undergo the subsequent maturation processes required to achieve fertilization. It is important to understand that while the results may correlate with "fertility," the assay is not a direct measure of fertility (Guzick et al. 2001; Smith et al. 1977; Brazil 2010). An understanding of the physiology and pathophysiology associated with ejaculation and semen collection is also critical to the interpretation of the results of semen analysis.

Routine semen analysis includes (a) physical characteristics of semen, including liquefaction, viscosity, pH, color, and odor, (b) specimen volume, (c) sperm concentration, (d) sperm motility and progression, (e) sperm morphology, (f) leukocyte quantification, and (g) fructose detection in cases where no spermatozoa are found and ejaculate volume is low (Esteves et al. 2011). Routine semen analysis is the main pillar in male fertility investigation. In order to establish consistency in laboratory procedures, the WHO first published a manual for the examination of human semen and semen-cervical mucus interaction in 1980. The WHO criteria of 1987 and 1992 (World Health Organization 1987, 1992; Kruger et al. 1988) which classify more sperm in the normal category are also widely used in the routine semen evaluation. True reference ranges have not been established for semen parameters. The WHO manual also identified standards to exclude influences, such as the health of patient over the previous spermatogenic cycle, length of sexual abstinence, time, and temperature. The manual has been regularly updated (1980, 1987, 1992, and 1999). The addition of normal reference values in the WHO manuals has been of significant help in establishing some consistency of what constitutes a normal value. The WHO Laboratory Manual for the Examination and Processing of Human Semen serves as the basis for semen analysis in most of the recognized laboratories throughout the world. Table 5.1 shows the cutoff values of various parameters as per the previous WHO manuals.

5.3 Semen Collection

Semen must be collected after a standardized period of abstinence, usually 3 days (2–4 days), and the period must be indicated in the laboratory report. The time of collection, when the semen was liquefied, must be reported, as a delay of longer than an hour may adversely affect sperm motility (World Health Organization 2010). The standardization is essential to minimize fluctuations in semen quality, especially sperm count and sperm motility, due to short/long abstinence.

Table 5.1 Changes in cutoff reference values in WHO guidelines

Semen characteristics	WHO 1980	WHO 1987	WHO 1992	WHO 1999	WHO 2010[a]
Volume (ml)	ND	≥2	≥2	≥2	1.5
Sperm count (10^6/ml)	20-200	≥20	≥20	≥20	15
Total sperm count (10^6)	ND	≥40	≥40	≥40	39
Total motility (% motile)	≥60	≥50	≥50	≥50	40
Progressive motility[b]	≥ 2[c]	≥25 %	≥25 % (grade a)	≥25 % (grade a)	32 % (a+b)
Vitality (% alive)	ND	≥50	≥75	≥75	58
Morphology (% normal forms)	80.5	≥50	≥30[d]	(14)[e]	4[f]
Leukocyte count (10^6/ml)	<4.7	<1.0	<1.0	<1.0	<1.0

Reproduced from Esteves et al. (2012)
ND=not defined
[a]Lower reference limits generated from the lower fifth centile value
[b]Grade a = rapid progressive motility (>25 μm/s); grade b = slow/sluggish progressive motility (5–25 μm/s). Normal=50 % motility (grades a+b) or 25 % progressive motility (grade a) within 60 min of ejaculation
[c]Forward progression (scale 0–3)
[d]Arbitrary value
[e]Value not defined but strict criterion is suggested
[f]Strict (Tygerberg) criterion

5.4 Macroscopic Evaluation of Semen

Semen samples can show substantial variation in physicochemical properties including color and odor. Pathologically, seminal discoloration may be due to fresh blood, drugs (pyridium), jaundice, or contamination of semen with urine (e.g., bladder neck dysfunction). The complete semen analysis includes analysis of the semen volume, pH, liquefaction or non-liquefaction, and viscosity.

Volume The normal volume of ejaculate after 2–7 days of sexual abstinence ranges from 2 to 6 ml. However, there are other possibilities as follows (Vasan 2011; Bornman and Aneck-Hahn 2012):

1. Aspermia: No ejaculate after orgasm.
2. Hypospermia: Less than 0.5 ml of semen. This can be due to improper collection, hypogonadism, partial retrograde ejaculation, and congenital bilateral absence of the vas deferens (CBAVD), and obstruction of lower urinary tract may yield low volume.
3. Hyperspermia: More than 6 ml of semen. This can be attributed to prolonged abstinence or excessive secretion from the accessory sex glands and also occurs in cases of male accessory gland infection (World Health Organization 2010).

pH The main component of semen is a coagulated alkaline fluid that comes from the seminal vesicles. This fluid along with the sperm from the vas deferens empties through the ejaculatory duct. Prostatic fluid, the second largest component of seminal volume, generally has a relatively acidic pH of 6.5 and combines with the seminal fluid and sperm in the urethra. Prostatic fluid does not traverse the ejaculatory ducts. Normal semen pH is in the range of 7.2–8.2 and it tends to increase with time after ejaculation. Changes in pH of semen are usually due to inflammation of the prostate or seminal vesicles. A low volume sample with measured pH below 7.0 indicates obstruction of the ejaculatory ducts.

Liquefaction Liquefaction of semen depends on coagulation of proteins found in the seminal fluid as well as the liquefaction by prostate-specific antigen, a proteolytic enzyme, secreted by the prostate. This process may take up to 60 min. If complete liquefaction does not occur after 60 min, it should be noted. Exact liquefaction time is of no diagnostic importance unless > 2 h elapse without any change. The clinical significance of abnormalities in liquefaction is still controversial (Keel 1990). Failure to liquefy is usually a sign of inadequate secretion of the proteolytic enzymes – fibrinolysin, fibrinogenase, and aminopeptidase – by the prostate (Amelar 1962). On the other hand, absence of coagulation may indicate ejaculatory duct obstruction or congenital absence of seminal vesicles.

Semen Viscosity Viscosity measures the resistance of the seminal fluid to flow. High viscosity may interfere with determination of sperm motility, concentration, and antibody coating of spermatozoa. Normally, semen coagulates upon ejaculation and usually liquefies within 15–20 min. Semen that remains a coagulum is termed non-liquefied, whereas that which pours in thick strands instead of drops is termed hyperviscous. Importantly, liquefaction should be differentiated from viscosity, as abnormalities in viscosity can be the result of abnormal prostate function and/or the use of an unsuitable type of plastic container. Viscosity of semen is noted after liquefaction, although the clinical significance of hyperviscous semen is controversial. There is no correlation between seminal hyperviscosity and semen cultures, leukocytes, or presence of sperm antibodies; however, worse outcomes after in vitro fertilization (IVF) with seminal hyperviscosity have been observed (Munuce et al. 1999; Esfandiari et al. 2008). Sperm processing prior to intrauterine insemination (IUI) can be considered, if there is a clinical concern for hyperviscosity.

5.5 Microscopic Sperm Analysis

Sperm Concentration Concentration of sperm in unstained preparations of fresh/washed semen sample is determined using, preferably, a phase-contrast microscope with volumetric dilution and hemocytometry. Sperm count is typically reported as concentration (millions of sperm per milliliter) as well as total sperm count (sperm concentration × ml of semen) in the ejaculate. Normozoospermia, oligozoospermia, and azoospermia are diagnosed based upon total sperm count. Azoospermia refers to the absence of sperm in the seminal plasma. Prior to the diagnosis of azoospermia, the sample should be centrifuged and the pellet examined for the presence of sperm. Oligozoospermia (also often called oligospermia) refers to seminal plasma concentration < 15 million/ml. This finding can accompany a variety of defects and has implications for the type of assisted reproductive options that can be utilized, as there are significant reductions in pregnancy rates (Smith et al. 1977).

Motility The efficient passage of spermatozoa through cervical mucus is dependent on rapid-progressive motility, that is, spermatozoa must have a forward progression of a minimum of 25 μm/s (Björndahl 2010; Lindholmer 1974). Reduced sperm motility can be a symptom of disorders related to male accessory sex gland secretion and the sequential emptying of these glands. Rapid and slow-progressive motility is calculated by the speed at which sperm moves with flagellar movement in a given volume as a percentage (range 0–100 %) by counting 200 sperms and classified as follows:

A. (Rapid progressive motility: > 25 μm/s at 37 °C and > 20 μm/s at 20 °C
   Note: 25 μm is approximately equal to 5 head lengths or half a tail length).
B. Slow or sluggish progressive motility
C. Nonprogressive motility (<5 μm/s)
D. Immotile

A normal semen analysis must contain at least 50 % grade A and B progressively motile spermatozoa (Table 5.1). If greater than 50 % of sperms are immotile, then the sperms should be checked for viability. Persistent poor motility is a good predictor of failure in fertilization, an outcome that is actually more important when making decisions regarding a couple's treatment options (Aitken et al. 1985).

Vitality Supravital staining differentiates between live and dead sperm and is assessed when sperm motility is < 50 %. A large proportion of vital, but immotile, sperm may indicate structural defects in the sperm tail (World Health Organization 1999) or Kartagener's syndrome. A high percentage of immotile, nonviable (dead) sperm may indicate epididymal pathology (World Health Organization 2010). Antisperm antibodies (ASA) may also be present, if the immotile sperms are dead (Björndahl et al. 2010a).

Morphology The staining of a seminal smear (Papanicolaou Giemsa, Shorr, and Diff-Quik) allows the quantitative evaluation of normal and abnormal sperm morphological forms in an ejaculate. Smears can be scored for morphology using the World Health Organization (WHO) classification or by Kruger's strict criteria classification (Menkveld et al. 1990). WHO method classifies abnormally shaped spermatozoa into specific categories based on specific head, tail, and mid-piece abnormalities, which is based on the appearance of sperm recovered from postcoital cervical mucus or from the surface of zona pellucida (>30 % normal forms). In contrast, Kruger's strict criteria classifies sperm as normal only if the sperm shape falls within strictly defined parameters of shape, and all borderline forms are considered abnormal (>14 % normal forms).

1. *Head defects*: Large, small, tapered, pyriform, round, amorphous, vacuolated (>20 % of the head area occupied by unstained vacuolar areas) heads with small acrosomal area (<40 % of head area), double heads, or any combination of these
2. *Neck and mid-piece defects:* Bent neck; asymmetrical insertion of mid-piece into the head; thick, irregular mid-piece; abnormally thin mid-piece; or any combination of these
3. *Tail defects*: Short, multiple, hairpin, broken, bent, kinked, coiled tails, or any combination of these
4. *Cytoplasmic droplets*: Greater than one-third of the area of a normal sperm head

Morphology should be used along with other parameters, and not as an isolated parameter, when determining clinical implications. It is important to realize that, in general, pregnancy is possible with low morphology scores and that both motility and morphology have demonstrated prognostic value, as do combinations of parameters (Van Waart et al. 2001; Keegan et al. 2007). The clinical implications of poor morphology scores remain highly controversial. The initial studies using rigid criteria reported that patients undergoing in vitro fertilization (IVF) who had greater than 14 % normal forms had better fertilization rates (Coetzee et al. 1998). Later studies reported that most impairment in fertilization rates occurred with morphology scores of less than 4 % (Menkveld et al. 1990).

Morphology is a particularly challenging parameter to interpret because of the subjective nature of the classification and the presence of multiple classification systems, as well as controversy about the implications of various morphological features. There are studies correlating fertilization rates with morphology scores and other studies which show no relationship between morphology scores and IVF results (Deck and Berger 2000; Schlegel 1997). As there are a number of scoring methodologies, the clinician should explore and adopt a particular methodology and reporting for their laboratory. In spite of the controversy about overall morphology scores, absence of acrosomes or globozoospermia is highly predictive of failure of fertilization (Male Infertility Best Practice Policy Committee of the American Urological Association and Practice Committee of the American Society for Reproductive Medicine 2006).

In view of these findings, it is beneficial for the physician to have a detailed analysis of the morphological defects in addition to the percentage of normal forms. In the case of globozoospermia, treatment with intracytoplasmic sperm injection (ICSI) can be more successful compared to IUI (Baker et al. 1994). For some morphology, such as pin head or short tailed, sperms fail to have pronuclei fusion leading to failure of even ICSI (Dunson et al. 2004). Overall, there is significant difficulty with defining the relationship between morphology and pregnancy rates, especially with the management of patients with low morphology scores (Abbey et al. 1992).

The current evidence suggests that, in general, sperm morphology scores should not be used in isolation to make patient management decisions.

5.6 Computer-Aided Sperm Analysis (CASA)

Advances in technology and the use of fluorescent DNA stains have facilitated development of computer-aided sperm analysis (CASA). Determination of sperm concentration and concentration of progressively motile spermatozoa has been possible due to the availability of advanced tail detection algorithms (Zinaman et al. 1996; Garrett et al. 2003). CASA can be used for routine diagnostic applications when specimen is prepared with proper care and adequate quality control procedures are in place. CASA systems with semiautomated morphology units are available and can be used to measure sperm concentration, motility, kinematics, and morphology with high precision. Studies have also shown the significance of CASA sperm concentration and kinematic parameters in the determination of in vitro and in vivo fertilization rates (Garrett et al. 2003; Liu et al. 1991; Barratt et al. 1993). Progress in digital image analysis has brought about greater objectivity and improved precision to quantitative assessment of sperm morphology (Garrett and Baker 1995).

Manual semen analysis lacks the ability to measure the kinematics of sperm motion. CASA is potentially useful because of its capacity to analyze sperm motion (sperm head and flagellar kinetics), some of which have been shown to be related to IVF outcome (Fréour et al. 2010). Important kinematic parameters are as follows:

A. *Curvilinear velocity*: Curvilinear velocity (VCL) is the measure of the rate of travel of the centroid of the sperm head over a given time period.
B. *Average path velocity*: Average path velocity (VAP) is the velocity along the average path of the spermatozoon.
C. *Straight-line velocity*: Straight-line velocity (VSL) is the linear or progressive velocity of the cell.
D. *Linearity*: Linearity of forward progression (LIN) is the ratio of VSL to VCL and is expressed as percentage.
E. *Amplitude of lateral head displacement*: Amplitude of lateral head displacement (ALH) of the sperm head is calculated from the amplitude of its lateral deviation about the cell's axis of progression or average path.

Although CASA is very accurate for determining the details of sperm kinetics, manual assessment of semen is much more accurate in discerning among debris, crystals, and immotile and dead sperm heads. Therefore, manually assessed sperm concentrations and number of immotile spermatozoa are much more reliable than corresponding data obtained by CASA, provided individual is adequately trained with appropriate internal and external quality control measures (Makler 1978; Ginsburg and Armant 1990).

5.7 Other Markers

The secretion of zinc by the prostate is androgen dependent, and a level of < 2.4 μmol/ejaculate indicates a low contribution of the fluid to the ejaculate, incomplete collection of the ejaculate, prostatic inflammation, or androgen insufficiency (Björndahl et al. 2010b). Fructose is another androgen-dependent secretion emanating mainly from the seminal vesicles, with a small contribution from the epithelial cell of the secretory epithelium in the ampulla of the vas deferens. Seminal fructose is used as a marker of the seminal vesicles and < 13.0 μmol/ejaculate is considered abnormal. This is seen in hypogonadal men after a short abstinence time, and where ejaculation or emission of fluid is impaired, such as in neuromuscular diseases, after surgery, in cases of drug use, and in obstruction in the ejaculatory ducts, or with inflammation in the vesicles or prostate that may hinder emission (Bornman and Aneck-Hahn 2012).

Infection of the male reproductive tract can directly or indirectly cause infertility (Mortimer 1994a). Pyospermia is a laboratory finding categorized as the abnormal presence of leukocytes in human ejaculate and may indicate genital tract inflammation (Anderson 1995). Polymorphonuclear (PMN) leukocytes are the primary sources of reactive oxygen species (ROS) that cause inflammation, and peroxidase staining is used to detect their presence (Wolff et al. 1992).

Presence of agglutinated clumps of moving sperm in the semen sample could hamper the passage of sperm through the cervical mucus, and zonal binding and passage (Mortimer 1994b). Such clumps are formed by the exposure of spermatozoa to systemic immune defense system, due to the release of antisperm antibodies (ASA). ASA can also cause cell death and immobilized sperm cells. Detection of ASA bound to the surface of motile sperm is carried out by the mixed agglutination reaction assay (MAR test; only for IgGs) and the immuno-bead binding assay (for IgA, IgG, and IgMs) (Jarow and Sanzone 1992).

5.8 Sperm Functional Tests

Tests of Sperm Capacitation Capacitation is a series of biochemical and structural changes that spermatozoa go through to undergo acrosome reaction (AR) and be able to fertilize. The process takes place in the female genital tract but can be induced in vitro by incubating spermatozoa with capacitation-inducing media. It is thought to have a role in preventing the release of lytic enzymes until spermatozoa reach the oocyte (Tesarik 1989). One of the signs of capacitation is the display of hyper-activation by spermatozoa. At the present time, the clinical value of sperm capacitation testing remains to be determined.

Tests of Hemizona and Zona Pellucida Binding The interaction between spermatozoa and the zona pellucida is a critical event leading to fertilization and reflects multiple sperm functions (i.e., completion of capacitation as manifested by the ability to bind to the zona pellucida and to undergo ligand-induced AR) (Oehninger et al. 1994; Liu and Baker 2003; Consensus workshop on advanced diagnostic andrology techniques. ESHRE (European Society of Human Reproduction and Embryology) Andrology Special Interest Group 1996). The most common sperm-zona pellucida binding tests currently utilized are the hemizona assay (or HZA) and a competitive intact-zona binding assay (Quintero et al. 2005; Fénichel et al. 1991). The HZA which uses non-fertilized oocytes is useful to determine the cause, in couples who have failed to fertilize during regular IVF. As the binding is species-specific, human zona must be used, thus limiting the utility of these assays (Fénichel et al. 1991; Cross et al. 1986). The induced AR assays appear to be equally predictive of fertilization outcome and are simpler in their methodologies. The use of a calcium ionophore to induce AR is currently the most widely used methodology (Henkel et al. 1993; Katsuki et al. 2005).

Sperm Penetration Assay This assay is also called as sperm capacitation index or zona-free hamster oocyte penetration assay. The concept of the sperm penetration assay was introduced by Yanagamachi (1972; Yanagimachi et al. 1976). It yields information regarding the fertilizing capacity of human spermatozoa by testing capacitation, AR, sperm/oolemma fusion, sperm incorporation into the ooplasm, and decondensation of the sperm chromatin during the process. However, penetration of the zona pellucida and normal embryonic development are not tested. The spermatozoa penetration assay (SPA) utilizes the golden hamster egg, which is unusual in that removal of its zona pellucida results in loss of all species specificity to egg penetration. Thus, a positive SPA does not guarantee fertilization of intact human eggs nor their embryonic development, whereas a negative SPA has not been found to correlate with poor fertilization in human IVF (Yanagimachi et al. 1976). The acrosin assay, an indirect measure of sperm's penetrating capability, measures acrosin, which may be responsible for penetration of the zona pellucida and also triggering the AR (Rogers and Brentwood 1982). Measurement of acrosin is thought to correlate with sperm binding to and penetration of the zona pellucida (Cross et al. 1986; Cummins et al. 1991).

Tests of Sperm DNA Damage Mammalian fertilization involves the direct interaction of the sperm and the oocyte, fusion of the cell membranes, and union of male and female gamete genomes. Although a small percentage of spermatozoa from fertile men also possess detectable levels of DNA damage, which is repaired by oocyte cytoplasm, there is evidence to show that the spermatozoa of infertile men possess substantially more DNA damage that may adversely affect reproductive outcomes (Evenson et al. 1999; Zini et al. 2001). There appears to be a threshold of sperm DNA damage which can be repaired by oocyte cytoplasm (i.e., abnormal chromatin packaging, protamine deficiency) beyond which embryo development and pregnancy are impaired (Ahmadi and Ng 1999; Cho et al. 2003).

A. *DNA damage – direct tests*
   (a) Terminal deoxynucleotidyl transferase-mediated deoxyuridine triphosphate (dUTP) nick end-labeling (TUNEL) assay
   (b) COMET assay

B. *DNA damage – indirect tests*
   (a) Sperm chromatin structure assay (SCSA)
   (b) Sperm chromatin dispersion assay
   (c) Sperm fluorescence in situ hybridization analysis (FISH)

Overall, studies suggest that there is no significant relationship between sperm DNA damage and fertilization rate or pregnancy outcomes at IVF or IVF/ICSI (Bungum et al. 2007; Payne et al. 2005; Zini et al. 2005; Borini et al. 2006; Benchaib et al. 2007). However, there is evidence to suggest that sperm DNA damage is associated with poor pregnancy outcome after standard IVF (Lin et al. 2008; Frydman et al. 2008). Sperm FISH analysis may be useful in (a) infertile men with sex chromosome numerical anomalies, prior to ICSI; (b) infertile men with structural chromosome anomalies, prior to ICSI; (c) infertile men with severe oligozoospermia, prior to ICSI; and (d) couples with a history of recurrent miscarriages and trisomic pregnancies.

Assessment of Reactive Oxygen Species Reactive oxygen species, (ROS) also referred to as free radicals, are formed as a by-product of oxygen metabolism. Contaminating leukocytes are the predominant source of ROS in these suspensions (Aitken et al. 1989a, b). They can be eradicated by enzymes (e.g., catalase or glutathione peroxidase) or by nonenzymatic antioxidants, such as albumin, glutathione, and hypotaurine, as well as by vitamins C and E. Small amounts of ROS may be necessary for the initiation of critical sperm functions, including capacitation and AR. On the other hand, a high ROS level produces a state known as oxidative stress that can lead to biochemical or physiologic abnormalities with subsequent cellular dysfunction or cell death. Significant levels of ROS can be detected in the semen of 25 % of infertile men, whereas fertile men do not have a detectable level of semen ROS (Aitken et al. 1989b, 1991; Agarwal et al. 2006). Sperm ROS can be measured by using cellular probes coupled with flow cytometry by the detection of chemiluminescence (Marchetti et al. 2002). Briefly, this is done by incubating fresh semen or sperm suspensions with a redox-sensitive, light-emitting probe (e.g., luminol) and by measuring the light emission over time with a luminometer. The clinical value of semen ROS determination in predicting IVF outcome remains unproven, but identifying oxidative stress as an underlying cause of sperm dysfunction has the advantage for suggesting possible therapies. Administration of antioxidants has been attempted in several trials with mixed results. Currently, there are no established semen ROS cutoff values that can be used to predict reproductive outcomes (Agarwal et al. 2005, 2008).

Sperm Proteomics Sperm proteomics, an experimental technique, used extensively in several branches of medicine, may identify some of the molecular targets implicated in sperm dysfunction (Aitken and Baker 2008). Sperm proteomics allows comparison of protein structure of normal and defective spermatozoa (Aitken 2010).

5.9 Pre-2010 WHO Guidelines

Prior to 2010, semen analyses were performed mainly according to the WHO guidelines (World Health Organization 1992) to obtain volume, pH, sperm concentration, motility, and morphology. Sperm concentration was determined with the use of a Makler counting chamber. Motility was expressed as the percentage of motile spermatozoa and their mean speed, or motility quality (on a scale of 1–6, where 1 stands for immotile and 6 for very fast progressive motile, i.e., 100 μm/s). For sperm morphology evaluation, two slides were prepared of each sample after incubation of the semen samples with trypsin (10 min at room temperature); one slide was used for routine morphology evaluation by WHO criteria and the other for strict criteria evaluation. For evaluation according to WHO criteria, smears were flame-fixed and stained with methylene blue/eosin. At least 100 cells were examined per slide, with a final magnification of x1000. Each slide was evaluated independently by two technicians. There should not be any statistically significant difference (by Pearson's correlation matrix analysis) between the results of the two observers. The slides for evaluation by strict criteria were stained according to the Papanicolaou method and evaluated (Menkveld et al. 1990). In addition to the morphology evaluation according to strict criteria, the acrosome index (AI) and teratozoospermia index (TZI) were also determined (World Health Organization 1992; Menkveld and Kruger 1996).

Teratozoospermia Index The TZI is an indication of the number of abnormalities present per abnormal spermatozoon. According to the 1992 WHO manual (World Health Organization 1992), each abnormal spermatozoon can have one to four abnormalities, viz., a head abnormality, a neck/mid-piece abnormality, a tail abnormality, or the presence of a cytoplasmic residue. These abnormalities can occur as a single defect or in a combination of two, three, or all four abnormalities simultaneously. The classification of spermatozoa for the TZI is recorded simultaneously, on a five-key laboratory counter, with the recording of spermatozoa as normal or abnormal, in specific classes. The total number of abnormalities recorded are added together and divided by the total number of abnormal spermatozoa, i.e., 100 minus the percentage of morphologically normal spermatozoa.

Acrosome Index Sperm acrosomal morphology was evaluated by light microscopy at ×1250 oil magnification based on acrosomal size and form as well as staining characteristics (Menkveld and Kruger 1996). Results were expressed as the AI (% normal acrosomes). For the evaluation of acrosome morphology, the same principles as for the evaluation of normal sperm morphology according to strict criteria are applicable. For an acrosome to be regarded as normal, the acrosome must have a smooth normal oval shape, with the same dimensions as for a normal spermatozoon. Acrosomes must be well-defined and comprising about 40–70% of the normal-sized sperm head. The post-acrosomal part of the sperm head can be abnormal, but the rest of the spermatozoon must be normal; thus no neck/mid-piece and tail abnormalities and no cytoplasmic residue may be present. If the spermatozoon is classified as normal, the acrosome must always be classified as normal. The acrosome evaluation can be performed simultaneously with the routine morphology evaluation and the TZI, with the use of two laboratory counters. As with the normal sperm morphology, at least 100 spermatozoa are evaluated. The repeatability of the AI is be determined and should be within acceptable limits.

Reference Intervals Reference intervals are the most widely used tool for the interpretation of clinical laboratory results. Reference interval development has classically relied on concepts elaborated by the International Federation of Clinical Chemistry Expert Panel on Reference Values during the 1980s. These guidelines involve obtaining and classifying samples from a healthy population of at least 120 individuals and then identifying the outermost 5 % of observations to use in defining limits for two-sided or one-sided reference intervals. Pre-2010 WHO guidelines were based on data obtained from laboratories that used different methodologies and examined different male populations, not supported by standardized methods or without the definition of fertile population. The male population studied included men without proven paternity, patients of human reproduction clinics that sought treatment, semen donors, and vasectomy candidates. Semen donors can be fertile and vasectomy candidates are very likely to be fertile, although there is no data about how long it took for their partners to get pregnant (Cooper et al. 2010). The cutoff point of 20×10^6/ml was suggested as the lower normal value for sperm concentration in an ejaculate (World Health Organization 1999). However, there are studies indicating sperm concentrations of subfertile men to be less than 13.5×10^6/ml (Guzick et al. 2001) and 31.2×10^6/ml for fertility status (Nallella et al. 2006). Therefore, caution must be exercised with interpretation of the semen analysis based upon the reference values as men may be infertile with "normal" semen parameters or alternatively can be fertile with markedly "abnormal" semen profiles. There is likely no upper limit of semen morphology, motility, or count as pregnancy rates appear to generally increase with increasing numbers as well as improved sperm morphology and motility (Garrett et al. 2003).

Sperm Morphology The clinical implications of poor morphology scores remain highly controversial. Initial studies evaluating the utility of strict sperm morphology in predicting fertilization rates during IVF used a score of greater than 14 % for normal. However, subsequent studies reported fertilization rates were lowest for patients with morphology scores of less than 4 %. Pregnancy rates have also been reported to be suboptimal with lower scores (Coetzee et al. 1998), but some recent studies have reported no relationship of morphology to IVF results (Keegan et al. 2007). The relationship between morphology scores and pregnancy rates with (IUI) (Van Waart et al. 2001; Spiessens et al. 2003; Shibahara et al. 2004) and intercourse (Guzick et al. 2001; Gunalp et al. 2001) have been examined; however, there has been no consensus on thresholds and management implications of poor morphology scores. Certain rare morphological abnormalities, such as sperm without acrosomes (globozoospermia), are highly predictive of failure to fertilize ova, yet in most cases fertilization and pregnancy are possible even with very low morphology scores. Although most clinicians utilize strict morphology in everyday practice, most studies have not addressed the significance of isolated low morphology in patients with otherwise normal semen parameters.

5.10 Need for Revised Guidelines

Human semen is very different from other body fluids, mainly because of its heterogeneity. Heterogeneity leads to several negative effects on the quality of the semen analysis. Some of the problems with the interpretation of semen analysis arise from the fact that production of spermatozoa is known to vary in the same individual and that semen analysis technique is poorly standardized. Many conditions including the duration of ejaculatory abstinence, activity of the accessory sex glands, analytical errors, and inherent biological variability account for the discrepancies (Berman et al. 1996; Carlsen et al. 2004; Sanchez-Pozo et al. 2013; Hamada et al. 2012). Analysis on multiple ejaculates from the same individual is recommended before characterizing a man as normal or infertile due to the large within-subject variation in sperm parameters (Keel 2006). In one study, the within-subject variability of 20 healthy subjects assessed over a 10-week follow-up ranged from 10.3 to 26.8 % (Alvarez et al. 2003). Concentration showed the highest within-subject variation (26.8 %), followed by morphology (19.6 %) and progressive motility (15.2 %), whereas vitality had the lowest variation (10.3 %). For these reasons, it would not be suitable to take the results of a single semen specimen as a surrogate for a man's ability to father a child, unless it is at extremely low levels (Jequier 2005). Hence, it is prudent that clinicians request at least two semen specimens following 2–5 days of ejaculatory abstinence to allow a better understanding of the baseline semen quality status of a given individual (Berman et al. 1996; Carlsen et al. 2004; Sanchez-Pozo et al. 2013). In view of the intra- and interindividual variations in semen quality, population-based reference values are expected to have better utility in assessments of fertility (Esteves 2014). In addition, conventional semen analysis does not test for the diverse array of biological properties of spermatozoa that are responsible to bring about pregnancy. Table 5.1 displays the changes in semen analysis reference values in different editions of the WHO manual. Following publication of WHO 2010 manual, several semen analysis parameters and their recommended ranges prescribed by new guidelines became the topic of intense discussion. In this section, each of them is considered in some detail.

Sperm Motility Surprisingly, 2010 WHO manual abandons the distinction between slow- and rapid-progressive spermatozoa. The reasoning for this change appears to be primarily based on the observation that poorly trained technicians cannot distinguish between the two categories in a repeatable and reliable manner (Mortimer 1994c). In fact, the quality of sperm motility is a prime factor to be considered in a semen analysis (MacLeod and Gold 1951). In addition, proper training and achievement of intra- and interobserver standardization is essential to assess

Table 5.2 Distribution of values, lower reference limits, and their 95 % CI for semen parameters from fertile men whose partners has a time-to-pregnancy of 12 months or less

		Centiles										
Parameter	N	2.5	(95 % CI)	5	(95 % CI)	10	25	50	75	90	95	97.5
Semen volume (ml)	1941	1.2	(1.0–1.3)	1.5	(1.4–1.7)	2	2.7	3.7	4.8	6	6.8	7.6
Sperm concentration (10^6/ml)	1859	9	(8–11)	15	(12–16)	22	41	73	116	169	213	259
Total number (10^6/ml)	1859	23	(18–29)	39	(33–46)	69	142	255	422	647	802	928
Total motility (PR + NP,%)[a]	1781	34	(33–37)	40	(38–42)	45	53	61	69	75	78	81
Progressive motility (PR, %)[a]	1780	28	(25–29)	32	(31–34)	39	47	55	62	69	72	75
Normal forms (%)	1851	3	(2.0–3.0)	4	(3.0–4.0)	5.5	9	15	24.5	36	44	48
Vitality (%)	428	53	(48–56)	58	(55–63)	64	72	79	84	88	91	92

Reproduced from Cooper et al. (2010)

[a]*PR* progressive motility (WHO, 1999 grades a + b), *NP* nonprogressive motility (WHO, 1999 grade c). The values are from unweighted raw data. For a two-sided distribution the 2.5th and 97.5th centiles provide the reference limits; for a one-sided distribution, the fifth centile provides the lower reference limit

sperm motility. The arguments posited by the WHO have been refuted elsewhere (Björndahl 2010; Eliasson 2010). Very importantly, there are clinical data both from manual sperm motility assessments and computer-aided sperm analysis showing the distinction of rapidly progressive spermatozoa to be biologically, and hence clinically, important. This evidence ranges from the ability of spermatozoa to penetrate cervical mucus (Aitken et al. 1985; Mortimer et al. 1986) and in vivo conceptions (Comhaire et al. 1988; Barratt et al. 1992) to clinical outcome studies in donor insemination (Irvine and Aitken 1986), IUI (Bollendorf et al. 1996), and IVF (Bollendorf et al. 1996; Sifer et al. 2005). Even with regard to ICSI, the straight-line velocity of the individual spermatozoa subsequently injected into the oocyte has been shown to have a significant effect on fertilization outcome (Van den Bergh et al. 1998). In view of these evidences, it is scientifically and clinically inappropriate to abandon the differentiation of rapid- and slow-progressive spermatozoa.

Sperm Morphology WHO 2010 manual has fully adopted the Tygerberg Strict Criteria for normal sperm morphology (Menkveld et al. 1990). These criteria are based on the typical morphology of spermatozoa that are able to migrate through cervical mucus and bind to the zona pellucida, even though in "normal" men only a small proportion of spermatozoa correspond to the typical morphology (Menkveld et al. 2011). As a consequence, an extra measure that includes the different types of abnormalities can provide additional useful information by identifying men with more severe disturbances in sperm form and related function, e.g., the multiple anomalies index (MAI) (Jouannet et al. 1988) and the teratozoospermia index (TZI) (Menkveld et al. 1998; Mortimer et al. 1990; Mortimer and Menkveld 2001).

The TZI is an indirect indication of (i) the risk of what appeared to be normal spermatozoa actually having defects that were invisible at the level of observation and (ii) just how badly affected spermiogenesis was in the man and hence how impaired his sperm fertilizing ability might be (Mortimer and Menkveld 2001). The TZI can provide extra information in cases where there are very few morphological normal forms, as presence of 4 or 6 % normal forms is considered to reflect a major difference in clinical significance. TZI would be highly pertinent when interpreting sperm morphology assessments based on counts of just 200 spermatozoa, and there will not be a statistically significant difference between 4 and 6 % normal form values at 95 % confidence interval (Björndahl et al. 2010a).

In the 2010 WHO manual, the assessment of multiple sperm defects has been relegated to "Optional Procedures," although calculation of the TZI has been corrected to be out of four instead of three, as erroneously used in the 4th edition (World Health Organization 1999). Even if only % normal spermatozoa is reported, the actual assessment procedure should include all the characteristics/criteria needed for TZI since recording the prevalence of the four categories of morphological deviations is essential for quality control (internal and external) purposes. In terms of clinical application of the TZI, the consensus-based *WHO Manual for the Standardized Investigation, Diagnosis and Management of the Infertile Male* (Rowe et al. 2000) has commented that, together with the introduction of the Tygerberg

Strict Criteria in the 1999 WHO laboratory manual, the TZI had been included to provide additional information to facilitate discrimination of the extent of impairment of sperm functional potential in men with very low numbers of normal spermatozoa. In addition, applicable reference values based on the four defect category TZI could be have been included in the manual.

Retention of the Use of Nomenclature Terms The WHO 2010 manual retains the use of nomenclature terms such as oligozoospermia. Such terms simply classify the perceived quality of the semen but do not identify, or even suggest, biological cause or real fertility potential (Eliasson 1977, 2010; Eliasson et al. 1970; Bostofte et al. 1981) and hence are not very helpful. Many experts have discussed the possible reference values and such nomenclature, and probably the most useful approach is to provide three interpretation categories: normal, doubtful, and pathological or not normal (Guzick et al. 2001; Björndahl 2010; Eliasson 1977).

Multiple Methods and Nonlinear Method Presentation WHO 2010 still includes multiple methods for performing some of the tests, with poor explanations of their relative merits or otherwise, e.g., determination of low sperm concentrations in semen, alternative stains for sperm morphology assessment (e.g., Diff-Quik™), and the use of eosin without a counterstain for sperm vitality assessment. Some of the methods (e.g., sperm concentration) are also presented in a complex manner (World Health Organization 2010). These issues diminish the practical usefulness and will delay adoption of the WHO 2010 guidelines. Lack of clear step-by-step protocols for easy implementation and routine use, information on the limitations of the methods, etc., make it harder for a laboratory to adapt a method into its standard operating procedure.

Inconsistencies and Errors There are several errors and inconsistencies in WHO 2010. One method particularly affected by this is the determination of sperm vitality using eosin-nigrosin staining: (1) The cutoff to perform a vitality assessment has been changed from 50 % immotile spermatozoa (World Health Organization 1992, 1999) to "less than about 40 % progressively motile spermatozoa" (World Health Organization 2010). The change is illogical since nonprogressively motile spermatozoa are clearly still "live," and (2) the interpretation criteria for eosin staining has been changed arbitrarily so that "light pink heads are considered alive" (World Health Organization 2010). This is contrary to papers on eosin exclusion staining for mammalian sperm vitality going back 60 years. The standard criterion is that any degree of pink coloration indicates that a spermatozoon is not "live" (Mortimer 1994a) with the sole, strict, exception of the "leaky neck" staining artifact where faint pink coloration might be seen in the very posterior region of the sperm head (Björndahl et al. 2003, 2004). The revised criterion in WHO 2010 is clearly wrong and will affect the results obtained.

Unnecessary Extra Work In WHO 2010, it is stated that both sperm vitality and sperm morphology assessments must be made in duplicate, evaluating 200 spermatozoa in each replicate "in order to achieve an acceptably low sampling error" (World Health Organization 2010). These requirements represent substantial extra work for what are unestablished improvements in accuracy and/or precision in the final results. Indeed, Menkveld has previously established the adequacy of a single assessment of sperm morphology on 200 cells from a single slide (Menkveld et al. 1990), and with a binary endpoint such as vitality, any possible improvement will be minimal. Similarly, the improved method for determining low values of sperm concentration leads to substantial extra work to improve accuracy or precision, which may not provide any increase in clinical value to be useful from a diagnostic or prognostic perspective. For each of these changes, the WHO manual should have provided justifications for the substantial extra effort and hence costs involved.

Illogical Sperm Preparation Methods WHO 2010 still allows simple centrifugal washing of spermatozoa for "good-quality" semen samples. Unfortunately, one cannot be certain that an ejaculate is free from the attendant risks of reactive oxygen species damage (Aitken and Clarkson 1987, 1988; Mortimer 1991) without assessing both sperm morphology for spermatozoa with retained cytoplasm and verifying the absence of peroxidase-positive leukocytes. To achieve both of these between completion of semen liquefaction and the need to commence sperm preparation by 30 min post-ejaculation is clearly impossible on a routine basis (Björndahl et al. 2010a; Mortimer 2000). The density-gradient method mentioned in the WHO 2010 contains numerous errors. It requires the addition of 10 ml of a 10× medium to 90 ml of a "density-gradient medium" of silane-coated colloidal silica, although all commercially available silanized colloidal silica sperm preparation products since 1997 are already isotonic. The only colloidal silica product that is not already isotonic is Percoll (which is polyvinyl alcohol-coated silica) and it has been banned from clinical use by its manufacturer effective 1 January 1997 (Mortimer 2000). WHO 2010 perpetuates the incorrect colloid layers that have been in the WHO laboratory manual since 1992 (World Health Organization 1992), using a 72 % colloid-equivalent lower layer, which is too low in density (i.e., 1.1 g/ml). While this will provide an apparently higher yield, it only does so by allowing poorer quality spermatozoa into the pellet (Björndahl et al. 2010a; Mortimer 2000). Finally, WHO 2010 still recommends Ham's F10 medium for all sperm preparation methods, even after 15 years of a clear recommendation that it should not be used for this purpose due to its iron content (Gomez and Aitken 1996).

The Delusion of Suddenly Changed Limits Between Fertile and Subfertile men The part of WHO 2010 that has caught most attention in the field of reproductive medicine is the lowered reference limits calculated from results on semen provided by recent fathers and men in a general population. It appears that there is a common belief that the biology of subfertility has changed as a result of the lowering of the "normal/fertile" reference limits or ranges. There are, however, a number of problems related to the establishment of reference ranges based only on individuals without the disorder, i.e., men who are not subfertile (Björndahl 2011). Furthermore, since the data were collected during a long period of time, and external quality control had not been implemented in all contributing laboratories (Cooper et al. 2010), the validity of the suggested reference limits can be questioned. Due to the considerable overlap of results from fertile and subfertile men, a valid approach would be to identify three zones: (i) "normal results," i.e., a low probability of subfertility and high probability of fertility; (ii) "abnormal results," i.e., a high probability of subfertility and low probability of fertility; and (iii) "borderline results," i.e., no clear discrimination between subfertility and fertility (Björndahl 2010; Björndahl et al. 2010a). Dividing the range of results into these three zones is well established in andrology (Mortimer 1994a; Eliasson 1977), and the material presented in WHO 2010 provides no evidence that might contradict the validity of this principle.

A further concern regarding the origin of the WHO 2010 reference values is that the data came from studies on semen samples obtained after 2–7 days of abstinence, as has been advocated in all five editions of the WHO manual. This persistently ignores the fact that MacLeod and Gold (1952) clearly demonstrated that ejaculate volume, and sperm concentration in particular, increase considerably with each day of increasing abstinence: e.g., sperm concentration more than doubled when the abstinence increased from 3 to 10 days. Similar results have been reported by others (Mortimer et al. 1982). For the purpose of standardization, and especially comparisons between groups, it is therefore of the utmost importance that the prescribed period of abstinence before a semen analysis should be from 3 to 4 days (Björndahl et al. 2010a; Menkveld 2007). The fact that abstinence periods were not so standardized in the source studies for the WHO 2010 casts further doubt on the usefulness of the derived reference values.

In the most recent 2010 manual (World Health Organization 2010), the WHO has published new criteria for human semen characteristics that are markedly lower than those previously reported. It is noteworthy that the WHO manual reports reference values identified in fertile population rather than the minimum requirements for male fertility. The reference ranges have been identified based on the assessment of 4,500 men from 14 different countries whose partners were able to conceive within 12 months (Cooper et al. 2010). Cooper et al. have published updated reference values obtained from analyses of multi-country data from laboratories that have used the WHO standard methodology for semen analysis (World Health Organization 1987, 1992, 1999). For the first time, semen analysis results from recent fathers with known time-to-pregnancy (TTP), defined as months (or cycles) from stopping contraception to achieving a pregnancy, were analyzed. Raw data obtained from five studies of seven countries in three continents were pooled then assessed (Stewart et al. 2009; Slama et al. 2002; Swan et al. 2003; Jensen et al. 2001; Haugen et al. 2006; Auger et al. 2001). Approximately 1,900 men, who had fathered a child within 1 year of trying to initiate pregnancy, provided a sample of semen each for sperm counts, motility, and volume assessments. Data on sperm morphology were extracted from four studies comprising approximately 1,800 men, whereas sperm vitality, assessed by the eosin-nigrosin method, was obtained from approximately 400 men of two countries (Stewart et al. 2009; Swan et al. 2003; Haugen et al. 2006; Auger et al. 2001). The mean ± SD male age was 31 ± 5 years (range 18–53 y) and only ten men were over 45 years old. Participating laboratories practiced internal and external quality control and used standardized methods for semen analysis according to the WHO manual for the examination of human semen current at the time of the original studies (Cooper et al. 2010). The 95 % reference intervals are commonly referenced with the lower 2.5 and 5 percentile being used as limits for two- and one-sided distributions (Table 5.2). The fifth centile was proposed as the lower reference cutoff limit for "normality" (Cooper et al. 2010).

Data from three other groups have been used for comparison: (1) "unscreened" men from the general population or young volunteers participating in hormonal contraception studies, considered representatives of the general population (965 samples, 7 studies, 5 countries, 3 continents); (2) "screened" men from different origins, of unknown fertility but with semen analysis within reference values (934 samples, 4 studies, 4 countries, 3 continents, 2 WHO multinational studies); and (3) fertile men with unknown TTP, representing the group and all ranges of fecundity – normal or moderately or severely impaired (817 samples, 2 studies, 2 continents, 2 WHO multinational studies).

The assessment of progressive motility according to grades, as recommended by the previous WHO manuals, has been replaced by categorizing motile sperm as being "progressive" or "nonprogressive." In addition, the strict criterion for morphology assessment was incorporated as the standard method. The lower limits of these distributions were lower than the values presented in previous editions except for the total sperm number per ejaculate (World Health Organization 1987, 1992, 1999, 2010).

The very low cutoff value for sperm morphology of 4 % morphologically normal spermatozoa, as proposed in the new edition of the WHO manual on semen analysis, is in agreement with recently published values and reflects the trend of a decline in reported mean values for normal sperm morphology. The reduced value for morphologically normal spermatozoa over the years may be due to several factors. The first is the introduction of strict criteria for the evaluation of sperm morphology. Other reasons may include the introduction of additional criteria for sperm morphology abnormalities and the suggested decrease in semen parameters because of increasing negative environmental influences. The newly proposed very low normal value may not provide the strong predictive value for a males' fertility potential. However, certain morphology patterns and sperm abnormalities are now known to be of strong prognostic value. A good predictive value can be obtained by following the holistic, strict approach for sperm morphology and related parameter evaluation (Menkveld 2010).

5.11 Impact of 2010 WHO Guidelines

Several studies have evaluated consequences of revised reference limits and other parameters proposed in the 2010 WHO guidelines. Catanzariti et al. have reevaluated the results of semen analysis of 427 men using the new criteria. Almost 16 % of the patients, considered infertile according to the old criteria, were evaluated to be normal by the new classification and they would not need any treatment for infertility (Catanzariti et al. 2013). Their study also demonstrated that none of the patients that were previously considered normal changed to abnormal, according to the new classification, but some patients, about 15 %, changed from abnormal to normal by the new classification.

In a recent study by Baker et al., fertility categories were assigned as follows: BE (below WHO 2010 criteria), BTWN (above WHO 2010 criteria but below WHO 1999 criteria), and N (above WHO 1999 criteria) (Baker et al. 2015). A total of 82.3 % of initial semen tests were categorized as BE, and the predominance of this category was unchanged by publication of the WHO 2010 criteria. Men with initial semen analysis categorized as BTWN or N represented 16.2 and 1.5 % of the referral population, respectively. Subjects initially categorized as BTWN were more likely to change fertility categories, and overwhelmingly this migration was downward. Analysis of normal individual semen parameters revealed statistically worse mean concentration and motility when at least one other parameter fell below the WHO 2010 criteria (Baker et al. 2015).

Estaves et al. also mention about reclassification of data involving 982 men that had abnormal semen analysis results based on the 1990 WHO criteria. Approximately 39 % of these men would be reclassified as "normal" by the new 2010 criteria. Morphology itself accounted for over 50 % of the reclassifications (Esteves 2014).

Semen parameters below the WHO 2010 reference limits will be used to define male infertility and to recommend further evaluation and treatment. Such recommendation will not address the case of unexplained infertility presenting with at least two normal semen analysis and no identifiable causes after a thorough work-up including history, physical examination, and endocrine laboratory testing in the absence of female infertility (Hamada et al. 2012). The use of the new WHO 2010 reference values will lead to more men to be classified as "fertile." As a result, assessment of semen analysis alone as a surrogate measure for male fertility may lead to nondiagnosis or delayed diagnosis of male infertility.

The WHO 2010 reference limit will also impact recommendation for further treatment based on the results of semen analysis. Current guidelines propose treatment to men with clinical varicoceles in the presence of abnormal semen analyses (Male Infertility Best Practice Policy Committee of the American Urological Association and Practice Committee of the American Society for Reproductive Medicine 2004; Dohle et al. 2012; de Radiologia and Projeto Diretrizes da Associacao Medica Brasileira 2013; Practice Committee of American Society for Reproductive Medicine 2008), but the application of the new WHO reference values might lead to their ineligibility for treatment if their semen parameters are above the fifth centile. This may prevent them from achieving a substantial improvement in semen parameters and a greater chance of spontaneous pregnancy (Esteves 2014).

The threshold for normal sperm in terms of sperm morphology (strict criteria; Tygerberg method) has been lowered to 4 % in the WHO 2010 criteria compared to 14 % in the previous 1999 standards. Murray et al. have shown that 15.9–19.3 % of men would be reclassified as having normal morphology of > 4 % from having been abnormal in the past, i.e., < 14 % (Murray et al. 2012). This could lead to increased recommendation of intracytoplasmic sperm injection (ICSI) instead of conventional IVF or intrauterine insemination (IUI) as the pregnancy outcome of IVF and IUI are significantly lower when semen with low proportion of normal sperm is used (Van Waart et al. 2001; Coetzee et al. 1998). However, 5 % of the subject population used to determine the reference limits themselves had less than 4 % cutoff for normal sperm morphology. Medical disease associated with male infertility may also be missed with fewer men potentially being defined as infertile by the new reference values. Kolettis and Sabanegh (2001) found that 6 % of infertile men were found to have significant medical pathology detected by the infertility work-up.

5.12 Limitations of the 2010 WHO Standards

The significance of a cutoff value defining fertile from nonfertile men without knowledge of the overall clinical history is a concern (World Health Organization 1999, 2010). The values created in the 2010 WHO study were from 4,500 fertile men, and analyses of semen from infertile men were not performed. Therefore, WHO did not define men as infertile if they were below the one-sided 95 % confidence interval of fertile men. The value of semen analysis parameters themselves has been questioned with other functional sperm abnormalities potentially evident that are independent from the current measured parameters (Barratt et al. 2011; Esteves et al. 2012).

The assignment of 5th centile as a discriminating cutoff value in male reproductive potential is a new development. More specifically, the 5th-centile values for semen parameters were generated on the basis of broader statistical norms and not on the basis of any clinical outcomes from fertile and infertile men. In other words, there is no clear evidence that application of these values effectively segregates men on the basis of their fertility, yet that is exactly how these new ranges are being applied clinically all over the world. As noted by Niederberger (2011), although 5th-centile values are commonly used as cutoff markers in statistics, the ability of this arbitrarily assigned cutoff point to provide meaningful information about a male's fertility potential is questionable (Yerram et al. 2012).

There are pitfalls with reference limits and the proper use of such limits is essential for the interpretation of the results of semen analysis. It is critical to understand the statistical basis of reference ranges and cutoff limits and the importance of standardizing methods and practical laboratory training. Proper understanding of biological and physiological variability is also essential for the correct interpretation of semen analysis results. Understanding all the factors influencing semen analyses is of great importance for the development of the entire field of reproductive medicine (Björndahl 2011).

The reference population needs to be carefully defined for the intended clinical use of semen analysis. To determine appropriate reference intervals for use in male fertility assessment, a reference population of men with documented time-to-pregnancy of <12 months would be the most suitable. However, for epidemiological assessment, a reference population made up of unselected healthy men would be preferred. Currently, reference and decision limits derived for individual semen analysis test results are the interpretational tools of choice. In the long term, interpretation of semen analysis in combination with information from the female partner using multivariate methods will be necessary for the assessment of the likelihood of achieving a successful pregnancy in a subfertile couple (Boyd 2010).

Appropriate interpretation of the seminal analysis should be based on the dependability of the laboratory and the medical knowledge about the meaning of the seminal alterations. A recent study compared the evaluation of semen parameters from three laboratories, using the WHO recommendations for reporting sperm count, motility, and morphology. In a study by Montes et al., there was a statistical significant interlaboratory variability of the parameters studied ($p<0.001$). The observed mean coefficients of variation intra-observer (CVs) were 3.6 % for sperm count, 20.3 % for motility, and 9.4 % for sperm morphology (Rivera-Montes et al. 2013). Procedures for the quality control of semen analysis methods have been introduced recently. However, there are issues relating to the methodology of Cooper et al. (1999, 2002). Even with internal and external quality controls, semen analysis is operator dependent and subjective assessment, especially so for sperm morphology (Menkveld 2010; Keel et al. 2000).

The methodology employed to determine the reference ranges in WHO 2010 manual gives rise to important concerns on careful examination. It appears unsound to assume that the 2010 reference standards represented the distribution of fertile men across the globe (Esteves et al. 2012; Vieira 2013). The group of studied men represented a limited population of individuals who lived in large cities in the Northern hemisphere, but for a small subset of men from Australia. Of note it was the absence of men from densely populated areas in Asia, the Middle East, Latin America, and Africa. This fact precludes the examination of regional and racial discrepancies that could account for semen quality variability. The selection criteria were arbitrary, as stated by Cooper et al.: "laboratories and data were identified through the known literature and personal communication with investigators and the editorial group of the fifth edition of the WHO laboratory manual" (Cooper et al. 2010). The heterogeneity of human semen further diminishes the clinical significance of the WHO reference values. Data indicate that there are subtle variations in semen parameters between men in different geographic areas and even between samples from the same individual (Alvarez et al. 2003; Jorgensen et al. 2001).

The lowered 2010 WHO thresholds have also been attributed to the decline in sperm count caused by endocrine disruptors and other environmental pollutants, such as insecticides and pesticides (Handelsman 2001; Sadeu et al. 2010; Carlsen et al. 1992). However, the observed discrepancies are more likely to be associated with the methodological factors, such as patient selection criteria, the higher laboratory quality control standards, and the strict criteria for morphology assessment (Cocuzza and Esteves 2014).

Conclusions

What seems like a relatively small change has a large potential impact. This might actually result in previously subfertile men being classified as fertile by many providers, especially in idiopathic cases where the only feature may be the semen analysis to make a decision on male factor. This will affect reporting data for research or even demographics and outcomes. This may mislead and misrepresent the definition of male infertility and underrepresent the cause and subsequent work-up of infertility in a couple. In addition, better international standardization of the technical methodology, consensus on the interpretation of sperm morphology evaluation criteria, and standardized international external quality control (EQC) schemes are of utmost importance to formulate robust guidelines that will have good predictive value for fertility.

References

Abbey A, Halman LJ, Andrews FM. Psychosocial, treatment, and demographic predictors of the stress associated with infertility. Fertil Steril. 1992;57(1):122–8.

Agarwal A, Allamaneni SS, Nallella KP, George AT, Mascha E. Correlation of reactive oxygen species levels with the fertilization rate after *in vitro* fertilization: a qualified meta-analysis. Fertil Steril. 2005;84:228–31.

Agarwal A, Sharma RK, Nallella KP, Thomas Jr AJ, Alvarez JG, Sikka SC. Reactive oxygen species as an independent marker of male factor infertility. Fertil Steril. 2006;86:878–85.

Agarwal A, Makker K, Sharma R. Clinical relevance of oxidative stress in male factor infertility: an update. Am J Reprod Immunol. 2008;59:2–11.

Ahmadi A, Ng SC. Fertilizing ability of DNA-damaged spermatozoa. J Exp Zool. 1999;284:696–704.

Aitken RJ. Whither must spermatozoa wander? The future of laboratory seminology. Asian J Androl. 2010;12:99–103.

Aitken RJ, Baker MA. The role of proteomics in understanding sperm cell biology. Int J Androl. 2008;31:295–302.

Aitken RJ, Clarkson JS. Cellular basis of defective sperm function and its association with the genesis of reactive oxygen species by human spermatozoa. J Reprod Fertil. 1987;81: 459–69.

Aitken RJ, Clarkson JS. Significance of reactive oxygen species in defining the efficacy of sperm preparation techniques. J Androl. 1988;9:367–76.

Aitken RJ, Sutton M, Warner P, Richardson DW. Relationship between the movement characteristics of human spermatozoa and their ability to penetrate cervical mucus and zona-free hamster oocytes. J Reprod Fertil. 1985;73:441–9.

Aitken RJ, Clarkson JS, Fishel S. Generation of reactive oxygen species, lipid peroxidation and human sperm function. Biol Reprod. 1989a;41:183–7.

Aitken RJ, Clarkson JS, Hargreave TB, Irvine DS, Wu FC. Analysis of the relationship between defective sperm function and the generation of reactive oxygen species in cases of oligozoospermia. J Androl. 1989b;10:214–20.

Aitken RJ, Irvine DS, Wu FC. Prospective analysis of sperm-oocyte fusion and reactive oxygen species generation as criteria for the diagnosis of infertility. Am J Obstet Gynecol. 1991;164:542–51.

Alvarez C, Castilla JA, Martinez L, Ramirez JP, Vergara F, Gaforio JJ. Biological variation of seminal parameters in healthy subjects. Hum Reprod. 2003;18:2082–8.

Amelar RD. Coagulation, liquefaction and viscosity of human semen. J Urol. 1962;87:187–90.

Anderson DJ. Should male infertility patients be tested for leukocytospermia? Fertil Steril. 1995;63:246–8.

Auger J, Eustache F, Andersen AG, Irvine DS, Jorgensen N, Skakkebaek NE, et al. Sperm morphological defects related to environment, lifestyle and medical history of 1001 male partners of pregnant women from four European cities. Hum Reprod. 2001;16:2710–7.

Baker DJ, Paterson MA, Klaassen JM, Wyrick-Glatzel J. Semen evaluations in the clinical laboratory: how well are they being performed? Lab Med. 1994;25(8):509–14.

Baker K, Li J, Sabanegh E. Analysis of semen parameters in male referrals: impact of reference limits, stratification by fertility categories, predictors of change, and comparison of normal semen parameters in subfertile couples. Fertil Steril. 2015;103(1):59–65.e5.
Barratt CL, McLeod ID, Dunphy BC, Cooke ID. Prognostic value of two putative sperm function tests: hypo-osmotic swelling and bovine sperm mucus penetration test (penetrak). Hum Reprod. 1992;7:1240–4.
Barratt CLR, et al. Prognostic significance of computerized motility analysis for in vivo fertility. Fertil Steril. 1993;60:520–5.
Barratt CL, Mansell S, Beaton C, Tardif S, Oxenham SK. Diagnostic tools in male infertility-the question of sperm dysfunction. Asian J Androl. 2011;13:53–8.
Benchaib M, Lornage J, Mazoyer C, Lejeune H, Salle B, François Guerin J. Sperm deoxyribonucleic acid fragmentation as a prognostic indicator of assisted reproductive technology outcome. Fertil Steril. 2007;87:93–100.
Berman NG, Wang C, Paulsen CA. Methodological issues in the analysis of human sperm concentration data. J Androl. 1996;17:68–73.
Björndahl L. The usefulness and significance of assessing rapidly progressive spermatozoa. Asian J Androl. 2010;12:33–5.
Björndahl L. What is normal semen quality? On the use and abuse of reference limits for the interpretation of semen analysis results. Hum Fertil. 2011;14:179–86.
Björndahl L, Söderlund I, Kvist U. Evaluation of the one-step eosin-nigrosin staining technique for human sperm vitality assessment. Hum Reprod. 2003;18:813–6.
Björndahl L, Söderlund I, Johansson S, Mohammadieh M, Pourian MR, Kvist U. Why the recommendations for eosin-nigrosin staining techniques for human sperm vitality assessment must change. J Androl. 2004;25:671–8.
Björndahl L, Mortimer D, Barratt CR, et al. A practical guide to basic laboratory andrology. Cambridge: Cambridge University Press; 2010a.
Björndahl L, Mortimer D, Barratt CR, et al. A practical guide to basic laboratory andrology. Cambridge: Cambridge University Press; 2010b. p. 77–112.
Bollendorf A, Check JH, Lurie D. Evaluation of the effect of the absence of sperm with rapid and linear progressive motility on subsequent pregnancy rates following intrauterine insemination or in vitro fertilization. J Androl. 1996;17:550–7.
Borini A, Tarozzi N, Bizzaro D, Bonu MA, Fava L, Flamigni C, et al. Sperm DNA fragmentation: paternal effect on early post-implantation embryo development in ART. Hum Reprod. 2006;21:2876–81.
Bornman R, Aneck-Hahn N. The interpretation of a semen analysis. Continuing Medical Education. 2012;30(5):163–5.
Bostofte E, Serup J, Rebbe H. Hammen semen quality classification and pregnancies obtained during a twenty-year follow-up period. Fertil Steril. 1981;36:84–7.
Boyd JC. Defining laboratory reference values and decision limits: populations, intervals, and interpretations. Asian J Androl. 2010;12(1):83–90.
Brazil C. Practical semen analysis: from A to Z. Asian J Androl. 2010;12:14–20.
Bungum M, Humaidan P, Axmon A, Spano M, Bungum L, Erenpreiss J, et al. Sperm DNA integrity assessment in prediction of assisted reproduction technology outcome. Hum Reprod. 2007;22:174–9.
Carlsen E, Giwercman A, Keiding N, Skakkebaek NE. Evidence for decreasing quality of semen during past 50 years. BMJ. 1992;305:609–13.
Carlsen E, Petersen JH, Andersson AM, Skakkebaek NE. Effects of ejaculatory frequency and season on variations in semen quality. Fertil Steril. 2004;82:358–66.
Catanzariti F, Cantoro U, Lacetera V, Muzzonigro G, Polito M. Comparison between WHO (World Health Organization) 2010 and WHO 1999 parameters for semen analysis - interpretation of 529 consecutive samples. Arch Ital Urol Androl. 2013;85(3):125–9.
Cho C, Jung-Ha H, Willis WD, Goulding EH, Stein P, Xu Z, et al. Protamine 2 deficiency leads to sperm DNA damage and embryo death in mice. Biol Reprod. 2003;69:211–7.

Cocuzza M, Esteves SC. Shedding light on the controversy surrounding the temporal decline in human sperm counts: a systematic review. Scientific World J. 2014;2014:365691.

Coetzee K, Kruge TF, Lombard CJ. Predictive value of normal sperm morphology: a structured literature review. Hum Reprod Update. 1998;4:73–82.

Comhaire FH, Vermeulen L, Hinting A, Schoonjans F. Accuracy of sperm characteristics in predicting the in vitro fertilizing capacity of semen. J In Vitro Fert Embryo Transf. 1988;5:326–31.

Consensus workshop on advanced diagnostic andrology techniques. ESHRE (European Society of Human Reproduction and Embryology) Andrology Special Interest Group. Hum Reprod. 1996;11:1463–79.

Cooper TG, Atkinson AD, Nieschlag E. Experience with external quality control in spermatology. Hum Reprod. 1999;14(3):765–9.

Cooper TG, Björndahl L, Vreeburg J, Nieschlag E. Semen analysis and external quality control schemes for semen analysis need global standardization. Int J Androl. 2002;25(5):306–11.

Cooper TG, Noonan E, von Eckardstein S, Auger J, Baker HW, Behre HM, et al. World Health Organization reference values for human semen characteristics. Hum Reprod Update. 2010;16(3):231–45.

Cross NL, Morales P, Overstreet JW, Hanson FW. Two simple methods for detecting acrosome-reacted human sperm. Gamete Res. 1986;15:213–26.

Cummins JM, Pember SM, Jequier AM, Yovich JL, Hartmann PE. A test of the human sperm acrosome reaction following ionophore challenge. Relationship to fertility and other seminal parameters. J Androl. 1991;12:98–103.

Deck AJ, Berger RE. Should vasectomy reversal be performed in men with older female partners? J Urol. 2000;163(1):105–6.

Dohle GR, Diemer T, Kopa Z, Krausz C, Giwercman A, Jungwirth A, et al. European association of urology guidelines on vasectomy. Eur Urol. 2012;61:159–63.

Dunson DB, Baird DD, Colombo B. Increased infertility with age in men and women. Obstet Gynecol. 2004;103(1):51–6.

Eliasson R. Semen analysis and laboratory workup. In: Cockett ATK, Urry RL, editors. Male infertility. Workup, treatment and research. New York: Grune & Stratton; 1977. p. 169–88.

Eliasson R. Semen analysis with regard to sperm number, sperm morphology and functional aspects. Asian J Androl. 2010;12:26–32.

Eliasson R, Hellinga G, Lubcke F, Meyhöfer W, Nierman H, Steeno O, et al. Empfehlungen zur Nomenklatur in der Andrologie. [Recommendations regarding nomenclature in Andrology.] Andrologie. 1970;2:186–187.

Esfandiari N, Burjaq H, Gotlieb L, Casper RF. Seminal hyperviscosity is associated with poor outcome of *in vitro* fertilization and embryo transfer: a prospective study. Fertil Steril. 2008;90:1739–43.

Esteves SC. Clinical relevance of routine semen analysis and controversies surrounding the 2010 World Health Organization criteria for semen examination. Int Braz J Urol. 2014;40:443–53.

Esteves SC, Miyaoka R, Agarwal A. An update on the clinical assessment of the infertile male. Clinics. 2011;66(4):691–700.

Esteves SC, Zini A, Aziz N, Alvarez JG, Sabanegh Jr ES, Agarwal A. Critical appraisal of World Health Organization's new reference values for human semen characteristics and effect on diagnosis and treatment of subfertile men. Urology. 2012;79(1):16–22.

Evenson DP, Jost LK, Marshall D, Zinaman MJ, Clegg E, Purvis K, et al. Utility of the sperm chromatin structure assay as a diagnostic and prognostic tool in the human fertility clinic. Hum Reprod. 1999;14:1039–49.

Fénichel P, Donzeau M, Farahifar D, Basteris B, Ayraud N, Hsi BL. Dynamics of human sperm acrosome reaction: relation with *in vitro* fertilization. Fertil Steril. 1991;55:994–9.

Fréour T, Jean M, Mirallié S, Dubourdieu S, Barrière P. Computer-Assisted Sperm Analysis (CASA) parameters and their evolution during preparation as predictors of pregnancy in intrauterine insemination with frozen-thawed donor semen cycles. Eur J Obstet Gynecol Reprod Biol. 2010;149:186–9.

Frydman N, Prisant N, Hesters L, Frydman R, Tachdjian G, Cohen-Bacrie P, et al. Adequate ovarian follicular status does not prevent the decrease in pregnancy rates associated with high sperm DNA fragmentation. Fertil Steril. 2008;89:92–7.

Garrett C, Baker HWG. A new fully automated system for the morphometric analysis of human sperm heads. Fertil Steril. 1995;63:1306–17.

Garrett C, et al. Automated semen analysis: "zona pellucida preferred" sperm morphology and straight line velocity are related to pregnancy rates in subfertile couples. Hum Reprod. 2003;18:1643–9.

Ginsburg KA, Armant DR. The influence on chamber characteristics on the reliability of sperm concentration and movement measurements obtained by manual and video-micrographic analysis. Fertil Steril. 1990;53:882–7.

Gomez E, Aitken J. Impact of in vitro fertilization culture media on peroxidative damage to human spermatozoa. Fertil Steril. 1996;65:880–2.

Gunalp S, Onculoglu C, Gurgan T, et al. A study of semen parameters with emphasis on sperm morphology in a fertile population: an attempt to develop clinical thresholds. Hum Reprod. 2001;16:110–4.

Guttmacher A. Factors affecting normal expectancy of conception. J Am Med Assoc. 1956;161:855–60.

Guzick DS, Overstreet JW, Factor-Litvak P, Brazil CK, Nakajima ST, Coutifaris C, et al. Sperm morphology, motility, and concentration in fertile and infertile men. N Engl J Med. 2001;345:1388–93.

Hamada A, Esteves SC, Nizza M, Agarwal A. Unexplained male infertility: diagnosis and management. Int Braz J Urol. 2012;38:576–94.

Handelsman DJ. Estrogens and falling sperm counts. Reprod Fertil Dev. 2001;13:317–24.

Haugen TB, Egeland T, Magnus O. Semen parameters in Norwegian fertile men. J Androl. 2006;27:66–71.

Henkel R, Müller C, Miska W, Gips H, Schill WB. Determination of the acrosome reaction in human spermatozoa is predictive of fertilization *in vitro*. Hum Reprod. 1993;8:2128–32.

Irvine DS, Aitken RJ. Predictive value of in-vitro sperm function tests in the context of an AID service. Hum Reprod. 1986;1:539–45.

Jarow JP, Sanzone JJ. Risk factors for male partner antisperm antibodies. J Urol. 1992;148:1805–7.

Jensen TK, Slama R, Ducot B, Suominen J, Cawood EH, Andersen AG, et al. Regional differences in waiting time to pregnancy among fertile couples from four European cities. Hum Reprod. 2001;16:2697–704.

Jequier AM. Is quality assurance in semen analysis still really necessary? A clinician's viewpoint. Hum Reprod. 2005;20:2039–42.

Jequier AM. Semen analysis: a new manual and its application to the understanding of semen and its pathology. Asian J Androl. 2010;12:11–3.

Jorgensen N, Andersen AG, Eustache F, et al. Regional differences in semen quality in Europe. Hum Reprod. 2001;16:1012–9.

Jouannet P, Ducot B, Feneux D, Spira A. Male factors and the likelihood of pregnancy in infertile couples. I. Study of sperm characteristics. Int J Androl. 1988;11:379–94.

Katsuki T, Hara T, Ueda K, Tanaka J, Ohama K. Prediction of outcomes of assisted reproduction treatment using the calcium ionophore-induced acrosome reaction. Hum Reprod. 2005;20:469–75.

Keegan BR, Barton S, Sanchez X, Berkeley AS, Krey LC, Grifo J. Isolated teratozoospermia does not affect in vitro fertilization outcome and is not an indication for intracytoplasmic sperm injection. Fertil Steril. 2007;88:1583–8.

Keel BA. The semen analysis. In: Keel B, Webster B, editors. CRC handbook of the laboratory diagnosis and treatment of infertility. Boca Raton: CRC Press; 1990. p. 27–69.

Keel BA. Within- and between-subject variation in semen parameters in infertile men and normal semen donors. Fertil Steril. 2006;85:128–34.

Keel BA, Quinn P, Schmidt CF, Serafy NT, Serafy NT, Schalue TK. Results of the American association of bioanalysts national proficiency testing programme in andrology. Hum Reprod. 2000;15(3):680–6.

Kolettis PN, Sabanegh ES. Significant medical pathology discovered during a male infertility evaluation. J Urol. 2001;166(1):178–80.

Kruger TF, Acosta AA, Simmons KF, et al. Predictive value of abnormal sperm morphology in *in vitro* fertilization. Fertil Steril. 1988;49:112–7.

Lin MH, Kuo-Kuang Lee R, Li SH, Lu CH, Sun FJ, Hwu YM. Sperm chromatin structure assay parameters are not related to fertilization rates, embryo quality, and pregnancy rates in *in vitro* fertilization and intracytoplasmic sperm injection, but might be related to spontaneous abortion rates. Fertil Steril. 2008;90:352–9.

Lindholmer C. The importance of seminal plasma for human sperm motility. Biol Reprod. 1974;10:533–42.

Liu DY, Baker HW. Disordered zona pellucida-induced acrosome reaction and failure of *in vitro* fertilization in patients with unexplained infertility. Fertil Steril. 2003;79:74–80.

Liu DY, et al. Relationship between sperm motility assessed with the Hamilton thorn motility analyzer and fertilization rates in vitro. J Androl. 1991;12:231–9.

MacLeod J, Gold RZ. The male factor in fertility and infertility. III. An analysis of motile activity in the spermatozoa of 1000 fertile men and 1000 men in infertile marriage. Fertil Steril. 1951;2:187–204.

MacLeod J, Gold RZ. The male factor in fertility and sterility V. Effect of continence on semen quality. Fertil Steril. 1952;3:297–315.

Makler A. A new chamber for rapid sperm count and motility determination. Fertil Steril. 1978;30:313–8.

Male Infertility Best Practice Policy Committee of the American Urological Association, Practice Committee of the American Society for Reproductive Medicine. Report on varicocele and infertility. Fertil Steril. 2004;82(1):S142–5.

Male Infertility Best Practice Policy Committee of the American Urological Association, Practice Committee of the American Society for Reproductive Medicine. Report on optimal evaluation of the infertile male. Fertil Steril. 2006;86(5 Suppl 1):S202–9.

Marchetti C, Obert G, Deffosez A, Formstecher P, Marchetti P. Study of mitochondrial membrane potential, reactive oxygen species, DNA fragmentation and cell viability by flow cytometry in human sperm. Hum Reprod. 2002;17:1257–65.

Menkveld R. Chapter 9: The basic semen analysis. In: Oehninger S, Kruger TF, editors. Male infertility. Diagnosis and treatment. Oxford: Informa Healthcare; 2007. p. 141–70.

Menkveld R. Clinical significance of the low normal sperm morphology value as proposed in the fifth edition of the WHO laboratory manual for the examination and processing of human semen. Asian J Androl. 2010;12(1):47–58.

Menkveld R, Kruger FT. Basic semen analysis. In: Acosta AA, Kruger TF, editors. Human spermatozoa in assisted reproduction. Carnforth: Parthenon Publishing; 1996. p. 53–71.

Menkveld R, Stander FS, Kotze TJ, Kruger TF, van Zyl JA. The evaluation of morphological characteristics of human spermatozoa according to stricter criteria. Hum Reprod. 1990;5:586–92.

Menkveld R, Stander FSH, Kruger TF. Comparison between acrosome index and teratozoospermia index as additional criteria to sperm morphology in the prediction of expected in-vitro fertilization outcome. Hum Reprod. 1998;13:52.

Menkveld R, Holleboom CAG, Rhemrev JPT. Measurement and significance of sperm morphology. Asian J Androl. 2011;13:59–68.

Mortimer D. Sperm preparation techniques and iatrogenic failures of *in-vitro* fertilization. Hum Reprod. 1991;6:173–6.

Mortimer D. Semen microbiology and virology. In: Practical laboratory andrology. Oxford: Oxford University Press; 1994a. p. 127–33.

Mortimer D. Antisperm antibodies. In: Practical laboratory andrology. Oxford: Oxford University Press; 1994b. p. 111–25.

Mortimer D. Practical laboratory andrology. Oxford: Oxford University Press; 1994c.

Mortimer D. Sperm preparation methods. J Androl. 2000;21:357–66.

Mortimer D, Menkveld R. Sperm morphology assessment – historical perspectives and current opinions. J Androl. 2001;22:192–205.

Mortimer D, Templeton AA, Lenton EA, Coleman RA. Influence of abstinence and ejaculation-to analysis delay on semen analysis parameters of suspected infertile men. Arch Androl. 1982;8:251–6.

Mortimer D, Pandya IJ, Sawers RS. Relationship between human sperm motility characteristics and sperm penetration into human cervical mucus *in vitro*. J Reprod Fertil. 1986;78:93–102.

Mortimer D, Mortimer ST, Shu MA, Swart R. A simplified approach to sperm-cervical mucus interaction testing using a hyaluronate migration test. Hum Reprod. 1990;5:835–41.

Munuce MJ, Bregni C, Carizza C, Mendeluk G. Semen culture, leukocytospermia and the presence of sperm antibodies in seminal hyperviscosity. Arch Androl. 1999;42:21–8.

Murray KS, James A, McGeady JB, Reed ML, Kuang WW, Nangia AK. The effect of the new 2010 World Health Organization criteria for semen analyses on male infertility. Fertil Steril. 2012;98(6):1428–31.

Nallella KP, Sharma RK, Aziz N, Agarwal A. Significance of sperm characteristics in the evaluation of male infertility. Fertil Steril. 2006;85:629–34.

Niederberger CS. Semen and the curse of cutoffs. J Urol. 2011;185(2):381–2.

Oehninger S, Blackmore P, Morshedi M, Sueldo C, Acosta AA, Alexander NJ. Defective calcium influx and acrosome reaction (spontaneous and progesterone-induced) in spermatozoa of infertile men with severe teratozoospermia. Fertil Steril. 1994;61:349–54.

Payne JF, Raburn DJ, Couchman GM, Price TM, Jamison MG, Walmer DK. Redefining the relationship between sperm deoxyribonucleic acid fragmentation as measured by the sperm chromatin structure assay and outcomes of assisted reproductive techniques. Fertil Steril. 2005;84:356–64.

Practice Committee of American Society for Reproductive Medicine. Report on varicocele and infertility. Fertil Steril. 2008;90:S247–9.

Quintero I, Ghersevich S, Caille A, Munuce MJ, Daniele SM, Morisoli L. Effects of human oviductal *in vitro* secretion on spermatozoa and search of sperm-oviductal proteins interactions. Int J Androl. 2005;28:137–43.

Rivera-Montes AM, Rivera-Gallegos A, Rodríguez-Villasana E, Juárez-Bengoa A, Díaz-Pérez M de los A, Hernández-Valencia M. Estimate of the variability in the evaluation of semen analysis. Ginecol Obstet Mex. 2013;81(11):639–44.

Rogers B, Brentwood J. Capacitation, acrosome reaction and fertilization. In: Zaneveld L, Chattterton T, editors. Biochemistry of mammalian reproduction. New York: Wiley; 1982. p. 203.

Rowe J, Comhaire FH, Hargreave TB, Mahmoud AMA. WHO manual for the standardized investigation, diagnosis and management of the infertile male. Cambridge: Cambridge University Press; 2000.

Sadeu JC, Hughes CL, Agarwal S, Foster WG. Alcohol, drugs, caffeine, tobacco, and environmental contaminant exposure: reproductive health consequences and clinical implications. Crit Rev Toxicol. 2010;40:633–52.

Sanchez-Pozo MC, Mendiola J, Serrano M, Mozas J, Bjorndahl L, Menkveld R, et al. Proposal of guidelines for the appraisal of SEMen QUAlity studies (SEMQUA). Hum Reprod. 2013;28:10–21.

Schlegel PN. Is assisted reproduction the optimal treatment for varicocele-associated male infertility? A cost-effectiveness analysis. Urology. 1997;49(1):83–90.

Shibahara H, Obara H, Ayustawati, et al. Prediction of pregnancy by intrauterine insemination using CASA estimates and strict criteria in patients with male factor infertility. Int J Androl. 2004;27:63–8.

Sifer C, Sasportes T, Barraud V, Poncelet C, Rudant J, Porcher R, et al. World Health Organization grade 'a' motility and zona-binding test accurately predict IVF outcome for mild male factor and unexplained infertilities. Hum Reprod. 2005;20:2769–75.

Sigman M, Lipshultz LI, Howards SS. Office evaluation of the subfertile male. In: Lipshultz LI, Howards SS, Niederberger CS, editors. Infertility in the male. 4th ed. New York: Cambridge University Press; 2009. p. 153–76.

Slama R, Eustache F, Ducot B, Jensen TK, Jorgensen N, Horte A, et al. Time to pregnancy and semen parameters: a cross-sectional study among fertile couples from four European cities. Hum Reprod. 2002;17:503–15.

Smith KD, Rodriguez-Rigau LJ, Steinberger E. Relation between indices of semen analysis and pregnancy rate in infertile couples. Fertil Steril. 1977;28:1314–9.

Sociedade Brasileira de Urologia & Colegio Brasileiro de Radiologia; Projeto Diretrizes da Associacao Medica Brasileira: Varicocele. Available from: http://www.projetodiretrizes.org.br/8_volume/40-Varicocele.pdf. Cited 5 Oct 2013.

Spiessens C, Vanderschueren D, Meuleman C, et al. Isolated teratozoospermia and intrauterine insemination. Fertil Steril. 2003;80:1185–9.

Stewart TM, Liu DY, Garrett C, Jorgensen N, Brown EH, et al. Associations between andrological measures, hormones and semen quality in fertile Australian men: inverse relationship between obesity and sperm output. Hum Reprod. 2009;24:1561–8.

Swan SH, Brazil C, Drobnis EZ, Liu F, Kruse RL, Hatch M, et al. Geographic differences in semen quality of fertile U.S. Males. Environ Health Perspect. 2003;111:414–20.

Tesarik J. Appropriate timing of the acrosome reaction is a major requirement for the fertilizing spermatozoon. Hum Reprod. 1989;4:957–61.

Thonneau P, Marchand S, Tallex A, Ferial ML, Ducot B, Lansac J, et al. Incidence and main causes of infertility in a resident population (1,850,000) of three French regions (1988–1989). Hum Reprod. 1991;6:811–6.

Van den Bergh M, Emiliani S, Biramane J, Vannin AS, Englert Y. A first prospective study of the individual straight line velocity of the spermatozoon and its influences on the fertilization rate after intracytoplasmic sperm injection. Hum Reprod. 1998;13:3103–7.

Van Waart J, Kruger TF, Lombard CJ, Ombelet W. Predictive value of normal sperm morphology in intrauterine insemination (IUI): a structured literature review. Hum Reprod Update. 2001;7:495–500.

Vasan SS. Semen analysis and sperm function tests: how much to test? Indian Journal of Urology. 2011;27(1):41–8.

Vieira M. New World Health Organization reference values for semen analysis: where do we stand? Einstein (Sao Paulo). 2013;11(2):263–4.

Wolff H, Panhans A, Zebhauser M, Meurer M. Comparison of three methods to detect white blood cells in semen: leukocyte esterase dipstick test, granulocyte elastase enzyme-immunoassay, and peroxidase cytochemistry. Fertil Steril. 1992;58:1260–2.

World Health Organization. WHO laboratory manual for the examination of human semen and sperm-cervical mucus interaction. 2nd ed. Cambridge: Cambridge University Press; 1987.

World Health Organization. WHO laboratory manual for the examination of human semen and sperm-cervical mucus interaction. 3rd ed. Cambridge: Cambridge University Pres; 1992.

World Health Organization. WHO laboratory manual for the examination of human semen and sperm-cervical mucus interaction. 4th ed. Cambridge: Cambridge University Press; 1999.

World Health Organization. WHO laboratory manual for the examination and processing of human semen. 5th ed. Cambridge: Cambridge University Press; 2010.

Yanagimachi R. Penetration of guinea-pig spermatozoa into hamster eggs *in vitro*. J Reprod Fertil. 1972;28:477–80.

Yanagimachi R, Yanagimachi H, Rogers B. The use of zona-free animal ova as a test-system for the assessment of the fertilizing capacity of human spermatozoa. Biol Reprod. 1976;15:471–6.

Yerram N, Sandlow JI, Brannigan RE. Clinical implications of the new 2010 WHO reference ranges for human semen characteristics. J Androl. 2012;33(3):289–90.

Zinaman MJ, et al. Evaluation of computer-assisted semen analysis (CASA) with IDENT stain to determine sperm concentration. J Androl. 1996;17:288–92.

Zini A, Bielecki R, Phang D, Zenzes MT. Correlations between two markers of sperm DNA integrity, DNA denaturation and DNA fragmentation, in fertile and infertile men. Fertil Steril. 2001;75:674–7.

Zini A, Meriano J, Kader K, Jarvi K, Laskin CA, Cadesky K. Potential adverse effect of sperm DNA damage on embryo quality after ICSI. Hum Reprod. 2005;20:3476–80.

Azoospermia: Diagnosis and Management

6

Satya Srini Vasan

6.1 Introduction

Azoospermia is one of the major reproductive disorders which causes male infertility in humans; however, the etiology of this disease is largely unknown. The reliable diagnosis of the absence of spermatozoa in a semen sample is an important criterion not only for diagnosing male infertility but also for ascertaining the success of vasectomy and for determining the efficacy of hormonal contraception (Aziz 2013).

The traditional definition of azoospermia is ambiguous, which has ramifications on the diagnostic criteria. The 5th edition of the World Health Organization (WHO) manual (World Health Organization 2010) defines Azoospermia as: "no spermatozoa are found in the sediment of a centrifuged sample" (Eliasson 1981). The American Urological Association has adopted a more detailed definition: "no sperm after centrifugation at 3000 × g for 15 min and examination of the pellet" (Male Infertility Best Practice Policy Committee of the American Urological Association 2006). Thus, the accurate assessment of very low sperm counts is particularly important to avoid labeling severely oligozoospermic men as azoospermic. Some of the important features of analyses of azoospermic semen samples are described in the following section.

Azoospermic samples and those with very low sperm counts appear less opaque. Although a low semen volume is more likely to be due to the incomplete collection of the ejaculate, it may also be due to obstruction of the ejaculatory duct, retrograde ejaculation, or congenital bilateral absence of the vas deferens (CBAVD) (de la Taille et al. 1998; Daudin et al. 2000). A characteristically low pH of 6.8 (normal pH 7.2) could also indicate CBAVD, as a consequence of dysplasia or the absence of the seminal

S.S. Vasan, DNB (Surgery, Urology)
Department of Andrology, Manipal Ankur Andrology and Reproductive Services,
422, 20th Main, I Block, Rajajinagar, Bangalore 560010, India
e-mail: vasan@manipalankur.com

K. Gunasekaran, N. Pandiyan (eds.), *Male Infertility*,
DOI 10.1007/978-81-322-3604-7_6

vesicles. Semen volume and pH are important for determining the differential diagnosis of the cause of azoospermia. Therefore, attention to detail is necessary when deviations from the normal value are encountered in the routine semen analysis.

When no spermatozoa are observed in replicate wet preparations, the semen sample should be centrifuged, and the pellet should be examined for the presence of sperm. WHO manual (World Health Organization 2010) recommends centrifugation at 3000 × g for 15 min at room temperature for all samples in which no spermatozoa are detected. The semen analysis should be performed according to the 2010 World Health Organization guidelines, and at least two semen samples, obtained more than 2 weeks apart, should be examined.

6.2 Evaluation of the Azoospermic Male

Complete evaluation of a suspected case of azoospermia should include a complete medical and surgical history, physical examination, and endocrine evaluation. Medical history of childhood illnesses (such as viral orchitis or cryptorchidism) and genital trauma, medications and allergies, and an inspection of past infections are important to ascertain the cause of infertility. Infertility could be due to gonadotoxin exposures and prior radiation therapy or chemotherapy. A general physical examination is an essential part of the evaluation of an azoospermic man. The presence of clinical varicocele should be investigated and correctly classified, as high-grade varicocele could be more frequently related to azoospermia (Cocuzza et al. 2013). Appropriate sexual development and possible androgen deficiency must be assessed. Palpation of the testes and measurement of their size is mandatory, as a decreased testicular size indicates impaired spermatogenic potential (Lipshultz and Corriere 1977). In the vast majority of patients, obstructive azoospermia may be easily distinguished from nonobstructive azoospermia through a thorough analysis of clinical diagnostic parameters, such as FSH levels (Cocuzza et al. 2013).

An endocrinologic evaluation of patients who have severe male factor infertility will be useful to determine specific diagnoses and treatment strategies. Determination of serum testosterone and FSH levels of men with sperm counts of less than 10 million/mL will be sufficient to detect a vast majority of clinically significant endocrinopathies (Sigman and Jarow 1997). The information obtained from a complete endocrine profile may help to elucidate the etiology.

6.3 Etiologies of Azoospermia

The etiologies of azoospermia can be grouped into three general categories: pretesticular, testicular, and posttesticular. Pretesticular causes of azoospermia are endocrine abnormalities that adversely affect spermatogenesis. Testicular etiologies involve intrinsic disorders of spermatogenesis inside the testes. These two categories together constitute the condition termed nonobstructive azoospermia (NOA). The posttesticular causes of azoospermia include obstruction of the ductal system at any location of the male reproductive tract and are termed obstructive azoospermia (OA). The treatment strategies and success rates for each of these conditions are different and range from correction of the defect to restore fertility to locate and extract sperm for use in assisted reproductive techniques (ARTs).

Pretesticular causes of azoospermia are mostly due to pathological endocrine conditions. It is very uncommon and prevalent to the extent of 3 % of infertile men (Sigman and Jarow 1997). Some of the etiologies include congenital or acquired hypogonadotropic hypogonadism. The pathophysiology involves a defect at the level of the hypothalamic secretion of gonadotropin-releasing hormone (GnRH). Acquired causes include pituitary tumors and trauma and the use of anabolic steroids. Hyperprolactinemia leading to inhibition of secretion of GnRH (Burrows et al. 2002) and androgen resistance due to mutation of the androgen receptor gene (Mak and Jarvi 1996) are the other pretesticular causes.

Testicular etiologies are intrinsic disorders of spermatogenesis. Direct testicular pathology may be due to varicocele-induced testicular damage, undescended testes, testicular torsion, mumps orchitis, gonadotoxic effects from medications, genetic abnormalities, and idiopathic causes. Chromosome alterations responsible for disruption of spermatogenesis are found in 15 % of azoospermic and 5 % of oligospermic men and represent one of the most common genetic defects in infertile men (Pandiyan and Jequier 1996; Peschka et al. 1999).

Posttesticular causes of azoospermia are due either to the obstruction of sperm delivery or ejaculatory dysfunction. The obstruction may be at different sites, such as vas deferens, epididymis, or ejaculatory duct, and depends on the presence of pathological conditions, such as the absence of the vasa deferentia, and disorders of ejaculation. The clinical management of obstructive azoospermia depends on its cause and ranges from surgical correction of the obstruction that may lead to natural conception, to retrieval of sperm directly from the epididymis or testis, followed by the use of ART (Practice Committee of American Society for Reproductive Medicine 2008).

Male factor infertility can result from an underlying medical condition that is often treatable but could possibly be life threatening. It can also be based only on seminal parameters without a physical exam. This behavior may lead to a delay in both the exact diagnosis and in possible specific infertility treatment. In recent years, male factor infertility has been exponentially rising due to a comprehensive evaluation of reproductive male function and improved diagnostic tools. Despite this improvement in diagnosis, azoospermia is always the most challenging topic associated with infertility treatment. Several conditions that interfere with spermatogenesis, reduce sperm production and quality can lead to azoospermia. Azoospermia may also occur because of a reproductive tract obstruction. Optimal management of patients with azoospermia requires a full understanding of the disease etiology (Cocuzza et al. 2013).

Many studies have been conducted to understand the underlying causes of NOA and to develop new therapeutic strategies for patients with NOA. In a recent morphological study, Sertoli cells isolated from NOA patients had a series of abnormal ultrastructural features compared with the normal control Sertoli cells: (i) existence of small and spindle-shaped nuclei, (ii) smaller diameter, (iii) deficient nucleolus or endoplasmic reticulum, and (iv) more vacuoles. Spectral intensities in Sertoli cells of NOA patients were distinct at four typical Raman peaks compared with the control Sertoli cells. In phenotype, SCF, BMP4, and GDNF transcripts and proteins were significantly lower in Sertoli cells of NOA patients than in the control Sertoli cells (Ma et al. 2013). In a study from Czech Republic, lower concentrations of homocysteine and cobalamin (but not folate) were found in azoospermic seminal plasma than in normozoospermic. Folate and cobalamin were higher in seminal plasma from OA than in NOA patients (Crha et al. 2010).

Comparison of expression of progesterone (PR) and estrogen receptors (ER alpha) in testicular tissue from OA and NOA patients has been studied by immunofluorescence and Western blot (Han et al. 2009). In patients with NOA due to maturation arrest (MA) and Sertoli cell only (SCO) syndrome, the expression of PR was reduced in all cell types as compared to that in the OA patients. ERalpha was expressed principally in the OA testis, but was decreased in MA testis and enhanced in the SCO testis. Thus, PR and ER alpha may be involved in the pathogenesis of MA and SCO phenotype in patients with infertility.

Male fertility problems range from diminished production of sperm, or oligozoospermia, to non-measurable levels of sperm in semen, or azoospermia, which is diagnosed in nearly 2 % of men in the general population. Testicular biopsy is the only definitive diagnostic method to distinguish between obstructive (OA) and nonobstructive (NOA) azoospermia and to identify the NOA subtypes of hypospermatogenesis, maturation arrest, and Sertoli-cell-only syndrome. Rare foci of sperm production may be found in up to 60 % of men with NOA. Sperm production, if present, is minimal for sperm appearance in the ejaculate. Given that there are no treatment options to restore fertility, sperm retrieval is the only alternative to find testicular sperm that can be used for in vitro fertilization (IVF). Among sperm acquisition methods, micro-surgical testicular sperm extraction (micro-TESE) has higher success rate at obtaining sperm compared with testicular sperm extraction and testicular sperm aspiration. In general, no major differences were noted in short-term neonatal outcomes and congenital malformation rates between children from fathers with NOA and OA (Esteves and Agarwal 2013).

6.4 Obstructive Azoospermia

Obstructive azoospermia can be due to several factors, the most common being congenital bilateral absence of the vas deferens. Other etiologies included an idiopathic cause, an iatrogenic condition due to surgical causes, ejaculatory duct obstruction, trauma, retrograde ejaculation, and vas deferens occlusion. Posttesticular sperm maturation requires a specific luminal environment in the epididymis, which is created, in part, by the blood-epididymis barrier. However, recent microarray studies have shown that epididymal cellular junctions appear to be altered in OA (Dube et al. 2010).

Ejaculatory duct obstruction (EDO) is a rare cause of OA and accounts for approximately 1 % of patients presenting with male infertility. It should be suspected when the patient has low-volume, acidic semen that contains no sperm.

Absence of fructose in the semen supports the diagnosis, as fructose is present in the secretions from the seminal vesicles. Occasionally, pain at the time of ejaculation is reported. Physical examination may reveal enlarged seminal vesicles or a midline nodule in the prostate, but frequently, the rectal exam is unremarkable. Testicular volume is usually normal, and vasa deferentia are present. Laboratory studies will confirm normal gonadotropin and testosterone levels. Retrograde ejaculation should be ruled out by examining post-ejaculatory urine for sperm. Transrectal ultrasound is a useful tool for confirming the diagnosis and further defining the causative factor. Sonography can also demonstrate dilation of the ejaculatory ducts, calcifications within the ejaculatory ducts, or prostate, utricle, or Mullerian duct cysts that can occlude the ejaculatory ducts. Traditional treatment consists of transurethral resection of the ejaculatory ducts (TURED) (Yurdakul et al. 2008).

Congenital bilateral absence of the vas deferens (CBAVD) is often caused by a mutation in the cystic fibrosis transmembrane conductance regulator (CFTR) gene. This condition is suspected based on the absence of palpable vas deferens at the time of physical examination. The caput of the epididymis is present, and the testicles should be of a normal size and consistency; however, the seminal vesicles are absent or hypoplastic in a majority of patients (Kuligowska and Fenlon 1998). Unilateral or bilateral vasal hypoplasia or unilateral absence of the vas may be an indicator of obstructive azoospermia, as a high percentage of these patients will have anomalies of the contralateral seminal vesicle. Surgical reconstruction may be a viable treatment for some patients with unilateral vasal agenesis or hypoplasia. CBAVD is not amenable to surgical reconstruction, but sperm is readily retrievable from these patients via percutaneous (PESA) or microsurgical (MESA) epididymal aspiration, testicular sperm aspiration (TESA), or simple open biopsy (TESE).

Epididymitis is a common genitourinary condition, and an infectious etiology should always be considered in men with this diagnosis. Gonorrhea, chlamydia, trichomonas, brucellosis, BCG, ureaplasma, mycoplasma, coliforms bacteria, adenovirus, and enterovirus have all been reported as causes of epididymitis. Regardless of the etiology, epididymitis can cause an intense inflammatory reaction, leading to secondary scarring and obstruction of the epididymis. Physical examination may reveal enlarged or indurated epididymides and a transition point suggesting the site of obstruction. Semen volumes are typically normal, and white cells are not necessarily present in the ejaculate. The incidence of postinfectious epididymal obstruction is thought to be low in developed countries due to prompt treatment, but it may account for a disproportionately large percentage of OA in developing countries (Ho et al. 2009). Scrotal exploration and microsurgical reconstruction are a viable option for postinfectious epididymal obstruction.

Iatrogenic injury or injury to the vas during surgical procedures has been well described and presents a unique challenge to fertility specialists. Vasal injury has been attributed to a variety of inguinal, scrotal, and pelvic surgeries, including herniorrhaphy, hydrocelectomy, appendectomy, and renal transplant. Surgical reconstruction is possible in many cases of iatrogenic injury to the vas in the scrotum or inguinal canal. Some factors, such as age and obstructive interval, are likely to impact postoperative outcomes after vasal reconstruction for etiologies of OA.

6.4.1 Treatment of OA

Obstructive azoospermia (OA) is defined as the absence of spermatozoa in the ejaculate despite normal spermatogenesis. It is a common cause of male infertility and can result from infection, congenital anomalies, or iatrogenic injury and accounts for 6.1–13.6 % of patients presenting for fertility evaluation (Aziz et al. 2006; Jequier 1985). Microsurgical vasal reconstruction is a suitable and cost-effective treatment for many cases of OA, this approach may not be feasible or desired in some cases, and such couples will require sperm retrieval paired with in vitro fertilization (Baker and Sabanegh 2013). This process requires several considerations and decisions to be made, including the cause and duration of obstruction, choice of sperm retrieval technique, and whether to use fresh or frozen-thawed sperm. Sperm retrieval can be achieved by percutaneous (PESA) or microsurgical (MESA) epididymal sperm aspiration, testicular sperm aspiration (TESA), or simple open biopsy (TESE).

Use of spermatozoa obtained by PESA in ICSI is a viable treatment for men with OA (Jiang et al. 2013). Spermatozoa can be retrieved from the testis and epididymis of men with OA and used for ICSI. In some cases, the use of testicular spermatozoa altered the embryonic development, and the use of epididymal spermatozoa should be preferred, irrespective of the etiology of OA (Buffat et al. 2006).

Percutaneous sperm retrieval is a highly effective method for collecting sperm in men with OA. Successful sperm retrieval was achieved in over 85 % of the cases using PESA, but more than one aspiration was often required (Esteves et al. 2013). In cases of failed PESA, TESA was adequate to obtain sperm in nearly all cases. Motile spermatozoa were obtained in approximately 73 % of the cases after the first or second PESA aspiration, and TESA has been performed as a rescue procedure after failed PESA in approximately 14 % of the individuals (Esteves et al. 2013). ICSI outcomes using spermatozoa collected by PESA or TESA are similar, suggesting that the reproductive potential of those gametes is independent of their source in OA. However, epididymal spermatozoa are easier to handle in the IVF laboratory compared with testicular sperm, and it is more likely that there will be excess sperm for freezing in case of epididymal retrieval (Miyaoka and Esteves 2013).

Some studies have indicated the risks of using nonejaculated spermatozoa in assisted reproduction techniques. In cases of OA, the epididymal sperm may be immature or senescent because of the long stay in the obstructed epididymis and lead to genetic risks when it is used for fertilization (O'Connell et al. 2002). On the other hand, testicular sperm can have the potential risk of incomplete genomic imprinting, incomplete chromatin condensation, and incomplete protamination (Golan et al. 1996; Tesarik et al. 1998). However, a recent Dutch multicenter study has dispelled some of these concerns. Assessment of children born from ICSI cycles, using retrieved epididymal sperm in comparison with those born from ICSI or IVF using ejaculated sperm, did not reveal any disparities in terms of incidence of stillbirths, malformations, motor performance, or mental-language development (Woldringh et al. 2011).

6.5 Nonobstructive Azoospermia

The initial evaluation of NOA needs to resolve the following issues: (1) confirming azoospermia, (2) differentiating obstructive from nonobstructive etiology, (3) assessing for the presence of reversible factors, and (4) evaluating for the presence of genetic abnormalities. An elevated follicle-stimulating hormone (FSH) level or an absence of normal spermatogenesis by testicular histology in the presence of azoospermia is generally considered sufficient evidence of a nonobstructive etiology. NOA has been identified with the Sertoli-cell-only syndrome. Other etiologies included an idiopathic cause, Klinefelter syndrome, maturation arrest, Y-chromosome microdeletion, cryptorchidism, trauma, exogenous testosterone supplementation, and other genetic disorders.

Hormone analysis forms the cornerstone of further evaluation and management of NOA and serves two important functions. The first function is to identify a distinct subset of men who have hypogonadotropic hypogonadism (low FSH), in which azoospermia results from an inadequate stimulation of the testis by gonadotropins. The second function is to predict the success of medical therapy and of surgical sperm retrieval. The American Urological Association recommends estimation of serum FSH and testosterone as the initial hormonal assessment (American Urological Association 2012).

6.5.1 Treatment of NOA

NOA is diagnosed in approximately 10% of infertile men. It represents a failure of spermatogenesis within the testis and, from a management standpoint, is due to either a lack of appropriate stimulation by gonadotropins or an intrinsic testicular impairment. The former category of patients has hypogonadotropic hypogonadism and benefits from specific hormonal therapy. These men show a remarkable recovery of spermatogenic function with exogenously administered gonadotropins or gonadotropin-releasing hormone. This category of patients also includes some individuals whose spermatogenic potential has been suppressed by excess androgens or steroids, and they also benefit from medical management. Hypogonadotropic hypogonadism is one of the few causes of NOA that have shown a consistent response to medical management (Hoffman and Crowley 1982; Belchetz et al. 1978). Gonadotropin therapy is begun at the time the patient wishes to father a child, and 3–6 months of treatment are usually sufficient to induce spermatogenesis (Vicari et al. 1992; Finkel et al. 1985). Therapy is initiated with human chorionic gonadotropin (hCG) at 2,000 IU subcutaneously three times per week or 2,500 IU twice a week and supplemented with FSH (menopausal, purified, or recombinant) at 37.5–150 IU three times a week after 3–6 months. hCG is sufficient to initiate spermatogenesis, but FSH is required to complete the spermiogenesis, particularly in patients with congenital abnormalities (Kumar 2013). An alternative method for treating hypogonadotropic hypogonadism is with a pulsatile injection of 5–20 μg of

GnRH, administered every 2 h subcutaneously. GnRH therapy reliably corrected the hypogonadism, with a reversal of azoospermia (Sykiotis et al. 2010).

The enzyme aromatase, present in the adipose tissue, liver, testis, and skin, is responsible for converting testosterone and other androgens to estradiol in men. Estradiol suppresses pituitary LH and FSH secretion and also directly inhibits testosterone biosynthesis. This results in an imbalance in the testosterone and estradiol (T/E) ratio, which may be reversible. Aromatase inhibitors have the potential to block the conversion of androgens to estradiol. The two types of aromatase inhibitors are steroidal (testolactone) and nonsteroidal (anastrozole, letrozole). Both of these groups of agents have been studied for potential therapeutic roles in NOA. The other, larger category of NOA consists of men with an intrinsic testicular impairment where empirical medical therapy yields little benefit. The primary role of medical management in these men is to improve the quantity and quality of sperm retrieved from their testis for in vitro fertilization. Gonadotropins and aromatase inhibitors show promise in achieving this end point (Kumar 2013).

Locating and retrieving spermatozoa in men with NOA remains a clinical challenge, largely because sperm production in these men can be patchy or focal in nature. Rare foci of sperm production may be found in up to 60 % of men with NOA. Sperm production, if present, is minimal for sperm appearance in the ejaculate. Given that there are no treatment options to restore fertility, sperm retrieval is the only alternative to find testicular sperm. The retrieved sperm can then be used for in vitro fertilization (IVF). Fertilization and pregnancies have been achieved with spermatozoa recovered from the seminiferous tubules. The most common methods for retrieving testicular sperm are testicular sperm aspiration (TESA), or needle/fine-needle aspiration (FNA), and testicular sperm extraction (TESE) by open testicular biopsy. A systematic review of the available sperm retrieval techniques has been published by Donoso et al. (2007) and efficacy of the techniques has been compared (Hauser et al. 2006). The optimal technique for sperm extraction should be minimally invasive and avoid destruction of testicular function, without compromising the chance to retrieve adequate numbers of spermatozoa to perform ICSI.

FNA is highly informative, minimally invasive and is associated with fewer complications than other commonly used approaches for sperm detection. As it is challenging to find foci of sperm production, strategies such as FNA mapping have been developed to find spermatozoa. FNA mapping has gained considerable attraction as an informative, "testis-sparing" technique for sperm detection in NOA. With knowledge of sperm presence and location prior to sperm retrieval, FNA maps can help clinicians tailor sperm retrieval to optimize time, effort, and extent of procedures needed to procure spermatozoa in difficult cases (Beliveau and Turek 2011). Inhibin B and FSH have been evaluated as predictors of the recovery of sperm in testicular fine-needle aspirate in men with azoospermia (Goulis et al. 2008).

Microdissection TESE (micro-TESE), performed with an operative microscope, is widely considered to be the best method for sperm retrieval in NOA, as larger and opaque tubules, presumably with active spermatogenesis, can be directly identified, resulting in higher spermatozoa retrieval rates with minimal tissue loss and low postoperative complications. Micro-TESE, in combination with ICSI, is applicable in all cases of NOA, including Klinefelter syndrome (KS). In addition, short- and long-term complications of micro-TESE in NOA and KS patients need to be considered (Ishikawa 2012; Everaert et al. 2006).

Among sperm acquisition methods, micro-TESE has higher success rates at obtaining sperm compared with testicular sperm extraction and testicular sperm aspiration. Micro-TESE allowed the identification and extraction of sperm-containing seminiferous tubules with minimum tissue excision and marked reduction in time of processing of testicular specimens for sperm injection (Esteves 2013). Despite the improved success rate of sperm by micro-TESE methods, it becomes necessary to stimulate spermatogenesis in some NOA cases. This has been achieved by hormonal stimulation by using human chorionic gonadotropin (hCG) injections for 4–5 months prior to retrieval. The hCG stimulation was found to be effective in men with hypospermatogenesis (Shiraishi et al. 2012). Use of letrozole (2.5 mg per day) has also been found to improve sperm count in NOA patients with normal serum FSH (Cavallini et al. 2011). Clomiphene citrate has also been administered to enhance the availability of sperm prior to surgical retrieval in NOA patients (Hussein et al. 2005).

Testicular sperm retrieval techniques associated with intracytoplasmic sperm injection are currently used for the treatment of NOA patients, but reliable clinical and laboratory prognostic factors of sperm recovery are still absent. There are no reliable positive prognostic factors that guarantee sperm recovery for patients with NOA. The only negative prognostic factor is the presence of AZFa and AZFb microdeletions (Glina and Vieira 2013).

Numerous studies on NOA have reported that varicocelectomy not only can induce spermatogenesis but can also increase the sperm retrieval rate; however, the value of varicocelectomy in patients with NOA still remains controversial (Inci and Gunay 2013).

Another novel technique used for the identification of spermatogenesis in NOA is the use of ^{1}H magnetic resonance spectroscopy (MRS), a noninvasive imaging tool that can identify and localize spermatogenesis in the testis. Phosphocholine (PC) and taurine tissue concentrations were significantly different between normal and NOA testicular tissue. Mean PC concentrations were three times higher in normal testes compared with NOA (SCO). A predictive model for sperm presence was developed based on tissue concentrations of PC (Aaronson et al. 2010).

6.6 Genetic Studies of Azoospermia

Azoospermia due to obstructive and nonobstructive mechanisms is a common manifestation of male infertility accounting for 10–15 % of such cases. Known genetic factors are responsible for approximately 1/3 of cases of azoospermia. Genetic factors explain 21–29 % of azoospermia (Lee et al. 2011), whereas 12–41 % of azoospermic cases are idiopathic and most likely related to unknown genetic factors (Hernandez Uribe et al. 2001). Azoospermia of a genetic origin is primarily caused by a wide array of genetic disorders, such as chromosomal abnormalities,

Table 6.1 Genetic diseases and abnormalities that result in azoospermia

Obstructive azoospermia of genetic origin
Cystic fibrosis
Congenital bilateral absence of the vas deferens (CBAVD)
Congenital unilateral absence of the vas deferens (CUAVD)
Congenital bilateral epididymal obstruction and normal vasa
Young syndrome
Nonobstructive azoospermia of genetic origin
Genetic pretesticular causes of NOA
Hypothalamic hypogonadotropic hypogonadism
Congenital hypogonadotropic hypogonadism
Adult-onset genetic hypothalamic hypogonadotropic hypogonadism
Pituitary disorders associated with hypogonadism
Generalized anterior pituitary hormone deficiency
Selective gonadotropin deficiency
Genetic testicular disorders affecting spermatogenesis and androgen production
Klinefelter syndrome
XX male syndrome
Mutation in X-linked USP 26
X-linked SOX3 mutation
Bilateral anorchia
Noonan syndrome
45 X/46XY mosaicism (mixed gonadal dysgenesis)
Genetic testicular disorders affecting spermatogenesis
Y-chromosome microdeletion
Autosome translocations
Monogenic disorders
Multifactorial disorders (e.g., cryptorchidism)
Genetic testicular disorders affecting androgen production or action
Androgen receptor mutation
Steroidogenic acute regulatory protein StAR mutation
3BHSD type 2 deficiency
SRD5A2 mutation
Dysfunctional cell regulatory pathways
Epigenetic defects
Genetic abnormities at the primordial germ cell level

Reproduced from Hamada et al. (2013)

monogenic disorders, multifactorial genetic diseases, and epigenetic disorders. These conditions constitute the genetic basis of reproductive failure. Table 6.1 summarizes the genetic basis of azoospermia at the posttesticular (obstructive azoospermia), pretesticular, and testicular (nonobstructive azoospermia) levels.

Among the OA of genetic origin, CBAVD is the most frequent condition (Tuttelmann et al. 2011). Cystic fibrosis (CF) is a life-threatening autosomal recessive disease in which the failure is due to a mutation in the cystic fibrosis transmembrane conductance regulator (CFTR) gene. The CFTR gene is expressed in the epithelial cell of exocrine tissues, such as the head of the epididymis and the vas deferens. CFTR has a role in sperm maturation in the epididymis, as this protein is necessary for fluid absorption and facilitation of sperm capacitation and fertilization ability (Wong 1998; Chan et al. 2009). Epididymal malformations are common manifestation of CF; seminal vesicles anomalies and obstructed ejaculatory ducts are also common. CBAVD accounts for at least 6–25 % of cases of OA and approximately 2 % of infertility cases (Oates and Amos 1994; Patrizio and Leonard 2000). CFTR is mutated in 60–90 % of patients with CBAVD (Ferlin et al. 2007a). The most common CFTR mutation found in men with CBAVD is a combination of ΔF508/R117H, which accounts for 40 % of the cases (Ratbi et al. 2007; Jezequel et al. 2000). CFTR mutations have also been observed in men with CUAVD.

NOA is the most severe form of azoospermia that can be caused by many factors, such as heat, radiation, drugs, varicocele, infections, and cancer, in addition to genetic factors. Genetic etiologies contribute significantly to the development of this disorder and are responsible for 21–28 % of cases (Lee et al. 2011; Hernandez Uribe et al. 2001; Hamada et al. 2013; Donohue and Fauver 1989). The genetic factors are further classified as pretesticular and testicular causes. The genetic pretesticular etiology encompasses hereditary hypothalamic-pituitary abnormalities resulting in small testes that exhibit an immature histological pattern. In these cases, immature Sertoli cells or spermatogonia type A and the absence of Leydig cells are often observed.

Genetic testicular causes of NOA include the following: (i) chromosomal abnormalities, (ii) Y-chromosome microdeletions, (iii) failure of the primordial germ cells to reach the developing gonads, (iv) lack of differentiation of the primordial germ cells to spermatogonia, and (v) male germ line mutations that affect spermatogenesis.

6.6.1 Y-Chromosome Microdeletion

The long and short arms of the Y-chromosome contain many genes that regulate spermatogenesis and testis development, respectively. Microdeletions on the long arm of the Y-chromosome (Yq) are well correlated with male infertility. Yq microdeletions are detected in approximately 13 % of men with NOA and in 5 % of men with severe oligozoospermia (sperm counts lower than 5 million/mL) (Reijo et al. 1995; McLachlan et al. 1998). A microdeletion is defined as a chromosomal deletion that spans several genes but that is small in size and cannot be detected using conventional cytogenetic methods (e.g., karyotyping). The region at Yq11 is referred to as the "azoospermia factor" (AZF) region. The AZF region is further subdivided into three subregions that are termed AZFa, AZFb, and AZFc. The most common aberrations in the AZF region are multiple gene deletions in the AZFb and AZFc subregions (Ferlin et al. 2007b), which can produce a wide range of infertility phenotypes.

Three regions in the long arm of the Y-chromosome, known as AZFa, AZFb, and AZFc, are involved in the most frequent patterns of Y-chromosome microdeletions. These regions contain a high density of genes that are thought to be responsible for impaired spermatogenesis. In 2003, the Y-chromosome sequence was mapped, and microdeletions are now classified according to the palindromic structure of the euchromatin that is composed of a series of repeat units called amplicons. Although it has been shown that the AZFb and AZFc are overlapping regions, the classical AZF regions are still used to describe the deletions in clinical practice (Sadeghi-Nejad and Farrokhi 2007). Y-chromosome microdeletions are among the major causes of male infertility.

Both the European Academy of Andrology (EAA) and the European Molecular Genetics Quality Network (EMQN) have recommended the use of sY84 and sY86 markers for the detection of azoospermia factor a (AZFa) microdeletion during DNA testing for male infertility (Wu et al. 2011). Detection of various subtypes of these deletions has a prognostic value in predicting the potential success of testicular sperm retrieval for assisted reproduction. Men with azoospermia and AZFc deletions may have retrievable sperm in their testes. However, with ICSI, there is a risk of transmission of these microdeletions to the male offsprings (Mau Kai et al. 2008). There is a high-frequency genetic abnormality, such as Y-chromosome microdeletions in patients of NOA, and a risk of passing the genetic defects to their offspring. Consequently, there is need for genetic testing and counseling of NOA patients prior to ART. The genetic testing may also be useful in prognosis and choice of ART technique. A high prevalence of Y-chromosome microdeletions have been observed in Middle Eastern (28.41 %) (Alhalabi et al. 2013), Ukrainian (35 %) (Pylyp et al. 2013), Brazilian (18.8 %) (Mafra et al. 2011), and Iranian patients (66.67 % of AZFb) (Mirfakhraie et al. 2011), but the incidence seems to be low in Slovak azoospermic patients (Behulova et al. 2011). Genetic anomalies in patients with severe oligozoospermia and azoospermia have also been detected in eastern Turkey. A prospective study detected Y-chromosome microdeletions, especially of the AZFc locus to the extent of 64 % (Ceylan et al. 2010). The most frequent deletions were in the AZFc region (50 %) in Thai men with azoospermia and comparable with infertile men from other Asian and Western countries (Vutyavanich et al. 2007).

About 10 % of cases of male infertility are due to the presence of microdeletions within the long arm of the Y-chromosome (Yq). Despite the large literature covering this critical issue, very little is known about the pathogenic mechanism leading to spermatogenesis disruption in patients carrying these microdeletions. Testicular gene expression profiling of patients carrying an AZFc microdeletion has been carried out by employing a microarray assay techniques. Results indicated a down-regulation of several genes related to spermatogenesis that are mainly involved in testicular mRNA storage. If that several forms of infertility can be triggered by a common pathogenic mechanism, that is likely related to alterations in testicular mRNA storage due to lack of testicular DAZ gene expression (Gatta et al. 2010).

Maturation arrest (MA) refers to failure of germ cell development leading to clinical NOA. Although the azoospermic factor (AZF) region of the human Y-chromosome is clearly implicated in some cases, thus far very little is known about which individual Y-chromosome genes are important for complete male germ cell development. Stahl et al. (2012) have attempted to identify single genes on the Y-chromosome that may be implicated in the pathogenesis of NOA associated with MA in the American population. Based on the genotype-phenotype analysis of 132 men with Y-chromosome microdeletions, they identified CDY2 and HSFY as the genes for which differences in expression were observed between the MA and OA. Men with OA had 12-fold and 16-fold higher relative expression of CDY2 and HSFY transcripts, respectively, compared to MA. CDY2 and HSFY were also underexpressed in patients with Sertoli-cell-only syndrome. These observations suggest that CDY2 and HSFY are important for sperm maturation, and their impaired expression could be implicated in the pathogenesis of MA.

Genetic mechanisms implicated as a cause of male infertility are poorly understood. Meiosis is unique to germ cells and essential for reproduction. The synaptonemal complex is a critical component for chromosome pairing, segregation, and recombination. Hormad1 is essential for mammalian gametogenesis. Mutational analysis of all HORMAD1 coding regions in Japanese men revealed meiotic arrest in the early pachytene stage, and synaptonemal complexes could not be visualized. By the sequence analysis, three polymorphism sites, SNP1 (c. 163A>G), SNP2 (c. 501 T>G), and SNP3 (c. 918C>T), have been found in exons 3, 8, and 10. SNP1 and SNP2 were associated with human azoospermia caused by complete early maturation arrest ($P<0.05$) (Miyamoto et al. 2012a). In similar studies, SEPTIN12 and UBR2 gene have also been found to be associated with increased susceptibility to azoospermia caused by meiotic arrest (Miyamoto et al. 2011, 2012b). Mutations in PRDM9 (MEISETZ) gene have also been implicated in Japanese NOA patients (Irie et al. 2009; Miyamoto et al. 2008).

Specimens from testicular biopsies of men with NOA have been used to investigate the expression of spermatogenesis-related genes MND1, SPATA22, GAPDHS, and ACR. Analysis of the expression of spermatogenic genes in human testes with abnormal spermatogenesis showed different expression patterns in patients from the three groups: hypospermatogenesis (HS), maturation arrest (MA), and Sertoli-cell-only syndrome (SCO) groups. Fertilization rates were similar at 70 %, but pregnancy rates for ACR and GAPDHS genes were low at 6–8 % (Dorosh et al. 2013).

A genome-wide association study in Chinese population has revealed that variants within the HLA region are associated with risk for NOA (Zhao et al. 2012). They have detected variants at human leukocyte antigen (HLA) regions, HLA-DRA, rs3129878, and rs498422 to be independently associated with NOA.

Recently, a separate Chinese genome-wide association study (GWAS) (Hu et al. 2012) identified four autosomal single-nucleotide polymorphism (SNP) loci as being significantly associated with risk factors for NOA: rs12097821, rs2477686, rs10842262, and rs6080550. Although not significant, three of four SNPs (rs12097821, rs2477686, and rs10842262) have also showed associations in Japanese men. However, further larger case–control studies are required to establish whether the SNPs are genetic risk factors for NOA in these populations (Sato et al. 2013). C677T in the methylenetetrahydrofolate reductase (MTHFR) gene is also suggested as a genetic risk factor in Chinese men (A et al. 2007).

A genome-wide gene expression study by Okada et al. (2008) demonstrated that SNPs (rs6836703) of the ADP-ribosyltransferase 3 gene (ART3) were associated with NOA with highest significance. These findings clarify a molecular pathophysiology of NOA and suggest a novel therapeutic target in the treatment of NOA. MicroRNAs (miRNAs) are a class of small noncoding RNA molecules. The expression of miRNAs is altered in testicular tissues of patients with NOA, suggesting a role of miRNAs in regulating spermatogenesis (Lian et al. 2009).

Nonetheless, at least 40 % of cases are currently categorized as idiopathic and may be linked to unknown genetic abnormalities. It is recommended that various genetic screening tests are performed in azoospermic men, given that their results may play vital role in not only identifying the etiology but also in preventing the iatrogenic transmission of genetic defects to offspring via advanced assisted conception techniques (Hamada et al. 2013).

6.7 Prognostic Factors of Sperm Retrieval

Introduction of intracytoplasmic sperm injection (ICSI) has brought hope for men with severe male infertility and provided a chance for them to become biological fathers. ICSI and other assisted reproduction techniques require testicular spermatozoa to be extracted to fertilize oocytes. Sperm retrieval is conducted with testicular aspiration or biopsy for testicular sperm extraction (TESE). Despite the current use of TESE, reliable clinical and laboratory prognostic factors of sperm recovery are still absent. Currently, several prognostic factors such as testis size, follicle-stimulating hormone (FSH), inhibin beta, the etiology of infertility, and genetic alterations are utilized; however, the histological testicular pattern remains the best predictor of sperm retrieval, but is associated with an invasive procedure (Glina et al. 2005).

Measurement of follicle-stimulating hormone (FSH) levels has been used as a predictor of sperm recovery, but its use remains controversial. Inhibins, anti-Mullerian hormone (AMH), and activins are glycoproteins that are transforming growth factors (TGF). Plasma levels of inhibin fraction B and seminal levels of AMH can be used as predictive parameters for sperm recovery in NOA (Deffieux and Antoine 2003). Other tests include the genetic detection of chromosome alterations. Y-chromosome microdeletions have also been used as a prognostic factor for sperm recovery. This possibility is based on the absence of mature sperm in azoospermic men with AZFa and AZFb microdeletions who underwent sperm retrieval techniques. Fortunately, AZFc is the Y microdeletion most often found in azoospermic men (60 %), and sperm can be retrieved for these patients. Therefore, the presence of AZFa or AZFb is a negative predictive factor for sperm retrieval in azoospermic men (Shefi and Turek 2006). The following section describes recent attempts toward development of prognostic markers that predict sperm retrieval in azoospermic patients.

Cell-free seminal mRNA (cfs-mRNA) exists in human ejaculate at high concentrations and with high stability and contains many tissue-specific transcripts secreted from the male reproductive system. Such cfs-mRNAs have been evaluated as candidates for noninvasive biomarkers for the presence of germ cells and of physio-pathological condition of complete obstruction in men with azoospermia. Li et al. (2012) have used the highly sensitive mRNA technology, to amplify the germ cell-specific (DDX4), seminal vesicle-specific (SEMG1), and prostate-specific (TGM4) mRNAs from cfs-mRNAs. TGM4 was detected in all participants. Consistent with their diagnosis, DDX4 was detected in all patients with MA or incomplete Sertoli-cell-only patients, but was absent in cases of complete Sertoli cell only, vasectomy, and congenital bilateral absence of the vas deferens (CBAVD), indicating absence of sperm. These results suggest that cfs-mRNA could be used as noninvasive biomarkers with high sensitivity.

More recently, the study of the seminal plasma proteome appears to offer the potential to identify biomarkers that may aid in the diagnosis of the causes of azoospermia. Many of the proteins in the seminal plasma are expressed in the testis and epididymis and are linked to fertility. Some of these proteins may be useful as noninvasive biomarkers to discriminate NOA from OA (Batruch et al. 2012). Drabovich et al. (2013) have identified two proteins, epididymis-expressed ECM1 and testis-expressed TEX101, which differentiated OA and NOA with high specificities and sensitivities. The performance of ECM1 was confirmed by enzyme-linked immunosorbent assay. On the basis of a cutoff level of 2.3 μg/ml derived from the current data, we could distinguish OA from normal spermatogenesis with 100 % specificity and OA from NOA with 73 % specificity, at 100 % sensitivity. Immunohistochemistry and an immunoenrichment mass spectrometry-based assay revealed the differential expression of TEX101 in distinct NOA subtypes. TEX101 semen concentrations differentiated Sertoli-cell-only syndrome from the other categories of NOA. They have proposed a simple two-biomarker decision tree for the differential diagnosis of OA and NOA and, in addition, for the differentiation of NOA subtypes. ECM1 and TEX101 clinical assays have the potential to replace most of the diagnostic testicular biopsies and facilitate the prediction of outcome of sperm retrieval procedures, thus increasing the reliability and success of assisted reproduction techniques (ART).

Genome-wide microRNA expression profiling of three validated seminal plasma miRNAs (sp-miRNAs) was examined in testicular tissues of patients with NOA and of fertile controls. miR-141, miR-429, and miR-7-1-3p are significantly increased in seminal plasma of patients with NOA compared with fertile controls. These sp-miRNAs could provide a novel noninvasive, semen-based test for NOA diagnosis, as they show reproducible and stable expression levels (Wu et al. 2013). In another study from Japan, expression levels of VASA, outer dense fiber-1 (ODF1), ODF2, and sperm mitochondria-associated cysteine-rich protein (SMCP) mRNAs in testicular tissue specimens were found to be significantly high in successful micro-TESE cases, compared to failed ones. Of these mRNAs, VASA mRNA expression was independently related to micro-TESE outcome and could be a useful adjunct parameter to predict sperm retrieval in NOA (Ando et al. 2012).

In NOA, testicular sperm extraction (TESE) is successful only in about 50 % of cases. A parameter for predicting TESE quality and pregnancy rates after ICSI of testicular spermatozoa has been devised by Boitrelle et al. (2011), based on multivariate analysis of total testicular volume (TTV), FSH and inhibin B levels, and TESE quality from a retrospective study. This score has been found to be a predictor of successful TESE, with a positive likelihood ratio of +3.01. When the score was <18.5, TESE was successful in 77.4 % of cases and "sperm-rich" (i.e., yielding >100 spermatozoa) in 91.1 % of cases; 42.8 % of couples took a baby home. Such a score can be useful in improving patient case and pre-ICSI counseling in cases of NOA.

In a novel attempt, Ma et al. (2011) have used leptin and artificial neural networks (ANNs) to predict the accuracy of sperm retrieval in NOA. Twelve factors, grouped into four sets, were recorded as the input variables for ANNs: (1) testicular volume, (2) semen volume, seminal pH, seminal alpha-glucosidase and fructose, (3) serum hormones including FSH, LH, total testosterone (TT), prolactin, estradiol, and (4) serum and seminal leptin. Different ANN models were constructed and their prediction accuracy was compared by receiver operating characteristic (ROC) curve analysis. ANN consisting of all four sets of factors had the largest area under the curve (AUC=0.83) and demonstrated significantly greater accuracy compared to FSH (AUC=0.63, $P<0.01$) and leptin (AUC=0.59, $P<0.01$).

Optimal cutoff value for FSH has been used to predict the presence of spermatogenesis in patients with NOA. In a comparative study of FSH levels in NOA patients with spermatogenesis and successful sperm retrieval, mean serum FSH was significantly higher than those failed in sperm retrieval (Chen et al. 2010). A cutoff value of 19.4 mIU/mL discriminated between the two groups with a sensitivity of 70 %. The positive predictive value for failed sperm retrieval could reach 100 %. Elevated plasma levels of FSH could be used as a reliable criterion for a trial of sperm retrieval from testes in artificial reproductive techniques. On the other hand, a meta-analysis of inhibin B as an indirect marker of spermatogenesis in NOA concluded that it cannot serve as a stand-alone marker (Toulis et al. 2010).

The detection of seminal haploid cells by flow cytometry (FCM) has been evaluated for the prognosis of TESE results (Koscinski et al. 2005). FCM was found to be more sensitive (100 versus 59 %) but less specific (67 versus 83.5 %) than cytology. FCM will provide another noninvasive technique to predict TESE results and improve the management of NOA patients.

Conclusions

An accurate diagnosis of the etiology of azoospermia is important prior to the initiation of the appropriate treatment. Nonobstructive azoospermia remains the most challenging diagnosis for andrologists. Thousands of single or multiple genes are involved in establishing the male fertility potential, and many others are yet to be revealed. In the current era of ART, however, genetic testing has emerged as tools of paramount importance in helping clinicians not only to explore the specific genetic background of a disease but also to take the necessary precautions to prevent the transmission of the disease to the offspring via ART.

Incorporating novel techniques, such as genomics, proteomics, and metabolomics, into infertility research may assist in the creation of a complete portrait of the genes that are involved in infertility and would allow for improvements in ART and the development of more targeted solutions (Hamada et al. 2012). Microarrays are emerging as valuable tools for the determination of the gene expression profiles of infertile phenotypes and the examination of spermatogenesis (Lin et al. 2006). Gene expression microarray studies could be used to characterize the gene expression signature for normal human spermatogenesis, which can be a valuable diagnostic marker. Proteins identified using 2D electrophoresis and mass spectrometry techniques could be used to create proteome maps in relation to sperm and seminal plasma (Johnston et al. 2005; Pilch and Mann 2006). The identification of protein biomarkers for male factor infertility will allow for unbiased comparisons of fertile and infertile males and will clarify the pathophysiology of the disease. An advantageous characteristic of genomic and proteomic technology is that the results provide a definitive characterization of infertile phenotypes.

Metabolites are small biomarkers that indicate the functionality of a cell and characterize certain diseases or physiological states. Determination of metabolite profiles for normal and infertile phenotypes may be useful in diagnosis and treatment of male factor infertility.

References

A ZC, Yang Y, Zhang SZ, Li N, Zhang W. Single nucleotide polymorphism C677T in the methylene-tetrahydrofolate reductase gene might be a genetic risk factor for infertility for Chinese men with azoospermia or severe oligozoospermia. Asian J Androl. 2007;9(1): 57–62.

Aaronson DS, Iman R, Walsh TJ, Kurhanewicz J, Turek PJ. A novel application of 1H magnetic resonance spectroscopy: non-invasive identification of spermatogenesis in men with non-obstructive azoospermia. Hum Reprod. 2010;25(4):847–52.

Alhalabi M, Kenj M, Monem F, Mahayri Z, Abou Alchamat G, Madania A. High prevalence of genetic abnormalities in Middle Eastern patients with idiopathic non-obstructive azoospermia. J Assist Reprod Genet. 2013;30(6):799–805.

American Urological Association. The optimal evaluation of the infertile male. Available from: http://www.auanet.org/content/media/optimalevaluation2010.pdf. Accessed 22 Feb 2012.

Ando M, Yamaguchi K, Chiba K, Miyake H, Fujisawa M. Expression of VASA mRNA in testis as a significant predictor of sperm recovery by microdissection testicular sperm extraction in patient with nonobstructive azoospermia. J Androl. 2012;33(4):711–6.

Aziz N. The importance of semen analysis in the context of azoospermia. Clinics. 2013;68(S1):35–8.

Aziz N, Agarwal A, Nallella KP, Thomas Jr AJ. Relationship between epidemiological features and aetiology of male infertility as diagnosed by a comprehensive infertility service provider. Reprod Biomed. 2006;12(2):209–14.

Baker K, Sabanegh E. Obstructive azoospermia: reconstructive techniques and results. Clinics. 2013;68(S1):61–73.

Batruch I, Smith CR, Mullen BJ, Grober E, Lo KC, Diamandis EP, et al. Analysis of seminal plasma from patients with non-obstructive azoospermia and identification of candidate biomarkers of male infertility. J Proteome Res. 2012;11(3):1503–11.

Behulova R, Varga I, Strhakova L, Bozikova A, Gabrikova D, Boronova I, et al. Incidence of microdeletions in the AZF region of the Y chromosome in Slovak patients with azoospermia. Biomed Pap Med Fac Univ Palacky Olomouc Czech Repub. 2011;155(1):33–8.

Belchetz PE, Plant TM, Nakai Y, Keogh EJ, Knobil E. Hypophysial responses to continuous and intermittent delivery of hypopthalamic gonadotropin-releasing hormone. Science. 1978; 202(4368):631–3.

Beliveau ME, Turek PJ. The value of testicular 'mapping' in men with non-obstructive azoospermia. Asian J Androl. 2011;13(2):225–30.

Boitrelle F, Robin G, Marcelli F, Albert M, Leroy-Martin B, Dewailly D, et al. A predictive score for testicular sperm extraction quality and surgical ICSI outcome in non-obstructive azoospermia: a retrospective study. Hum Reprod. 2011;26(12):3215–21.

Buffat C, Patrat C, Merlet F, Guibert J, Epelboin S, Thiounn N, et al. ICSI outcomes in obstructive azoospermia: influence of the origin of surgically retrieved spermatozoa and the cause of obstruction. Hum Reprod. 2006;21(4):1018–24.

Burrows PJ, Schrepferman CG, Lipshultz LI. Comprehensive office evaluation in the new millennium. Urol Clin North Am. 2002;29(4):873–94.

Cavallini G, Beretta G, Biagiotti G. Preliminary study of letrozole use for improving spermatogenesis in non-obstructive azoospermia patients with normal serum FSH. Asian J Androl. 2011;13(6):895–7. Remove this and letrazole !!.

Ceylan C, Ceylan GG, Serel TA. The azoospermia factor locus-c region was found to be related to Klinefelter syndrome in Turkish patients. Genet Mol Res. 2010;9(2):1229–33.

Chan HC, Ruan YC, He Q, Chen MH, Chen H, Xu WM, et al. The cystic fibrosis transmembrane conductance regulator in reproductive health and disease. J Physiol. 2009;587(Pt 10): 2187–95.

Chen SC, Hsieh JT, Yu HJ, Chang HC. Appropriate cut-off value for follicle-stimulating hormone in azoospermia to predict spermatogenesis. Reprod Biol Endocrinol. 2010;8:108.

Cocuzza M, Alvarenga C, Pagani R. The epidemiology and etiology of azoospermia. Clinics. 2013;68(S1):15–26.

Crha I, Kralikova M, Melounova J, Ventruba P, Zakova J, Beharka R, et al. Seminal plasma homocysteine, folate and cobalamin in men with obstructive and non-obstructive azoospermia. J Assist Reprod Genet. 2010;27(9–10):533–8.

Daudin M, Bieth E, Bujan L, Massat G, Pontonnier F, Mieusset R. Congenital bilateral absence of the vas deferens: clinical characteristics, biological parameters, cystic fibrosis transmembrane conductance regulator gene mutations, and implications for genetic counseling. Fertil Steril. 2000;74(6):1164–74.

de la Taille A, Rigot JM, Mahe P, Gervais R, Dumur V, Lemaitre L, et al. Correlation of genitourinary abnormalities, spermiogram and CFTR genotype in patients with bilateral agenesis of the vas deferens. Prog Urol. 1998;8(3):370–6.

Deffieux X, Antoine JM. Inhibins, activins and anti-Mullerian hormone: structure, signalling pathways, roles and predictive value in reproductive medicine. Gynecol Obstet Fertil. 2003;31(11):900–11.

Donohue RE, Fauver HE. Unilateral absence of the vas deferens. A useful clinical sign. JAMA. 1989;261(8):1180–2.

Donoso P, Tournaye H, Devroey P. Which is the best sperm retrieval technique for non-obstructive azoospermia? A systematic review. Hum Reprod Update. 2007;13(6):539–49.

Dorosh A, Tepla O, Zatecka E, Ded L, Koci K, Peknicova J. Expression analysis of MND1/GAJ, SPATA22, GAPDHS and ACR genes in testicular biopsies from non-obstructive azoospermia (NOA) patients. Reprod Biol Endocrinol. 2013;11:42.

Drabovich AP, Dimitromanolakis A, Saraon P, Soosaipillai A, Batruch I, Mullen B, et al. Differential diagnosis of azoospermia with proteomic biomarkers ECM1 and TEX101 quantified in seminal plasma. Sci Transl Med. 2013;5(212):212ra160.

Dube E, Hermo L, Chan PT, Cyr DG. Alterations in the human blood-epididymis barrier in obstructive azoospermia and the development of novel epididymal cell lines from infertile men. Biol Reprod. 2010;83(4):584–96.

Eliasson R. Analysis of semen. In: Burger H, de Kretser D, editors. The testis. New York: Raven; 1981. p. 381–99.

Esteves SC. Microdissection testicular sperm extraction (micro-TESE) as a sperm acquisition method for men with nonobstructive azoospermia seeking fertility: operative and laboratory aspects. Int Braz J Urol. 2013;39(3):440; discussion 441.

Esteves SC, Agarwal A. Reproductive outcomes, including neonatal data, following sperm injection in men with obstructive and nonobstructive azoospermia: case series and systematic review. Clinics (Sao Paulo). 2013;68 Suppl 1:141–50.

Esteves SC, Lee W, Benjamin DJ, Seol B, Verza Jr S, Agarwal A. Reproductive potential of men with obstructive azoospermia undergoing percutaneous sperm retrieval and intracytoplasmic sperm injection according to the cause of obstruction. J Urol. 2013;189(1):232–7.

Everaert K, De Croo I, Kerckhaert W, Dekuyper P, Dhont M, Van der Elst J, et al. Long term effects of micro-surgical testicular sperm extraction on androgen status in patients with non obstructive azoospermia. BMC Urol. 2006;6:9.

Ferlin A, Raicu F, Gatta V, Zuccarello D, Palka G, Foresta C. Male infertility: role of genetic background. Reprod Biomed Online. 2007a;14(6):734–45.

Ferlin A, Arredi B, Speltra E, Cazzadore C, Selice R, Garolla A, et al. Molecular and clinical characterization of Y chromosome microdeletions in infertile men: a 10-year experience in Italy. J Clin Endocrinol Metab. 2007b;92(3):762–70.

Finkel DM, Phillips JL, Snyder PJ. Stimulation of spermatogenesis by gonadotropins in men with hypogonadotropic hypogonadism. N Engl J Med. 1985;313(11):651–5.

Gatta V, Raicu F, Ferlin A, Antonucci I, Scioletti AP, Garolla A, et al. Testis transcriptome analysis in male infertility: new insight on the pathogenesis of oligo-azoospermia in cases with and without AZFc microdeletion. BMC Genomics. 2010;11:401.

Glina S, Vieira M. Prognostic factors for sperm retrieval in non-obstructive azoospermia. Clinics (Sao Paulo). 2013;68 Suppl 1:121–4.

Glina S, Soares JB, Antunes Jr N, Galuppo AG, Paz LB, Wonchockier R. Testicular histopathological diagnosis as a predictive factor for retrieving spermatozoa for ICSI in non-obstructive azoospermic patients. Int Braz J Urol. 2005;31(4):338–41.

Golan R, Cooper TG, Oschry Y, Oberpenning F, Schulze H, Shochat L, et al. Changes in chromatin condensation of human spermatozoa during epididymal transit as determined by flow cytometry. Hum Reprod. 1996;11(7):1457–62.

Goulis DG, Polychronou P, Mikos T, Grimbizis G, Gerou S, Pavlidou V, et al. Serum inhibin-B and follicle stimulating hormone as predictors of the presence of sperm in testicular fine needle aspirate in men with azoospermia. Hormones (Athens). 2008;7(2):140–7.

Hamada A, Esteves SC, Agarwal A. Genetics and male infertility. In: Dubey A, editor. Infertility – diagnosis, management & IVF. 1st ed. New Delhi: Jaypee Brothers Medical Publishers; 2012. p. 113–60.

Hamada AJ, Esteves SC, Agarwal A. A comprehensive review of genetics and genetic testing in azoospermia. Clinics. 2013;68(S1):39–60.

Han Y, Feng HL, Sandlow JI, Haines CJ. Comparing expression of progesterone and estrogen receptors in testicular tissue from men with obstructive and nonobstructive azoospermia. J Androl. 2009;30(2):127–33.

Hauser R, Yogev L, Paz G, Yavetz H, Azem F, Lessing JB, et al. Comparison of efficacy of two techniques for testicular sperm retrieval in nonobstructive azoospermia: multifocal testicular sperm extraction versus multifocal testicular sperm aspiration. J Androl. 2006;27(1):28–33.

Hernandez Uribe L, Hernandez Marin I, Cervera-Aguilar R, Ayala AR. Frequency and etiology of azoospermia in the study of infertile couples. Ginecol Obstet Mex. 2001;69:322–6.

Ho KL, Wong MH, Tam PC. Microsurgical vasoepididymostomy for obstructive azoospermia. Hong Kong Med J. 2009;15(6):452–7.

Hoffman AR, Crowley WF. Induction of puberty in Men by long-term pulsatile administration of low-dose gonadotropin-releasing hormone. New Engl J Med. 1982;307(20):1237–41.
Hu Z, Xia Y, Guo X, Dai J, Li H, Hu H, Jiang Y, Lu F, Wu Y, Yang X, Li H, Yao B, et al. A genome-wide association study in Chinese men identifies three risk loci for non-obstructive azoospermia. Nat Genet. 2012;44:183–6.
Hussein A, Ozgok Y, Ross L, Niederberger C. Clomiphene administration for cases of nonobstructive azoospermia: a multicenter study. J Androl. 2005;26(6):787–91; discussion 792–3.
Inci K, Gunay LM. The role of varicocele treatment in the management of non-obstructive azoospermia. Clinics (Sao Paulo). 2013;68 Suppl 1:89–98.
Irie S, Tsujimura A, Miyagawa Y, Ueda T, Matsuoka Y, Matsui Y, et al. Single-nucleotide polymorphisms of the PRDM9 (MEISETZ) gene in patients with nonobstructive azoospermia. J Androl. 2009;30(4):426–31.
Ishikawa T. Surgical recovery of sperm in non-obstructive azoospermia. Asian J Androl. 2012;14(1):109–15.
Jequier AM. Obstructive azoospermia: a study of 102 patients. Clin Reprod Fertil. 1985;3(1):21–36.
Jezequel P, Dubourg C, Le Lannou D, Odent S, Le Gall JY, Blayau M, et al. Molecular screening of the CFTR gene in men with anomalies of the vas deferens: identification of three novel mutations. Mol Hum Reprod. 2000;6(12):1063–7.
Jiang Y, Cao Q, Zhao X, Li L, Li S, Gao F. Percutaneous epididymal sperm aspiration and short time insemination in the treatment of men with obstructive azoospermia. J Assist Reprod Genet. 2013;30(9):1175–9.
Johnston DS, Wooters J, Kopf GS, Qiu Y, Roberts KP. Analysis of the human sperm proteome. Ann N Y Acad Sci. 2005;1061:190–202.
Koscinski I, Wittemer C, Rigot JM, De Almeida M, Hermant E, Defossez A. Seminal haploid cell detection by flow cytometry in non-obstructive azoospermia: a good predictive parameter for testicular sperm extraction. Hum Reprod. 2005;20(7):1915–20.
Kuligowska E, Fenlon HM. Transrectal US in male infertility: spectrum of findings and role in patient care. Radiology. 1998;207(1):173–81.
Kumar R. Medical management of non-obstructive azoospermia. Clinics. 2013;68(S1):75–9.
Lee JY, Dada R, Sabanegh E, Carpi A, Agarwal A. Role of genetics in azoospermia. Urology. 2011;77(3):598–601.
Li H, Wu C, Gu X, Xiong C. A novel application of cell-free seminal mRNA: non-invasive identification of the presence of germ cells or complete obstruction in men with azoospermia. Hum Reprod. 2012;27(4):991–7.
Lian J, Zhang X, Tian H, Liang N, Wang Y, Liang C, et al. Altered microRNA expression in patients with non-obstructive azoospermia. Reprod Biol Endocrinol. 2009;7:13.
Lin YH, Lin YM, Teng YN, Hsieh TY, Lin YS, Kuo PL. Identification of ten novel genes involved in human spermatogenesis by microarray analysis of testicular tissue. Fertil Steril. 2006;86:1650–8.
Lipshultz LI, Corriere Jr JN. Progressive testicular atrophy in the varicocele patient. J Urol. 1977;117(2):175–6.
Ma Y, Chen B, Wang H, Hu K, Huang Y. Prediction of sperm retrieval in men with non-obstructive azoospermia using artificial neural networks: leptin is a good assistant diagnostic marker. Hum Reprod. 2011;26(2):294–8.
Ma M, Yang S, Zhang Z, Li P, Gong Y, Liu L, et al. Sertoli cells from non-obstructive azoospermia and obstructive azoospermia patients show distinct morphology, Raman spectrum and biochemical phenotype. Hum Reprod. 2013;28(7):1863–73.
Mafra FA, Christofolini DM, Bianco B, Gava MM, Glina S, Belangero SI, et al. Chromosomal and molecular abnormalities in a group of Brazilian infertile men with severe oligozoospermia or non-obstructive azoospermia attending an infertility service. Int Braz J Urol. 2011;37(2):244–50; discussion 250–1.
Mak V, Jarvi KA. The genetics of male infertility. J Urol. 1996;156(4):1245–56; discussion 56–7.

Male Infertility Best Practice Policy Committee of the American Urological Association; Practice Committee of the American Society for Reproductive Medicine. Report on optimal evaluation of the infertile male. Fertil Steril. 2006;86(5 Suppl 1):S202–9.

Mau Kai C, Juul A, McElreavey K, Ottesen AM, Garn ID, Main KM, et al. Sons conceived by assisted reproduction techniques inherit deletions in the azoospermia factor (AZF) region of the Y chromosome and the DAZ gene copy number. Hum Reprod. 2008;23(7):1669–78.

McLachlan RI, Mallidis C, Ma K, Bhasin S, de Kretser DM. Genetic disorders and spermatogenesis. Reprod Fertil Dev. 1998;10(1):97–104.

Mirfakhraie R, Kalantar SM, Mirzajani F, Montazeri M, Salsabili N, Houshmand M. A novel mutation in the transactivation-regulating domain of the androgen receptor in a patient with azoospermia. J Androl. 2011;32(4):367–70.

Miyamoto T, Koh E, Sakugawa N, Sato H, Hayashi H, Namiki M, et al. Two single nucleotide polymorphisms in PRDM9 (MEISETZ) gene may be a genetic risk factor for Japanese patients with azoospermia by meiotic arrest. J Assist Reprod Genet. 2008;25(11–12):553–7.

Miyamoto T, Tsujimura A, Miyagawa Y, Koh E, Namiki M, Horikawa M, et al. Single nucleotide polymorphism in the UBR2 gene may be a genetic risk factor for Japanese patients with azoospermia by meiotic arrest. J Assist Reprod Genet. 2011;28(8):743–6.

Miyamoto T, Tsujimura A, Miyagawa Y, Koh E, Namiki M, Horikawa M, et al. Single-nucleotide polymorphisms in HORMAD1 may be a risk factor for azoospermia caused by meiotic arrest in Japanese patients. Asian J Androl. 2012a;14(4):580–3.

Miyamoto T, Tsujimura A, Miyagawa Y, Koh E, Namiki M, Horikawa M, et al. Single nucleotide polymorphisms in the SEPTIN12 gene may be associated with azoospermia by meiotic arrest in Japanese men. J Assist Reprod Genet. 2012b;29(1):47–51.

Miyaoka R, Esteves SC. Predictive factors for sperm retrieval and sperm injection outcomes in obstructive azoospermia: Do etiology, retrieval techniques and gamete source play a role? Clinics. 2013;68(S1):111–9.

O'Connell M, McClure N, Lewis SE. Mitochondrial DNA deletions and nuclear DNA fragmentation in testicular and epididymal human sperm. Hum Reprod. 2002;17(6):1565–70.

Oates RD, Amos JA. The genetic basis of congenital bilateral absence of the vas deferens and cystic fibrosis. J Androl. 1994;15(1):1–8.

Okada H, Tajima A, Shichiri K, Tanaka A, Tanaka K, Inoue I. Genome-wide expression of azoospermia testes demonstrates a specific profile and implicates ART3 in genetic susceptibility. PLoS Genet. 2008;4(2):e26.

Pandiyan N, Jequier AM. Mitotic chromosomal anomalies among 1210 infertile men. Hum Reprod. 1996;11(12):2604–8.

Patrizio P, Leonard DG. Mutations of the cystic fibrosis gene and congenital absence of the vas deferens. Results Probl Cell Differ. 2000;28:175–86.

Peschka B, Leygraaf J, Van der Ven K, Montag M, Schartmann B, Schubert R, et al. Type and frequency of chromosome aberrations in 781 couples undergoing intracytoplasmic sperm injection. Hum Reprod. 1999;14(9):2257–63.

Pilch B, Mann M. Large-scale and high-confidence proteomic analysis of human seminal plasma. Genome Biol. 2006;7:R40.

Practice Committee of American Society for Reproductive Medicine in collaboration with Society for Male Reproduction and Urology. The management of infertility due to obstructive azoospermia. Fertil Steril. 2008;90(5 Suppl):S121–4.

Pylyp LY, Spinenko LO, Verhoglyad NV, Zukin VD. Chromosomal abnormalities in patients with oligozoospermia and non-obstructive azoospermia. J Assist Reprod Genet. 2013;30(5):729–32.

Ratbi I, Legendre M, Niel F, Martin J, Soufir JC, Izard V, et al. Detection of cystic fibrosis transmembrane conductance regulator (CFTR) gene rearrangements enriches the mutation spectrum in congenital bilateral absence of the vas deferens and impacts on genetic counselling. Hum Reprod. 2007;22(5):1285–91.

Reijo R, Lee TY, Salo P, Alagappan R, Brown LG, Rosenberg M, et al. Diverse spermatogenic defects in humans caused by Y chromosome deletions encompassing a novel RNA-binding protein gene. Nat Genet. 1995;10(4):383–93.

Sadeghi-Nejad H, Farrokhi F. Genetics of azoospermia: current knowledge, clinical implications, and future directions. Part II: Y chromosome microdeletions. Urol J. 2007;4(4):192–206.

Sato Y, Jinam T, Iwamoto T, Yamauchi A, Imoto I, Inoue I, et al. Replication study and meta-analysis of human nonobstructive azoospermia in Japanese populations. Biol Reprod. 2013; 88(4):87.

Shefi S, Turek PJ. Sex chromosome abnormalities and male infertility: a clinical perspective. In: De Jonge C, Barrat C, editors. The sperm cell production, maturation, fertilization, regeneration. Cambridge: Cambridge University Press; 2006. p. 261–78.

Shiraishi K, Ohmi C, Shimabukuro T, Matsuyama H. Human chorionic gonadotrophin treatment prior to microdissection testicular sperm extraction in non-obstructive azoospermia. Hum Reprod. 2012;27(2):331–9.

Sigman M, Jarow JP. Endocrine evaluation of infertile men. Urology. 1997;50(5):659–64.

Stahl PJ, Mielnik AN, Barbieri CE, Schlegel PN, Paduch DA. Deletion or underexpression of the Y-chromosome genes CDY2 and HSFY is associated with maturation arrest in American men with nonobstructive azoospermia. Asian J Androl. 2012;14(5):676–82.

Sykiotis GP, Hoang XH, Avbelj M, Hayes FJ, Thambundit A, Dwyer A, et al. Congenital idiopathic hypogonadotropic hypogonadism: evidence of defects in the hypothalamus, pituitary, and testes. J Clin Endocrinol Metab. 2010;95(6):3019–27.

Tesarik J, Sousa M, Greco E, Mendoza C. Spermatids as gametes: indications and limitations. Hum Reprod. 1998;13:89–107.

Toulis KA, Iliadou PK, Venetis CA, Tsametis C, Tarlatzis BC, Papadimas I, et al. Inhibin B and anti-Mullerian hormone as markers of persistent spermatogenesis in men with non-obstructive azoospermia: a meta-analysis of diagnostic accuracy studies. Hum Reprod Update. 2010;16(6):713–24.

Tuttelmann F, Werny F, Cooper TG, Kliesch S, Simoni M, Nieschlag E. Clinical experience with azoospermia: aetiology and chances for spermatozoa detection upon biopsy. Int J Androl. 2011;34(4):291–8.

Vicari E, Mongioi A, Calogero AE, Moncada ML, Sidoti G, Polosa P, et al. Therapy with human chorionic gonadotrophin alone induces spermatogenesis in men with isolated hypogonadotrophic hypogonadism—long term follow-up. Int J Androl. 1992;15(4):320–9.

Vutyavanich T, Piromlertamorn W, Sirirungsi W, Sirisukkasem S. Frequency of Y chromosome microdeletions and chromosomal abnormalities in infertile Thai men with oligozoospermia and azoospermia. Asian J Androl. 2007;9(1):68–75.

Woldringh GH, Horvers M, Janssen AJWM, Reuser JJCM, de Groot SAF, Steiner K, et al. Follow-up of children born after ICSI with epididymal spermatozoa. Hum Reprod. 2011;26(7):1759–67.

Wong PY. CFTR gene and male fertility. Mol Hum Reprod. 1998;4(2):107–10.

World Health Organization. WHO laboratory manual for the examination and processing of human semen. 5th ed. Geneva: World Health Organization; 2010.

Wu Q, Chen G-W, Yan T-F, Wang H, Liu Y-L, Li Z, et al. Prevalent false positives of azoospermia factor a (AZFa) microdeletions caused by single-nucleotide polymorphism rs72609647 in the sY84 screening of male infertility. Asian J Androl. 2011;13(6):877–80.

Wu W, Qin Y, Li Z, Dong J, Dai J, Lu C, et al. Genome-wide microRNA expression profiling in idiopathic non-obstructive azoospermia: significant up-regulation of miR-141, miR-429 and miR-7-1-3p. Hum Reprod. 2013;28(7):1827–36.

Yurdakul T, Gokce G, Kilic O, Piskin MM. Transurethral resection of ejaculatory ducts in the treatment of complete ejaculatory duct obstruction. Int Urol Nephrol. 2008;40(2):369–72.

Zhao H, Xu J, Zhang H, Sun J, Sun Y, Wang Z, et al. A genome-wide association study reveals that variants within the HLA region are associated with risk for nonobstructive azoospermia. Am J Hum Genet. 2012;90(5):900–6.

Management of Infertile Men with Nonobstructive Azoospermia due to Spermatogenic Failure

7

Sandro C. Esteves

List of Abbreviations

ART	Assisted reproduction techniques
AZF	Azoospermia factor
EAA	European Association of Andrology
EMQN	European Molecular Genetics Quality Network
FSH	Follicle-stimulating hormone
hCG	Human chorionic gonadotropin
HH	Hypogonadotropic hypogonadism
ICSI	Intracytoplasmic sperm injection
ITT	Intratesticular testosterone
IVF	In vitro fertilization
LH	Luteinizing hormone
Micro-TESE	Microdissection testicular sperm extraction
NOA	Nonobstructive azoospermia
OA	Obstructive azoospermia
PCR	Polymerase chain reaction
SCOS	Sertoli cell-only syndrome
SCO	Sertoli cell only
SF	Spermatogenic failure
SRR	Sperm retrieval rates
SR	Sperm retrieval
STS	Sequence-tagged sites
TEFNA	Testicular fine-needle aspiration

S.C. Esteves, MD, PhD
Medical and Scientific Director, ANDROFERT, Andrology and Human Reproduction Clinic, Referral Center for Male Reproduction, Av. Dr. Heitor Penteado, 1464, 13075-460 Campinas, São Paulo, Brazil
e-mail: s.esteves@androfert.com.br

K. Gunasekaran, N. Pandiyan (eds.), *Male Infertility*,
DOI 10.1007/978-81-322-3604-7_7

TESA	Testicular sperm aspiration
TESE	Testicular sperm extraction
YCMD	Y chromosome microdeletion

7.1 Introduction

Men in reproductive age deliver, on average, 96 million sperm at each ejaculation (Cooper et al. 2010). Approximately 1 % of all men and 10–15 % of infertile males have azoospermia, defined as the complete absence of spermatozoa in the ejaculate without implying an underlying etiology (Esteves et al. 2011a; Aziz 2013). In approximately 2/3 of these men, azoospermia is associated with a spectrum of untreatable testicular disorders that results in spermatogenic failure (SF). Spermatogenic failure has been recognized as the most severe presentation of infertility in humans (Esteves and Agarwal 2013b). Although SF invariably results in infertility, it does not necessarily indicate absolute sterility. Infertility is defined as the inability of a sexually active couple with no contraception to achieve natural pregnancy within at least 1 year (World Health Organization 2000) and implies a reduced but not unattainable potential to achieve pregnancy. In contrast, sterility is denoted by permanent and complete inability to induce or achieve pregnancy. Of note, it has been shown that 30–60 % of men with SF have sparse areas exhibiting full spermatogenic activity within their dysfunctional testes. Sperm production, if present, is insufficient for sperm appearance in the ejaculate, and since there are no treatment options to restore fertility in these men, the only alternative is to attempt sperm retrieval with the aim of finding viable testicular sperm to be used for intracytoplasmic sperm injection (ICSI) (Esteves and Agarwal 2011; Esteves et al. 2011b; Silber 2000). Spermatozoa extracted from the testes of such men are capable of inducing normal fertilization and embryo development, as well as result in the production of healthy offspring with ICSI (Esteves et al. 2014; Belva et al. 2011; Carpi et al. 2009).

The management of men with spermatogenic failure seeking fertility has been a challenge for andrologists and reproductive medicine specialists alike. In this chapter, I present a personal perspective including the lessons I have learned after 15 years dealing with this male infertility condition (Esteves 2015). Figure 7.1 depicts

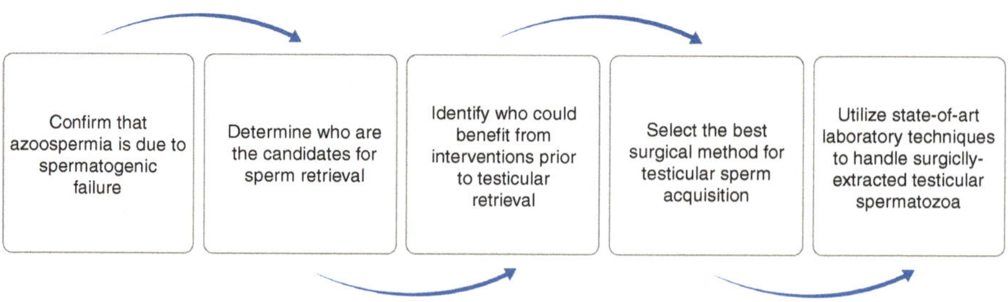

Fig. 7.1 Step-by-step approach for the clinical management of men with nonobstructive azoospermia seeking fertility (Adapted with permission from Esteves (2015))

an algorithm to guide clinicians on the management of azoospermic men with spermatogenic failure. I hope the information presented here could help healthcare practitioners to offer an even better service for men with spermatogenic failure seeking fertility.

7.2 Differential Diagnosis in Azoospermia

Azoospermia is defined based on the absence of spermatozoa in a given ejaculate. Proper laboratory technique is crucial to reduce analytical error and enhance precision when analyzing semen specimens (Aziz 2013; Esteves et al. 2012). Ejaculates of men with spermatogenic failure usually have normal volume and pH, which indicates both functional seminal vesicles and patent ejaculatory ducts. The lower reference limits for ejaculate volume and pH are 1.5 ml (fifth percentile, 95 % confidence interval 1.4–1.7) and 7.2, respectively (Cooper et al. 2010). Retrograde ejaculation should be suspected when a given ejaculate volume is <1 ml, and the diagnosis is confirmed by the finding of spermatozoa in the post-ejaculatory urine (Esteves et al. 2011a).

The assessment of an initially normal-volume azoospermic ejaculate should be immediately followed by the examination of the pelleted semen to exclude cryptozoospermia, which is defined by the presence of sperm only in the centrifuged pellet (Aziz 2013). In one study, centrifuging semen at the low speed of 200 *g* for 10 min revealed that 22.8 % of men diagnosed with azoospermia had spermatozoa in the semen pellet (Jaffe et al 1998). In addition, when supernatants resulting from low-speed centrifugation were centrifuged at higher speeds (>1000 *g*) for longer periods, spermatozoa were also detected (Corea et al. 2005). Thus, the accuracy of any centrifugation protocol of less than 1000 *g* in pelleting all the spermatozoa in an ejaculate is uncertain (Cooper et al. 2006). The importance of finding such minimal number of sperm is to allow assisted reproductive techniques (ART) to be performed with ejaculated sperm, thus avoiding the more invasive sperm retrieval methods. At our institution, we perform centrifugation at 3000 *g* for 15 min, which is followed by a careful examination of the pellet for the presence of sperm. Moreover, the diagnosis of azoospermia should be based on the examination of multiple semen specimens as transient azoospermia secondary to toxic, environmental, infectious, or iatrogenic conditions may occur (Castilla et al. 2006; Keel 2006). The examination of ejaculates on multiple occasions is also important given the large biological variability in semen specimens from the same individuals (Esteves et al. 2012; Castilla et al. 2006; Keel 2006). Patients should receive clear instructions on how to collect the entire ejaculate and to report the loss of any fraction of the sample. Determination of fructose, a major component of seminal vesicle secretion, is usually not necessary because the presence of a normal-volume ejaculate coupled with normal pH practically excludes any problem at the ejaculatory ducts or seminal vesicle level (Esteves et al. 2011a). In summary, azoospermia should be defined based on the absence of spermatozoa on multiple semen examinations after centrifugation of complete semen specimens using microscopic analysis.

History and physical examination and hormonal analysis (follicle-stimulating hormone and total testosterone serum levels) are undertaken to define the type of azoospermia. Together, these factors provide a >90 % prediction of the type of azoospermia (obstructive vs. nonobstructive). Obstructive azoospermia (OA) is attributed to a mechanical blockage that can occur anywhere along the reproductive tract, including the vas deferens, epididymis, and ejaculatory duct. OA is considered to be one of the most favorable prognostic conditions in male infertility since spermatogenesis is not disrupted, unlike spermatogenic failure (Esteves et al. 2013a; American Society for Reproductive Medicine and Society for Male Reproduction and Urology 2008). Etiology conditions associated with nonobstructive azoospermia (NOA) include genetic and congenital abnormalities, postinfections, exposure to gonadotoxins, medications, varicocele, trauma, endocrine disorders, and idiopathy. A detailed medical history should be obtained for any factor that may cause spermatogenic failure. Information not exclusive of the following areas should be collected: (a) previous diseases during childhood and puberty such as viral orchitis and cryptorchidism; (b) surgeries performed, especially those involving the pelvic and inguinal regions and genitalia; (c) genital traumas; (d) infections such as epididymo-orchitis and urethritis; (e) physical and sexual development; and (f) exposure to gonadotoxic agents such as radiotherapy, chemotherapy, and steroid abuse (Esteves et al. 2011a; Carpi et al. 2009).

Physical examination in men with spermatogenic failure usually reveals normal epididymides and palpable vasa deferentia. Small-sized testes (<15 ml in volume) are often encountered as approximately 85 % of the testicular parenchyma is involved in spermatogenesis. Nevertheless, testicular size is not a reliable clinical marker of sperm production. Men with spermatogenic maturation arrest, in whom spermatogenesis is hampered prior to its completion, have well-developed and normal-volume testes (Sokol and Swerdloff 1997; Hung et al. 2007).

The serum levels of follicle-stimulating hormone (FSH) are usually elevated, while testosterone is either low (<300 ng/dl) or within lower limits in men with spermatogenic failure (Gudeloglu and Parekattil 2013; Esteves et al. 2011a). FSH levels greater than twice the upper normal limit are a reliable indicator of spermatogenic failure (American Society for Reproductive Medicine and Society for Male Reproduction and Urology 2008). In one report, low testosterone levels were found in 45 % of the males with NOA who visited an infertility clinic (Sussman et al. 2008). In another study evaluating hormonal data of 736 men with NOA who were candidates for sperm retrieval, 346 (47 %) had baseline total testosterone (TT) levels <300 ng/dL (Reifsnyder et al. 2012). Low testosterone levels often reflect Leydig cell insufficiency, which is accompanied by elevated (or within upper limits) luteinizing hormone (LH) levels (Bobjer et al. 2012; Reifsnyder et al. 2012). Nevertheless, low testosterone levels in men with SF may also result from obesity and metabolic dysfunction (Kumar 2013). Obesity is associated with an increased serum estradiol levels due to the increased peripheral aromatization of C19 androgens (androstenedione, T) under the influence of aromatase, a product of the CYP19 gene, especially in individuals with tetranucleotide TTTA repeat polymorphism (TTTAn) present in intron 4 of the CYP19 gene (Hammoud et al. 2010). Elevated estradiol levels suppress pituitary LH and FSH secretion and also directly inhibit testosterone biosynthesis (Kumar 2013; Tchernof et al. 1995). Furthermore, Isidori et al. (1999) have demonstrated that excess circulating leptin may be an important contributor to the reduced androgen serum levels in male obesity. Their data have indicated that leptin has negative actions on steroidogenesis that are mediated by specific receptors in the Leydig cells. Low testosterone levels could also reflect an adaptation to changed SHBG levels and not testosterone deficiency. In fact, Strain et al. (1994) have reported that, during weight loss, serum SHBG levels increase at an average slope of 0.43 nmol/L per unit decrease in body mass index (BMI). Hence, the increased serum TT concentrations as seen after weight loss may be due to a combination of mechanisms that include (i) an increased binding capacity of SHBG, (ii) an increased amplitude of spontaneous LH pulses, (ii) a decreased androgen aromatization, and (iv) a decrease in circulating leptin and insulin concentrations. Surprisingly, a normal endocrine profile can be also found in men with spermatogenic failure. Control feedback of FSH and LH secretions is based on the number of spermatogonia and Leydig cells, respectively, which is well preserved in men with maturation arrest. It has been reported that patients with diffuse spermatogenic maturation arrest and 10 % of those diagnosed with Sertoli-cell-only syndrome (SCOS) present with nonelevated endogenous gonadotropins (Sokol and Swerdloff 1997; Hung et al. 2007).

Lastly, it is important to differentiate azoospermia due to spermatogenic failure from azoospermia due to hypogonadotropic hypogonadism (HH) as both conditions fall in the category of nonobstructive azoospermia (NOA). HH is an endocrine disorder characterized by failure of spermatogenesis due to lack of appropriate stimulation by gonadotropins, while spermatogenic failure comprises the most severe conditions associated with an intrinsic testicular impairment (Fraietta et al. 2013). Men with NOA due to HH have remarkably low levels of pituitary gonadotropins (FSH and LH levels below 1.2 mUI/ml) and androgens and usually have signs of absent or poor virilization. This category of NOA includes not only patients with congenital forms of HH but also men whose spermatogenic potential has been suppressed by excess exogenous androgen administration. Although it is out of my scope to discuss HH in detail, it is worth to mention that patients with HH, albeit rarely seen in the clinical settings, benefit from specific hormonal therapy and often show remarkable recovery of spermatogenic function with exogenously administered gonadotropins or gonadotropin-releasing hormone (Fraietta et al. 2013).

The "gold standard" test for confirmation of azoospermia due to SF is testicular biopsy and histopathology analysis. Hypospermatogenesis, germ cell maturation arrest, germ cell aplasia (Sertoli-cell-only syndrome), tubular sclerosis, or a combination of those is usually found on the histological examination of testicular biopsy specimens in spermatogenic failure. Biopsies can be performed using percutaneous or open methods. Histopathology results have been used not only to confirm the diagnosis of SF but also to predict the chances of finding testicular sperm on retrievals. In a recent study from our group evaluating 356 men with spermatogenic failure, patients with Sertoli-cell-only had lower sperm retrieval rates (19.5 %) compared with those with maturation arrest (40.3 %, $P=.007$), and both categories had lower sperm retrieval rates (SRR) compared with hypospermatogenesis (100.0 %,

$P<.001$; Esteves and Agarwal 2014). Although our data indicate that histopathology phenotypes have prognostic value, caution should be applied when interpreting results because an advanced site of sperm production can be found even in SCO, which represents the worst histopathology phenotype, in approximately 20 % of the cases (Esteves et al. 2014; Esteves and Agarwal 2014; Ashraf et al. 2013; Verza Jr and Esteves 2011). Removal of testicular tissue with the sole purpose of histopathology evaluation could potentially remove the rare foci of sperm production and thus jeopardize the chances of future retrieval attempts (Esteves et al. 2011b). Hence, we do not recommend routine testicular biopsy prior to sperm retrieval. We only perform testicular biopsies when a differential diagnosis between obstructive and non-obstructive azoospermia could not be established. In these cases, our approach is to perform the procedure either using a percutaneous or an open-"window" technique without testis delivery (Esteves et al. 2011a; Esteves and Verza 2012). Specimens should be placed in a fixative solution such as Bouin's, Zenker's, or glutaraldehyde; formalin should not be used as it may disrupt the tissue architecture. A fragment is taken for wet examination in addition to conventional histopathology analysis. When mature sperm is found on a wet examination, we routinely cryopreserve testicular spermatozoa using the liquid nitrogen vapor technique (Esteves and Verza 2012; Esteves and Varghese 2012).

In conclusion, proper laboratory techniques are needed to reduce the amount of analytical error and enhance sperm count precision when evaluating azoospermic specimens. The correct assessment of an initially azoospermic semen should be followed by the examination of multiple specimens after centrifugation to exclude cryptozoospermia, which is defined by presence of a very small number of live sperm in a centrifuged pellet. Accurate assessment of very low sperm counts is aimed to avoid labeling men with very low sperm counts as azoospermic, and it is particularly important in the current era of ART. History and physical examination and hormonal analysis are undertaken to define the type of azoospermia, which provide high diagnostic accuracy to discriminate azoospermia due to spermatogenic failure from obstructive azoospermia and hypogonadotropic hypogonadism (Table 7.1). Although the "gold standard" diagnostic test in azoospermia related to spermatogenic failure is testicular biopsy, removal of testicular tissue with the sole purpose of histopathology evaluation could potentially remove the rare foci of sperm production and thus jeopardize the chances of future retrieval attempts. Testicular biopsy prior to sperm retrieval is therefore not routinely recommended. Testicular biopsy can be performed in selected cases provided a wet prep examination and sperm cryopreservation is available.

7.3 Defining Who Are the Candidates for Sperm Retrieval

Owed to the untreatable nature of spermatogenic failure, sperm retrieval (SR) and ART are the only options for these men to generate their own biological offspring. Uncertainty of sperm acquisition, however, makes prognostic factors very desirable. Though factors such as etiology, testicular volume, serum levels of pituitary

Table 7.1 Interventions and recommended actions in the clinical management of azoospermic men with spermatogenic failure seeking fertility

Clinical management step	Interventions	Action taken	Interpretation
Differential diagnosis in azoospermia	Medical history, physical examination, endocrine profile (FSH and testosterone levels at a minimum; LH, prolactin, thyroid hormones, and estradiol are added as needed), and examination of pelleted semen in multiple occasions. Testicular biopsy could be considered in the few cases in which the differential diagnosis is not determined	Confirmation that azoospermia is due to spermatogenic failure and identification of men with severely impaired spermatogenesis with presence of few sperm in the ejaculate	A differential diagnosis between obstructive azoospermia, hypogonadotropic hypogonadism, and spermatogenic failure should be performed as treatment strategy and outcome vary according to the type of azoospermia
Determination of the individuals who are candidates for a sperm retrieval attempt	Y chromosome microdeletion screening using multiplex (PCR) blood test. The basic set of PCR primers recommended by the EAA/EMQN to be used in multiplex PCR reactions for the diagnosis of Yq microdeletion includes sY14 (SRY), ZFX/ZFY, sY84 and sY86 (AZFa), sY127 and sY134 (AZFb), and sY254 and sY255 (AZFc)	Deselect men with microdeletions involving subregions AZFa, AZFb, and AZFb+c	Approximately 10 % of men with azoospermia due to spermatogenic failure harbor microdeletions within the AZF region. The chances of sperm retrieval in men with YCMD involving the subregions AZFa, AZFb, and AZFb+c are virtually nil, and such patients should be counseled accordingly. The chances of a successful sperm retrieval in men with AZFc deletions range from 50 to 70 %. Genetic counseling should be offered to men with AZFc deletions because testicular spermatozoa used for ICSI will invariably transmit the deletion from father to son

(continued)

Table 7.1 (continued)

Clinical management step	Interventions	Action taken	Interpretation
Identification of the patients to whom interventions prior to testicular retrieval can be offered	Determination of the serum levels of total testosterone and estradiol	Medical treatment with gonadotropins, aromatase inhibitors, or clomiphene citrate should be considered for the patients with hypogonadism (TT < 300 ng/dL) or T/E ratio < 10	Patients should be counseled that the evidence of a positive effect of medical treatment is limited, and such interventions are at present considered empirical
	Physical examination to identify the presence of clinical varicocele and analysis of testicular biopsy results (if available)	Microsurgical repair of clinical varicocele	Microsurgical varicocele repair is associated with better outcome concerning recurrence and postoperative complications. Patients with testicular histopathology indicating Sertoli-cell-only are unlikely to benefit from varicocele repair. Evidence of a positive effect of varicocele repair is limited, and patients should be counseled accordingly
Selection of the most effective surgical method for testicular sperm acquisition	Analysis of testicular biopsy results (if available) and of whether sperm have been obtained in previous treatment and by which method	Microdissection testicular sperm extraction. Conventional testicular sperm extraction may be considered in cases of previous success with TESE, particularly when testicular histopathology indicates hypospermatogenesis	Micro-TESE in SF is associated with a more favorable sperm retrieval rate ranging from 42.9 to 63 % compared with 16.7–45 % in conventional TESE. The lower tissue removal facilitates sperm processing and lessens testicular damage
Application of state-of-the-art laboratory techniques to handle surgically extracted testicular spermatozoa	Extraction of a minimum volume of tissue by micro-TESE facilitates tissue processing and search for sperm. Testicular tissue preparation techniques include mechanical and enzymatic mincing and erythrocyte lysis	Sterile techniques, stable pH and temperature, and high laboratory air quality conditions useful to optimize micromanipulation efficiency and safety assurance Excess sperm not used for ICSI should be cryopreserved for future attempts	Spermatozoa collected from men with SF should be handled with great care because they are often compromised in quality and are more fragile than ejaculated counterparts. The reproductive potential of the gametes used for ICSI is differentially affected by SF

Adapted with permission from Esteves (2015)

ICSI intracytoplasmic sperm injection, *Micro-TESE* microdissection testicular sperm extraction, *PCR* polymerase chain reaction, *T/E* testosterone-to-estradiol ratio, *TESE* testicular sperm extraction, *TT* total testosterone gonadotropins, and testicular histopathology results reflect a global spermatogenic function, they cannot accurately discriminate individuals in whom foci of sperm production will be found upon SR. In an early series involving 60 men with SF, we determined the accuracy of commonly used prognostic parameters using a logistic regression analysis (Verza Jr and Esteves 2011). We confirmed that these parameters have low accuracy as the areas under the receiver-operating characteristic (ROC) curves of FSH, testosterone, and testicular volume for predicting a positive sperm extraction were 0.53, 0.59, and 0.52, respectively. In another study, Tournaye and cols. combined clinical and laboratory parameters, such as testicular volume and FSH levels and histopathology results, and found that diagnostic accuracy was only 74 % (Tournaye et al. 1997). Testicular sperm have been obtained in different etiology categories, including cryptorchidism, post-orchitis, Klinefelter syndrome, radio-/chemotherapy, and idiopathy, with variable success rates ranging from 25 to 70 % (Esteves et al. 2010; Schiff et al. 2005; Chan et al. 2001; Raman and Schlegel 2003; Esteves 2013). In summary, clinical parameters and endocrine profile are unreliable markers for determining the chances of sperm acquisition in men with azoospermia due to spermatogenic failure.

In contrast, the molecular diagnosis and subtyping of Y chromosome microdeletions (YCMD) have been shown to be useful preoperative biomarkers to determine the chances of sperm retrieval in men with azoospermia due to YCMD (Esteves and Agarwal 2011; Stahl et al. 2010; Krausz et al. 2000; Peterlin et al. 2002; Hopps et al. 2003; Simoni et al. 2008; Kleiman et al. 2011, 2012; Hamada et al. 2013). A microdeletion is a chromosomal deletion that usually spans over several genes but is small in size and cannot be detected using conventional cytogenetic methods such as karyotyping (Navarro-Costa et al. 2010; Hamada et al. 2013). The long arm of the Y chromosome contains a region at Yq11 that clusters 26 genes involved in spermatogenesis regulation (Simoni et al. 2008; Hamada et al. 2013; Repping et al. 2002; Krausz et al. 2014). This region is referred to as "azoospermia factor" (AZF) because microdeletions at this interval are often associated with azoospermia (Fig. 7.2). The application of molecular technology has allowed the recognition of three AZF subregions designated as AZFa, AZFb, and AZFc, each one including a major AZF candidate gene (Simoni et al. 2008; Krausz et al. 2014). It has been estimated that approximately 10 % of men with azoospermia due to spermatogenic failure harbor microdeletions within the AZF region that might explain their condition (Simoni et al. 2008; Krausz et al. 2014).

From the medical point of view, the following microdeletions have recurrently been found in men with spermatogenic failure (Krausz et al. 2014; Navarro-Costa et al. 2010): (i) AZFa, (ii) AZFb (P5/proximal P1), (iii) AZFbc (P5/distal P1 or P4/distal P1), and (iv) AZFc (b2/b4). The most frequent deletion subtypes comprise the AZFc region (~80 %) followed by AZFa (0.5–4 %), AZFb (1–5 %), and AZFbc (1–3 %) regions (Krausz et al. 2014). Deletions differentially affecting these AZF subregions cause a distinct disruption of germ cell development. AZFa deletions that remove the entire AZFa are invariably associated with the testicular histopathology phenotype of pure SCOS with no residual areas of active spermatogenesis. Although partial AZFa deletions have been described and may be eventually

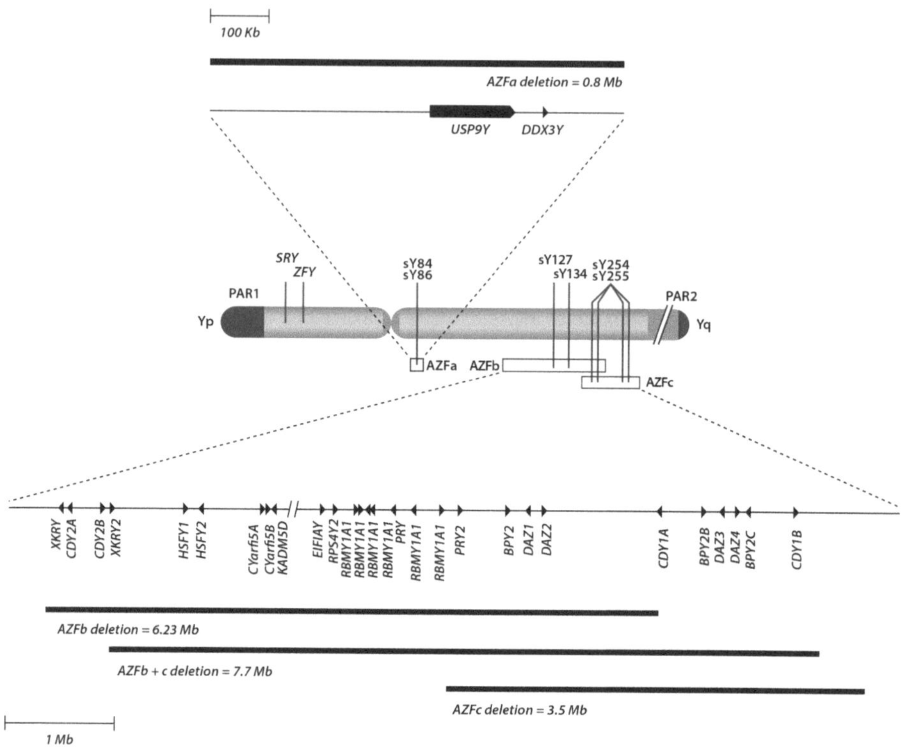

Fig. 7.2 Human Y chromosome map depicting the AZF subregions and gene content. The *AZFa* region maps from approximately 12.9–13.7 Mb of the chromosome and contains two single-copy genes, *USP9Y* and *DDX3Y*. *AZFb* spans from approximately 18–24.7 Mb of the chromosome and *AZFc* from approximately 23–26.7 Mb. Both regions contain multiple genes as depicted in the bottom of the figure. The location of the basic set of sequence-tagged sites primers to be investigated in azoospermic men with spermatogenic failure, according to the European Association of Andrology and the European Molecular Genetics Quality Network 2013 guidelines, is identified by *solid vertical lines*

associated with residual spermatogenesis, this event is extremely rare (Tyler-Smith and Krausz 2009). Hence, the diagnosis of a deletion in the AZFa region implies that the chances of retrieving testicular spermatozoa for ICSI are virtually nonexistent (Krausz et al. 2000; Hopps et al. 2003; Simoni et al. 2008; Kleiman et al. 2011; Vogt and Bender 2013). The clinical feature of complete AZFb and AZFbc (P5/proximal P1, P5/distal P1, P4/distal P1) deletions is similar to AZFa deletions as the chances of finding spermatozoa on attempts of sperm retrieval are close to zero (Krausz et al. 2000; Hopps et al. 2003; Kleiman et al. 2011). In AZFb and AZFbc deletions, the most common testicular histopathology phenotype is spermatogenic maturation arrest, but SCOS can also be found. Nevertheless, spermatid arrest and crypto-/oligozoospermia have been reported in three patients with a complete AZFb or AZbc deletions (Soares et al. 2012; Longepied et al. 2010). In addition, spermatozoa have been identified in rare cases of complete and partial AZFb and

AZFbc deletions (Kleiman et al. 2011). At present, however, given the difficulties to explain the biological nature of these unusual phenotypes, it is sound to assume that the diagnosis of complete deletions of AZFb or AZFbc (P5/proximal P1, P5/distal P1, P4/distal P1) implies that the chances of a successful testicular sperm retrieval are virtually zero (Krausz et al. 2014). In contrast, the chances of successful sperm retrieval in men with NOA and AZFc deletions are 50–70 % (Peterlin et al. 2002; Simoni et al. 2008). AZFc deletions are usually associated with residual spermatogenesis, and therefore testicular spermatozoa can be surgically retrieved and children can be conceived by ICSI (Kent-First et al. 1996; Mulhall et al. 1997; Kamischke et al. 1999; van Golde et al. 2001; Oates et al. 2002). The probability of fatherhood by ICSI seems to be unaltered by the presence of AZFc microdeletions (Peterlin et al. 2002; Kent-First et al. 1996; Mulhall et al. 1997; Kamischke et al. 1999; Oates et al. 2002; Cram et al. 2000). Notwithstanding, some authors have reported impaired embryo development in such cases (Simoni et al. 2008; van Golde et al. 2001). The male offspring born via ICSI from fathers with AZFc microdeletions will inherit the Yq microdeletion and as a result infertility. However, the exact testicular phenotype cannot be predicted as AZFc deletions may jeopardize Y chromosome integrity, predisposing to chromosome loss and sex reversal. There is a potential risk for the 45,X0 karyotype and to the mosaic phenotype 45,X/46,XY in these offspring, which may lead to spontaneous abortion or a newborn with genital ambiguity (Siffroi et al. 2000; Patsalis et al. 2000; Rajpert-De Meyts et al. 2011). Genetic counseling is therefore mandatory to provide information about the risk of conceiving a son with infertility and other genetic abnormalities.

Diagnostic testing for YCMD is based on a multiplex polymerase chain reaction (PCR) blood test aimed to amplify the AZFa, AZFb, and AZFc regions of the Y chromosome (Hamada et al. 2013). This technique primarily amplifies anonymous sequences of the Y chromosome using specific sequence-tagged sites (STSs) primers that are not polymorphic and are well known to be deleted in men affected by azoospermia according to the known, clinically relevant microdeletion pattern (Krausz et al. 2014). To obtain uniform results, it is necessary to follow validated guidelines, such as those issued by the European Association of Andrology (EAA) and the European Molecular Genetics Quality Network (EMQN) (Krausz et al. 2014). The basic set of PCR primers recommended by the EAA/EMQN to be used in multiplex PCR reactions for the diagnosis of Yq microdeletion includes sY14 (SRY), ZFX/ZFY, sY84 and sY86 (AZFa), sY127 and sY134 (AZFb), and sY254 and sY255 (AZFc) (Fig. 7.2). While the primer for the SRY gene is included as a control for the testis-determining factor on the short arm of the Y chromosome, the primers for the ZFX/ZFY gene act as internal controls because these primers amplify a unique fragment both in male and female DNA, respectively. A DNA sample from a fertile male and from a woman and a blank (water) control should be run in parallel with the set of primers. According to the current knowledge, once a deletion of both primers within a region is detected, the probability of a complete deletion is very high. The use of the aforementioned primer set enables the detection of almost all clinically relevant deletions and of over 95 % of the deletions reported in the literature in the three AZF regions (Krausz et al. 2014). However, as partial

AZFa, AZFb, and AZFbc deletions have been described and their phenotypic expression is milder than the complete ones (Krausz et al. 2000; Kleiman et al. 2011), the definition of the extension of the deletion is now recommended in sperm retrieval candidates and should be based on additional markers as described by Krausz and colleagues (2014).

In conclusion, patients with azoospermia due to spermatogenic failure who are candidates for sperm retrieval and ICSI should be screened for Y chromosome microdeletions because the diagnosis of a deletion has prognostic value and influences therapeutic options (Table 7.1). Retrieval attempts are not recommended in cases of complete deletion of the AZFa region. Sperm retrieval in azoospermic carriers of deletions of the AZFb or AZFbc regions may be eventually attempted. However, the patient should be fully informed about the very low/virtually zero chance to retrieve spermatozoa. Owed to reports of deletion carriers among men with nonidiopathic NOA, including cryptorchidism, post-chemo-/radiotherapy, varicocele, and Klinefelter syndrome, the presence of any of these diagnosis categories accompanied by azoospermia should be an indication for YCMD screening testing (Krausz et al. 1999; Mitra et al. 2006). Genetic counseling should be offered to men with AZFc deletions who are candidates for sperm retrieval because testicular spermatozoa used for ICSI will invariably transmit the deletion from father to son. Although the likely result is azoospermia, AZFc microdeletions might be associated with an increased risk of miscarriage and other genetic abnormalities in the offspring.

7.4 Defining Who Can Benefit from Interventions Prior to Sperm Retrieval

After identifying who are the candidates for SR by excluding those patients with complete AZFa, AZFb, and AZFbc microdeletions, the next step is to select the patients who could benefit from medical and surgical interventions prior to SR. While a positive clinical outcome has been observed after gonadotropin treatment in azoospermic men with hypogonadotropic hypogonadism, it is generally believed that medical therapy would be ineffective in SF due to the presence of high serum levels of gonadotropins. Treatments that could improve sperm production in men with SF are highly expected since nearly half of them will be halted in their attempt to conceive due to the absence of testicular sperm on retrievals (Kumar 2013; Esteves et al. 2011b, 2014; Carpi et al. 2009).

Given that approximately 50 % of men with azoospermia due to spermatogenic failure have hypogonadism, defined by low endogenous levels (<300 ng/dL) of total testosterone (Sussman et al. 2008; Reifsnyder et al. 2012), recent studies have examined the effect of therapies that could boost testosterone production as potential targets for medical intervention. Testosterone is essential for spermatogenesis (Quigley et al. 1995; McLachlan et al. 2002), and it has been shown that its levels are more than 100-fold greater in the testes as compared with the serum (Jarow et al. 2001). Although the mechanism by which testosterone regulates the spermatogenic process in humans is not fully understood, intratesticular testosterone action on target cells seems to involve a paracrine mechanism on androgen receptors (ARs) (Boukari et al. 2009; Kato et al. 2014). Enhancing testosterone production using medication could allow the restoration of adequate levels of intratesticular androgenic bioactivity that are essential to sustain spermatogenesis in combination with adequate Sertoli cell stimulation with FSH (Coviello et al. 2004). Drugs that have been utilized include clomiphene citrate, gonadotropins (human chorionic gonadotropin and FSH), and aromatase inhibitors (Ashraf et al. 2013; Schiff et al. 2005; Reifsnyder et al. 2012; Pavlovich et al. 2001; Ramasamy et al. 2009, 2012; Kumar 2013; Hussein et al. 2013).

Clomiphene citrate is a selective estrogen receptor modulator that competitively binds to estrogen receptors on the hypothalamus and pituitary gland. As a result, the pituitary perceives less estrogen, which leads to the secretion of both FSH and LH. The latter binds to LH receptors that are present in the Leydig cells and induces androgen secretion and a consequent rise in testosterone levels (Kumar 2013). Human chorionic gonadotropin (hCG) is a glycoprotein similar to the native LH, but with higher receptor affinity and half-life compared with LH (Kumar 2013; Leão and Esteves 2014). hCG binds to the same LH receptor at the Leydig cell level, thus stimulating the production of androgens. Aromatase inhibitors, on the other hand, block the aromatase enzyme present in the adipose tissue, liver, testis, and skin. The latter is responsible for converting testosterone and other androgens to estradiol. Aromatase inhibitors have been prescribed to obese and overweight infertile men who often have aromatase hyperactivity and consequently elevated estradiol levels (Hammoud et al. 2010). Estradiol suppresses pituitary LH and FSH secretion and also directly inhibits testosterone biosynthesis. This results in an imbalance in the testosterone and estradiol (T/E) ratio, which may be reversible by oral administration of aromatase inhibitors (Reifsnyder et al. 2012; Pavlovich et al. 2001). The aforementioned drug categories have been used in combination or alone.

In an early study including 43 men with SF associated with various etiologies, Pavlovich and colleagues reported an increase in T/E ratio after treatment with aromatase inhibitors, but none of the treated men experienced return of sperm into the ejaculate (Pavlovich et al. 2001). In a series involving 42 men with non-mosaic Klinefelter syndrome and azoospermia, Schiff and colleagues administered aromatase inhibitors alone or in combination with clomiphene citrate or hCG prior to sperm retrieval (Schiff et al. 2005). The authors observed an increased SR rate in men who had received medical therapy. In a later series from the same group also involving non-mosaic Klinefelter patients, the authors reported that the SR rates were increased by 1.4-fold in the men who responded to the medical therapy, defined by an absolute increase of 150 ng/dL of testosterone from baseline levels, compared to ones who did not (Ramasamy et al. 2009). In a recent study involving a large cohort of 442 men with azoospermia due to spermatogenic failure who received medication (clomiphene citrate and hCG) prior to SR, the investigators aimed at achieving 600–800 ng/dL serum testosterone posttreatment. In this study, SR rates were significantly higher in the group of patients who achieved the desired hormonal level post-medical therapy (57 vs. 33.6 %; Hussein et al. 2013). Contrary results, however, have been observed in a large cohort of unselected men with NOA treated with aromatase inhibitors, clomiphene citrate, and hCG (Reifsnyder et al. 2012). In this aforementioned series involving 736 men, the authors observed that SR rates were not significantly different between treated and untreated individuals (52 vs. 53 %) despite of a high positive response to medical therapy in terms of boosting endogenous testosterone levels.

Recently, Shinjo et al. (2013) demonstrated that the Leydig cells of men with SF produce increased amounts of intratesticular testosterone (ITT) in response to exogenous hCG stimulation even under a hypergonadotropic condition. The aforementioned authors studied a group of 20 men with SF and found that ITT levels were significantly higher after hCG treatment (pre, 273.6 ± 134.4; post, 1348.1 ± 505.4 ng/mL; $P < .0001$). LH secretion is characterized by the frequency, amplitude, and duration of its secretory pulses (Spratt et al. 1987). In men with SF, the relative amplitude of LH pulses is low because the basal LH levels are high (Shiraishi et al. 2012), thus indicating that the stimulation of Leydig and Sertoli cells by endogenous gonadotropins is paradoxically weak (Keenan and Veldhuis 2004). Not surprisingly, the percentage of Sertoli cells showing androgen receptors is significantly higher in the men with SF compared to those with normal spermatogenesis (23.7 % vs. 18 %, $p < 0.05$) (Kato et al. 2014).

Endogenous FSH is suppressed below preadolescent levels through a negative feedback mechanism of elevated serum testosterone in over half the azoospermic men with SF treated with hCG (Shiraishi et al. 2012). Such an effect could be beneficial since high plasma FSH levels, which cause downregulation of FSH receptors, impair tubular function. As a matter of fact, an improvement in Sertoli cell function was achieved after reduction of high FSH plasma concentration by administration of a GnRH analogue in men with severely impaired spermatogenesis (Foresta et al. 2004). Sertoli cells have been considered to be a major target for testosterone signaling via the activation of nuclear androgen receptors (Griswold 2005; Kato et al. 2014). The Sertoli cells support male germ cell development and survival, and their function can be restored by elevated intratesticular testosterone (O'Shaughnessy et al. 2010). Interestingly, Shinjo et al. (2013) showed that basal ITT was lower in men with SF who responded to hormonal treatment and had sperm retrieved than those who had not. Human chorionic gonadotropin treatment may not only increase intratesticular testosterone but also reset FSH action.

Although the exact mechanism underlying the beneficial effect of hCG therapy in men with SF remains unclear, it has been speculated that hCG acts by indirectly stimulating spermiogenesis as well as spermatogonia DNA synthesis in those patients with foci of hypospermatogenesis or late maturation arrest (Shinjo et al. 2013; Matthiesson et al. 2006; Aggarwal et al. 2009; Wistuba et al. 2010). These effects could result in the formation of well-differentiated seminiferous tubules that would be detected during sperm retrieval (Shiraishi et al. 2012).

Varicocele, found in approximately 5 % of men with SF, has also been a target for intervention prior to sperm retrieval (Miyaoka and Esteves 2012; Weedin et al. 2010). While it is still debatable whether varicocele is merely coincidental or contributory to spermatogenesis disruption, the surgical repair of clinical varicoceles, particularly using microsurgical techniques, has been carried out in an attempt to improve sperm production in such men (Miyaoka and Esteves 2012; Esteves and Glina 2005; Weedin et al. 2010). The goals are to allow the appearance of small quantities of sperm in the ejaculate or increase the chances of retrieving sperm from the testis. Sperm production restoration, albeit minimal, will facilitate sperm injection procedures. In an early study, we evaluated a group of 17 men with clinical varicocele and azoospermia due to SF who underwent microsurgical sub-inguinal varicocele repair (Esteves and Glina 2005). In a mean postoperative follow-up of 19 months, 35.3 % (6/17) of the patients had motile sperm in ejaculates with a mean sperm count of 0.8 million/ml (range 0.1–1.8). A testicular biopsy obtained for analysis revealed that the histopathology phenotype was associated with the surgical outcome. Viable sperm was identified in the ejaculates of 72.7 % (8/11) of the patients with hypospermatogenesis or maturation arrest, in contrast to none (0/6) of those with SCO (Esteves and Glina 2005). Subsequently, a meta-analysis of 11 case series-including our own-involving 233 patients with clinical varicocele and azoospermia showed similar results (Weedin et al. 2010). At a mean postoperative follow-up of 13 months, motile sperm was found in ejaculates of 39 % of the subjects. With a mean sperm count of 1.6 million/ml, natural and assisted conceptions were obtained in 26 % of the treated men. Analysis of testicular biopsies taken either prior or during varicocele repair revealed that hypospermatogenesis and maturation arrest were significantly more likely to be associated with the presence of sperm in the postoperative ejaculate compared with Sertoli-cell-only (odds ratio 9.4, CI 95 % 3.2–27.3; Weedin et al. 2010).

Although the aforementioned studies indicate that improvements in sperm production after varicocelectomy can be achieved in approximately one third of men with azoospermia, most of the treated individuals will either remain azoospermic or have inadequate number of sperm in the ejaculate for ICSI (Schlegel and Kaufmann 2004). In such cases, a sperm retrieval attempt will be the only alternative, and the validity of having had a varicocele operation has been examined. In one study, Schlegel and Kaufmann reported that 22 % of the patients had sperm on a post-varicocelectomy semen analysis at an average follow-up of 14.7 months, but only 9.6 % had motile sperm in the ejaculate to allow ICSI to be carried out without the need of a surgical sperm extraction (Schlegel and Kaufmann 2004). In this aforementioned retrospective study involving 138 patients, similar retrieval rates of 60 % per attempt were obtained regardless of whether or not varicocelectomy had been performed. In contrast, two retrospective series have shown that varicocelectomy applied to patients with SF and clinical varicocele is advantageous. Inci and colleagues, studying a group of 96 men, observed that retrieval rates were significantly higher in treated (53 %) compared with untreated men (30 %, $P=.03$), which represented a 2.6-fold increase in the chances of identifying sperm at a surgical retrieval attempt (odds ratio [OR], 2.63; 95 % confidence interval [CI] of 1.05–6.60; Inci et al. 2009). Along the same lines, in a study involving 66 men, Haydardedeoglu and cols. reported higher retrieval rates in men who have had varicocele repair prior to SR (61 %) compared with untreated men (38 %; $P<.01$;Haydardedeoglu et al. 2010).

In conclusion, interventions prior to SR including medical therapy to boost endogenous testosterone production and microsurgical varicocele repair can be offered to selected patients with azoospermia due to spermatogenic failure (Table 7.1). Although an overall beneficial effect has been observed, the evidence is currently limited and based mostly on case series. Hence, a firm conclusion on the role of medical and surgical intervention therapy in men with spermatogenic failure and azoospermia cannot be drawn yet. Randomized controlled trials are needed to assess the impact of such interventions on sperm production and sperm retrieval outcomes.

7.5 Defining What Is the Best Method of Sperm Retrieval for Azoospermic Men with Spermatogenic Failure

Sperm retrieval techniques should be aimed at offering the highest possible chance of obtaining an adequate number of good quality testicular sperm, which can be immediately used for ICSI or cryopreserved for future ICSI attempts. Retrieval methods should also minimize testicular damage, thus preserving androgen activity and the chance of repeated retrievals attempts.

Historically, the method of choice for sperm acquisition in azoospermia due to SF has been conventional testicular sperm extraction (TESE), with a mean reported SRR of 49.5 % (Donoso et al. 2007). In TESE, open single or multiple testicular biopsies are randomly taken, processed, and examined for the presence of sperm (Esteves et al. 2011b, 2013b; Carpi et al. 2009; Tournaye et al. 1997). Since prediction of both the existence and the geographic location of the islets of normal spermatogenesis is not possible prior to SR, more than one specimen is usually required until sperm is found. TESE with multiple biopsies resulted in higher SRR than fine-needle aspiration (TEFNA), a variation of testicular sperm aspiration (TESA), particularly in cases involving SCO and maturation arrest (Donoso et al. 2007). A disadvantage of TESE is that removal of large fragments of testicular tissue may jeopardize the already compromised androgen production, in a transient or permanent way, thus resulting in severe hypogonadism (Schlegel and Su 1997). Also, laboratory processing of such large quantities of testicular tissue taken by TESE is time consuming and labor intensive (Esteves and Verza 2012; Esteves and Varghese 2012; Schlegel 1999).

Microdissection testicular sperm extraction (micro-TESE) is a microsurgical method of sperm retrieval that has been proposed as a better alternative to TESE in cases of spermatogenic failure (Schlegel 1999). The reasons are the greater success at obtaining sperm, ranging from 43 % up to 70 %, and the lower tissue removal that facilitates sperm processing and lessens testicular damage (Esteves et al. 2011b, 2013b; Schlegel 1999; Okada et al. 2002; Amer et al. 2000; Tsujimura 2007; El-Haggar et al. 2007). The rationale of micro-TESE is to identify focal areas of sperm production within the testes, based on the size and appearance of the seminiferous tubules, with the aid of the operating microscope (Schlegel 1999). Such areas are selectively extracted thus allowing minimal tissue removal, which has been shown to be 50–70-fold less when compared with conventional TESE (Esteves et al. 2011b, 2013b; Schlegel 1999). The use of optical magnification also reduces the chances of vascular injury by proper identification of testicular blood supply, thus reducing the chances of hematoma formation and testicular devascularization (Esteves 2013). Although decrease in serum testosterone has been documented after removing testicular parenchyma by micro-TESE, especially in men with severely compromised androgen activity such as those with Klinefelter syndrome (Schiff et al. 2005), testosterone levels return to presurgical values in 95 % of the subjects within 18 months following surgery (Ramasamy et al. 2005).

For micro-TESE, a large incision is made in an avascular area of the tunica albuginea under 6–8X magnification, and the testicular parenchyma is widely exposed. The parenchyma is then dissected at 16– 25X magnification to enable the search and isolation of the seminiferous tubules that exhibit larger diameter in comparison with non-enlarged or collapsed counterparts. These enlarged tubules are more likely to contain germ cells and eventually normal sperm production (Fig. 7.3). Microsurgical-guided biopsies are performed by carefully removing such tubules, which are sent to the laboratory for examination. In addition to minimizing testicular damage, a smaller amount of tissue extracted facilitates laboratory processing and sperm search, thus increasing the process efficiency (Schlegel 1999; Amer et al. 2000; Tsujimura 2007; Esteves et al. 2011b, 2013b; Esteves and Varghese 2012; Ashraf et al. 2013; Esteves 2013).

In a controlled study from our group involving 60 men with SF, we compared SRR between micro-TESE and conventional single-biopsy TESE (Verza Jr and Esteves 2011). The SRR was significantly higher with micro-TESE (45vs. 25 %; $P=.005$) both overall and after stratifying the patients by testicular histopathology phenotype (hypospermatogenesis, 93 vs. 64 %; maturation arrest, 64 vs. 9 %; Sertoli-cell-only syndrome, 20 vs. 6 %; $P<.001$). Controlled studies have corroborated our results showing that micro-TESE is associated with a higher sperm recovery and lower complication rates (below 5 %) than conventional TESE (Okada et al.

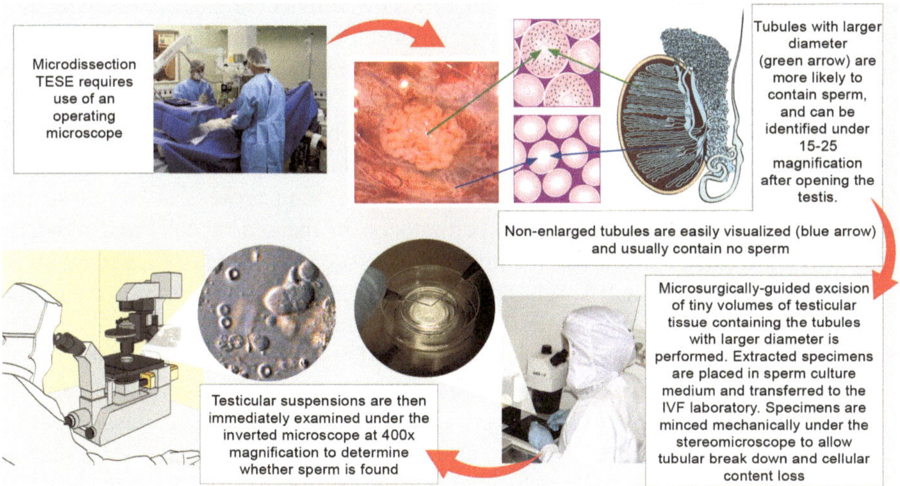

Fig. 7.3 Microdissection testicular sperm extraction. The flow chart illustrates the consecutive steps from the microsurgical procedure to the laboratory processing of testicular specimens (Reprinted with permission from Esteves (2015))

2002; Amer et al. 2000; Tsujimura 2007; El-Haggar et al. 2007). We have recently reported our updated experience involving 356 patients with SF who have undergone micro-TESE. SRR was 41.4 % overall (Esteves et al. 2014) and 100.0, 40.3, and 19.5 % according to the histopathology phenotypes of hypospermatogenesis, maturation arrest, and SCO, respectively (Esteves and Agarwal 2014). Micro-TESE has been shown to rescue approximately one third of the cases that failed in previous retrieval attempts with conventional TESE and TESA and is particularly useful for men with spermatogenic failure presenting the worst-case scenarios (Ashraf et al. 2013; Schlegel 1999). Lastly, a recent systematic review involving seven comparative studies and 1062 patients confirmed that micro-TESE in SF was associated with a more favorable sperm retrieval rate ranging from 42.9 to 63 % compared with 16.7 to 45 % in conventional TESE (Deruyver et al. 2014).

In conclusion, the efficiency of sperm retrieval in azoospermia due to SF varies according to the method of sperm acquisition. Micro-TESE should be the method of choice for SR in such cases because it not only increases the chance of retrieving testicular sperm for ICSI but also minimizes testicular damage (Table 7.1).

7.6 Laboratory Handling of Testicular Sperm

After sperm retrieval procedures, the extracted testicular parenchyma is immediately transferred to the embryology laboratory for sperm search. The laboratory handling of surgically retrieved gametes requires special attention because spermatozoa collected from men with NOA are often compromised in quality and are more fragile than ejaculated counterparts (Verza and Esteves 2008). Both sperm DNA fragmentation and aneuploidy rates are higher in testicular sperm obtained from men with spermatogenic failure compared with ejaculated sperm obtained from infertile men with various etiology categories (Vozdova et al. 2012; Meseguer et al. 2009). As a result, a lower fertilization, embryo development, and pregnancy rates have been achieved when the gametes retrieved from men with SF are used for ICSI (Esteves et al. 2014; Verza and Esteves 2008).

The extraction of a minimum volume of tissue by using advanced surgical techniques, such as micro-TESE, is advantageous because the processing of TESE specimens may be incredibly labor intensive. The searching process in large testicular tissue volumes may miss the rare spermatozoa in the sea of cells and noncellular elements. Hence, the lower the amount of tissue to be processed, the easier the sperm search (Esteves and Varghese 2012). Testicular tissue preparation techniques designed to increase sperm retrieval rates have been used to handle these specimens, including mechanical and enzymatic mincing. These methods ensure tubular wall break down and cellular content loss (Esteves and Varghese 2012; Aydos et al. 2005; Baukloh 2002). After proper disintegration of the seminiferous tubules, specimens are processed to eliminate surplus tissue elements and red blood cells. This step can be achieved by using erythrocyte lysing solution and density gradient centrifugation, respectively (Esteves and Varghese 2012; Ozkavukcu et al. 2014). Lastly, a series of Petri dishes are prepared containing oil-covered microdroplets of sperm culture media loaded with aliquots of processed testicular tissue. This offers the opportunity of an effective examination of the specimens by the embryologist, thus allowing the identification and retrieval of testicular spermatozoa (Esteves and Varghese 2012). This final step is carried out at the ICSI workstation. Throughout the aforesaid processes, the temperature and pH of working solutions should be kept constant. Moreover, state-of-the-art laboratory practice standards, including sterile techniques and laboratory air quality conditions, are of utmost importance to optimize micromanipulation efficiency and safety assurance (Esteves and Varghese 2012; Popal and Nagy 2013). At our center, we perform sperm retrieval and all related-laboratory steps involved in the handling of testicular specimens in controlled environments. The latter includes tissue processing, microinjection of surgically extracted sperm, culture of embryos generated from such procedures, and cryopreservation of gametes and embryos. Our facility, comprised of reproductive laboratories (IVF and andrology), an operating room where microsurgical sperm extractions and oocyte collections are carried out, and embryo transfer rooms, was constructed according to clean room standards for air particles and volatile organic compounds. Not surprisingly, we observed a significant increase in IVF treatment effectiveness after having implemented clean room technology (Esteves and Bento 2013).

After a successful SR in NOA, cryopreservation of surplus testicular sperm is highly recommended because such patients often require more than one ICSI attempt until a pregnancy is established, and repeated retrieval attempts are not always possible. Some centers prefer to retrieve and intentionally cryopreserve testicular sperm for future use, while others coordinate sperm retrieval and oocyte collection to occur simultaneously. In many cases, only immotile spermatozoa will be available for sperm injection after thawing, which could negatively impact ICSI outcomes. A comprehensive review of the advantages and disadvantages of performing sperm injections with fresh or frozen-thawed testicular sperm and the methods of selecting viable immotile sperm for ICSI can be found elsewhere (Esteves and Varghese 2012).

In conclusion, adherence to state-of-the-art laboratory techniques and quality control are recommended not only to avoid jeopardizing the sperm fertilizing potential but also to improve ICSI outcomes when handling testicular specimens extracted from men with azoospermia due to spermatogenic failure (Table 7.1).

7.7 Results of Assisted Reproductive Technology in Azoospermic Men with Spermatogenic Failure

The clinical outcomes of ICSI using surgically extracted testicular sperm from men with azoospermia due to SF are lower than ejaculated counterparts (Palermo et al. 1999; He et al. 2010; Esteves and Agarwal 2013a; Verza and Esteves 2008). The results are also lower when the former is compared with epididymal and testicular sperm obtained from men with obstructive azoospermia (OA), in whom spermatogenesis is not disrupted unlike spermatogenic failure (Esteves et al. 2014; He et al. 2010). These findings seems to be related to the higher tendency of these spermatozoa to carry deficiencies such as the ones related to the centrioles and genetic material, which ultimately affect the capability of the male gamete to activate the egg and trigger the formation and development of a normal zygote and a viable embryo (Vozdova et al. 2012; Meseguer et al. 2009).

In an early series involving 330 patients with different infertility conditions including 53 azoospermic men with SF, we examined the ICSI outcomes according to the source of spermatozoa and the type of azoospermia. We found that normal (2PN) fertilization rates were significantly lower when testicular sperm of men with SF was compared with ejaculated sperm, and with testicular/epididymal sperm of men with obstructive azoospermia (52.2, 71.1, and 73.6 % in SF, ejaculated sperm, and OA, respectively; $P<.05$). Embryo development and pregnancy rates are also negatively affected by SF (Verza Jr and Esteves 2011). In two recent series involving a larger cohort of azoospermic men with SF, we compared the outcomes of ICSI and analyzed the health of offspring according to the source of sperm and the type of azoospermia. In one study, 188 women underwent ICSI using sperm from partners with SF, and the outcomes were compared with a group of 182 and 465 women whose partners had OA and non-azoospermia male infertility, respectively. Live birth rates after ICSI were significantly lower in the SF group (21.4 %) compared with the OA (37.5 %) and ejaculated sperm (32.3 %) groups ($P=.003$). A total of 326 live births resulted in 427 babies born. Differences were not observed among the groups in gestational age, preterm birth, birth weight, and low birth weight, although we noted a tendency toward poorer neonatal outcomes in the azoospermia categories (Esteves and Agarwal 2013a). In another series, we compared 365 azoospermic men with SF who underwent micro-TESE with 40 men with SF who used donor sperm for sperm injections due to failed retrieval and 146 men with OA who underwent percutaneous sperm retrieval. The sperm retrieval rate in SF was 41.4 %, and the results were lower than the OA group (100 %; adjusted odds ratio, 0.033; 95 % CI, 0.007–0.164; $P<.001$). Live birth rates after sperm injections were lower in men with SF (19.9 %) compared with donor sperm (37.5 %; adjusted odds ratio, 0.377 (95 % CI, 0.233–0.609, $P<.001$)) and obstructive azoospermia (34.2 %; adjusted OR, 0.403 (95 % CI, 0.241–0.676, $P=.001$). Neither the miscarriage rates nor the newborn parameters (gestational age, birth weight, malformation rate, perinatal mortality) of infants conceived were significantly different among the groups (Esteves et al. 2014). Although the data on the health of resulting offspring after ICSI using sperm of men with azoospermia due to SF is reassuring, only five studies have compared to date the neonatal profile of such babies (Esteves et al. 2014; Esteves and Agarwal 2013a; Vernaeve et al. 2003; Fedder et al. 2007; Belva et al. 2011).

In conclusion, the chances of obtaining sperm on retrieval and achieving a live birth after ICSI are reduced in men with spermatogenic failure. The short-term profile of infants conceived after sperm injection does not seem to be negatively affected by spermatogenic failure.

7.8 Complete Aspermatogenesis: A Glance Toward the Future

Aspermatogenesis, defined as severe impairment of spermatogenesis in which germ cells are completely lacking or present only in an immature form, results in sterility in approximately 25–45 % of patients with spermatogenic failure (Aponte et al. 2013). In vitro fertilization with immature germ cells and in vitro culture of these cells have been proposed as an approach to overcome the cases where no mature spermatozoa are retrieved. ICSI with immature germ cells, including elongating and round spermatids, has yielded conflicting results, and despite deliveries of healthy offspring have been reported, the method has very low efficiency as currently used (Vloeberghs et al. 2013). In addition, there is uncertainty whether this approach can be considered a safe treatment option. Ethical and safety concerns related to potential transmission of genomic imprinted disorders have been raised leading to the ban of spermatid injection in the United Kingdom. Human spermatozoa are highly specialized cells with the purpose of not only delivering competent paternal DNA to the oocyte but also providing a robust epigenetic contribution to embryogenesis. The latter requires that chromatin contains layers of regulatory elements sufficient to drive genes toward activation or silencing upon delivery to the oocyte. Changes in epigenome are known to affect gene expression, and several genes participating in spermatogenesis are epigenetically regulated (Kumar et al. 2013).

Because assisted reproduction techniques require mature germ cells, research efforts are now focused on the differentiation of preexisting immature germ cells or the production/derivation of sperm from somatic cells. In this regard, biotechnology has been investigated as a valuable tool for rescuing fertility while maintaining biological fatherhood. Breakthrough advancement in this field has been accomplished by Japanese scientists who used stem cells from mouse embryos to create primordial germ cells, which differentiated into spermatozoa after testis transplantation in mice (Sato et al. 2011). In humans, formation of human haploid-like cells has already been obtained from pluripotent stem cells of somatic origin using the novel technique of in vitro sperm derivation. Haploidization is another technique under investigation as an option to create gametes based on biological cloning technology. Despite being promising, these methodologies are experimental, and the production of human gametes in the laboratory is a highly complex process which is yet to be fully translated to humans (Aponte et al. 2013).

In conclusion, biotechnology techniques have been investigated as an alternative to rescue fertility in men with complete aspermatogenesis. At present, these methods remain largely experimental and still require extensive research, which should address, among other concerns, ethical and biosafety issues, such as gamete epigenetic status, ploidy, and chromatin integrity.

Conclusions

The clinical management of azoospermic men with spermatogenic failure seeking fertility starts with a proper diagnosis workup that allows the differentiation between SF and other types of azoospermia. Azoospermia should be confirmed based on the absence of spermatozoa on multiple semen examinations after centrifugation using microscopic analysis. The combination of history and physical examination and hormonal analysis will differentiate with high accuracy spermatogenic failure from hypogonadotropic hypogonadism and obstructive azoospermia. Testicular biopsy with the sole purpose of histopathology diagnosis is not recommended because removal of testicular tissue might remove the rare foci of sperm production and thus jeopardize retrieval attempts.

Patients with azoospermia due to SF who are candidates for sperm retrieval should be screened for Y chromosome microdeletions because the diagnosis of a deletion has prognostic value and can influence therapeutic options. While retrieval attempts are not recommended in complete deletion of the AZFa region, SR in azoospermic carriers of AZFb or AZFbc deletions may be eventually attempted, but patients should be fully informed about the very low/virtually zero chance to retrieve sperm. The presence of AZFc deletions represents a good prognostic factor for positive sperm retrieval because this deletion subtype is usually associated with residual spermatogenesis. Nevertheless, genetic counseling should be offered to these men because testicular spermatozoa used for ICSI will invariably transmit the deletion from father to son.

Before a sperm retrieval attempt, medical therapy to boost endogenous testosterone production and microsurgical repair of clinical varicoceles can be offered to men with hypogonadism and clinical varicocele, respectively. Although some individuals will ejaculate minimal quantity of sperm after such interventions, the majority remains azoospermic and will require SR. Micro-TESE should be the method of choice for sperm retrieval in spermatogenic failure because it not only increases the chance of retrieving testicular sperm for ICSI but also minimizes testicular damage.

After sperm retrieval, the extracted testicular parenchyma is immediately transferred to the embryology laboratory for sperm search following tissue dissection. Adherence to state-of-the-art laboratory techniques and quality control are recommended not only to avoid jeopardizing the sperm fertilizing potential but also to improve ICSI outcomes when handling testicular specimens extracted from azoospermic men with SF. The chances of obtaining sperm on retrievals and achieving a live birth after ICSI are reduced in men with SF, but the short-term profile of infants conceived after sperm injection does not seem to be negatively affected by SF.

Biotechnology techniques of in vitro sperm generation remain largely experimental although they can become a valuable tool for rescuing fertility while maintaining biological fatherhood.

References

Aggarwal A, Misro M, Maheshwar A, Sehgal N, Nandan D. Adverse effects associated with persistent stimulation of Leydig cells with hCG in vitro. Mol Reprod Dev. 2009;76:1076–83.

Amer M, Ateyah A, Hany R, Zohdi W. Prospective comparative study between microsurgical and conventional testicular sperm extraction in non-obstructive azoospermia: follow-up by serial ultrasound examinations. Hum Reprod. 2000;15:653–6.

American Society for Reproductive Medicine, Society for Male Reproduction and Urology. Evaluation of the azoospermic male. Fertil Steril. 2008;90(Suppl):S74–7.

Aponte PM, Schlatt S, Franca LR. Biotechnological approaches to the treatment of aspermatogenic men. Clinics (Sao Paulo). 2013;68 Suppl 1:157–67.

Ashraf MC, Singh S, Raj D, Ramakrishnan S, Esteves SC. Micro-dissection testicular sperm extraction as an alternative for sperm acquisition in the most difficult cases of azoospermia: technique and preliminary results in India. J Hum Reprod Sci. 2013;6:111–23.

Aydos K, Demirel LC, Baltaci V, Unlü C. Enzymatic digestion plus mechanical searching improves testicular sperm retrieval in non-obstructive azoospermia cases. Eur J Obstet Gynecol Reprod Biol. 2005;120:80–6.

Aziz N. The importance of semen analysis in the context of azoospermia. Clinics (Sao Paulo). 2013;68 Suppl 1:35–8.

Baukloh V. Retrospective multicentre study on mechanic and enzymatic preparation of fresh and cryopreserved testicular biopsies. Hum Reprod. 2002;17:1788–94.

Belva F, De Schrijver F, Tournaye H, Liebaers I, Devroey P, Haentjens P, Bonduelle M. Neonatal outcome of 724 children born after ICSI using non-ejaculated sperm. Hum Reprod. 2011;26: 1752–8.

Bobjer J, Naumovska M, Giwercman YL, Giwercman A. High prevalence of androgen deficiency and abnormal lipid profile in infertile men with non-obstructive azoospermia. Int J Androl. 2012;35:688–94.

Boukari K, Meduri G, Brailly-Tabard S, Guibourdenche J, Ciampi ML, Massin N, Martinerie L, Picard JY, Rey R, Lombès M, Young J. Lack of androgen receptor expression in Sertoli cells accounts for the absence of anti-mullerian hormone repression during early human testis development. J Clin Endocrinol Metab. 2009;94:1818–25.

Carpi A, Sabanegh E, Mechanick J. Controversies in the management of nonobstructive azoospermia. Fertil Steril. 2009;91:963–70.

Castilla JA, Alvarez C, Aguilar J, Gonzalez-Varea C, Gonzalvo MC, Martinez L. Influence of analytical and biological variation on the clinical interpretation of seminal parameters. Hum Reprod. 2006;21:847–51.

Chan PTK, Palermo GD, Veeck LL, Rosenwaks Z, Schlegel PN. Testicular sperm extraction combined with intracytoplasmic sperm injection in the treatment of men with persistent azoospermia postchemotherapy. Cancer. 2001;92(6):1632–7.

Cooper TG, Hellenkemper B, Jonckheere J, Callewaert N, Grootenhuis AJ, Kersemaekers WM, Leung A, Wang C. Azoospermia: virtual reality or possible to quantify? J Androl. 2006; 27:483–90.

Cooper TG, Noonan E, von Eckardstein S, Auger J, Baker HW, Behre HM, Haugen TB, Kruger T, Wang C, Mbizvo MT, Vogelsong KM. World Health Organization reference values for human semen characteristics. Hum Reprod Update. 2010;16:231–45.

Corea M, Campagnone J, Sigman M. The diagnosis of azoospermia depends on the force of centrifugation. Fertil Steril. 2005;83:920–2.

Coviello AD, Bremner WJ, Matsumoto AM, Herbst KL, Amory JK, Anawalt BD, Yan X, Brown TR, Wright WW, Zirkin BR, Jarow JP. Intratesticular testosterone concentrations comparable with serum levels are not sufficient to maintain normal sperm production in men receiving a hormonal contraceptive regimen. J Androl. 2004;25:931–8.

Cram DS, Ma K, Bhasin S, Arias J, Pandjaitan M, Chu B, Audrins MS, Saunders D, Quinn F, deKretser D, McLachlan R. Y chromosome analysis of infertile men and their sons conceived through intracytoplasmic sperm injection: vertical transmission of deletions and rarity of de novo deletions. Fertil Steril. 2000;74:909–15.

Deruyver Y, Vanderschueren D, Van der Aa F. Outcome of microdissection TESE compared with conventional TESE in non-obstructive azoospermia: a systematic review. Andrologia. 2014; 2:20–4.

Donoso P, Tournaye H, Devroey P. Which is the best sperm retrieval technique for non-obstructive azoospermia? A systematic review. Hum Reprod Update. 2007;13:539–49.

El-Haggar S, Mostafa T, Abdel Nasser T, Hany R, Abgdel HA. Fine needle aspiration vs. mTESE in non-obstructive azoospermia. Int J Androl. 2007;31:595–601.

Esteves SC. Clinical management of infertile men with nonobstructiveazoospermia. Asian J Androl. 2015;17(3):459–70.

Esteves SC, Agarwal A. Novel concepts in male infertility. Int Braz J Urol. 2011;37:5–15.
Esteves SC, Agarwal A. Reproductive outcomes, including neonatal data, following sperm injection in men with obstructive and nonobstructive azoospermia: case series and systematic review. Clinics (Sao Paulo). 2013a;68 Suppl 1:141–50.
Esteves SC, Agarwal A. The azoospermic male: current knowledge and future perspectives. Clinics (Sao Paulo). 2013b;68 Suppl 1:1–4.
Esteves SC, Agarwal A. Re: Sperm retrieval rates and intracytoplasmic sperm injection outcomes for men with non-obstructive azoospermia and the health of resulting offspring. Asian J Androl. 2014;16:642.
Esteves SC, Bento FC. Implementation of air quality control in reproductive laboratories in full compliance with the Brazilian cells and germinative tissue directive. Reprod Biomed Online. 2013;26:9–21.
Esteves SC, Glina S. Recovery of spermatogenesis after microsurgical subinguinal varicocele repair in azoospermic men based on testicular histology. Int Braz J Urol. 2005;31:541–8.
Esteves SC, Hamada A, Kondray V, Pitchika A, Agarwal A. What every gynecologist should know about male infertility: an update. Arch Gynecol Obstet. 2012;286:217–29.
Esteves SC, Lee W, Benjamin DJ, Seol B, Verza Jr A, Agarwal A. Reproductive potential including neonatal outcomes of men with obstructive azoospermia undergoing percutaneous sperm retrieval and intracytoplasmic sperm injection according to the cause of obstruction. J Urol. 2013a;189:232–7.
Esteves SC, Miyaoka R, Agarwal A. An update on the clinical assessment of the infertile male. Clinics (Sao Paulo). 2011a;66:691–700.
Esteves SC, Miyaoka R, Agarwal A. Sperm retrieval techniques for assisted reproduction. Int Braz J Urol. 2011b;37:570–83.
Esteves SC, Miyaoka R, Orosz JE, Agarwal A. An update on sperm retrieval techniques for azoospermic males. Clinics (Sao Paulo). 2013b;68 Suppl 1:99–110.
Esteves SC, Prudencio C, Seol B, Verza S, Knoedler C, Agarwal A. Comparison of sperm retrieval and reproductive outcome in azoospermic men with testicular failure and obstructive azoospermia treated for infertility. Asian J Androl. 2014;16:602–6.
Esteves SC, Varghese AC. Laboratory handling of epididymal and testicular spermatozoa: what can be done to improve sperm injections outcome. J Hum Reprod Sci. 2012;5:233–43.
Esteves SC, Verza Jr S. PESA/TESA/TESE sperm processing. In: Nagy ZP, Varghese AC, Agarwal A, editors. Practical manual of in vitro fertilization. New York: Springer; 2012. p. 207–20.
Esteves SC, Verza S, Prudencio C, Seol B. Sperm retrieval rates (SRR) in nonobstructive azoospermia (NOA) are related to testicular histopathology results but not to the etiology of azoospermia. Fertil Steril. 2010;94(Suppl):S132. (abstract).
Esteves SC. Microdissection testicular sperm extraction (micro-TESE) as a sperm acquisition method for men with nonobstructive azoospermia seeking fertility: operative and laboratory aspects. Int Braz J Urol. 2013;39:440–1.
Fedder J, Gabrielsen A, Humaidan P, Erb K, Ernst E, Loft A. Malformation rate and sex ratio in 412 children conceived with epididymal or testicular sperm. Hum Reprod. 2007;22:1080–5.
Foresta C, Bettella A, Spolaore D, Merico M, Rossato M, Ferlin A. Suppression of the high endogenous levels of plasma FSH in infertile men are associated with improved Sertoli cell function as reflected by elevated levels of plasma inhibin B. Hum Reprod. 2004;19:1431–7.
Fraietta R, Zylberstejn DS, Esteves SC. Hypogonadotropic hypogonadism revisited. Clinics (Sao Paulo). 2013;68 Suppl 1:81–8.
Griswold MD. Perspective on the function of Sertoli cells. In: Skinner MK, Griswold MD, editors. Sertoli Cell Biology. San Diego: Elsevier Science. 2005. p. 15–8.
Gudeloglu A, Parekattil SJ. Update in the evaluation of the azoospermic male. Clinics (Sao Paulo). 2013;68 Suppl 1:27–34.
Hamada A, Esteves SC, Agarwal A. A comprehensive review of genetics and genetic testing in azoospermia. Clinics (Sao Paulo). 2013;68 Suppl 1:39–60.

Hammoud A, Carrell DT, Meikle AW, Xin Y, Hunt SC, Adams TD, Gibson M. An aromatase polymorphism modulates the relationship between weight and estradiol levels in obese men. Fertil Steril. 2010;94:1734–8.

Haydardedeoglu B, Turunc T, Kilicdag EB, Gul U, Bagis T. The effect of prior varicocelectomy in patients with nonobstructive azoospermia on intracytoplasmic sperm injection outcomes: a retrospective pilot study. Urology. 2010;75:83–6.

He X, Cao Y, Zhang Z, Zhao J, Wei Z, Zhao J, Wei Z, Zhou P, Cong L. Spermatogenesis affects the outcome of ICSI for azoospermic patients rather than sperm retrieval method. Syst Biol Reprod Med. 2010;56:457–64.

Hopps CV, Mielnik A, Goldstein M, Palermo GD, Rosenwaks Z, Schlegel PN. Detection of sperm in men with Y chromosome microdeletions of the AZFa, AZFb and AZFc regions. Hum Reprod. 2003;18:1660–5.

Hung AJ, King P, Schlegel PN. Uniform testicular maturation arrest: a unique subset of men with non-obstructive azoospermia. J Urol. 2007;178:608–12.

Hussein A, Ozgok Y, Ross L, Rao P, Niederberger C. Optimization of spermatogenesis-regulating hormones in patients with non-obstructive azoospermia and its impact on sperm retrieval: a multicentre study. BJU Int. 2013;111(3, pt B):E110–4.

Inci K, Hascicek M, Kara O, Dikmen AV, Gurgan T, Ergen A. Sperm retrieval and intracytoplasmic sperm injection in men with nonobstructive azoospermia, and treated and untreated varicocele. J Urol. 2009;182:1500–5.

Isidori AM, Caprio M, Strollo F, Moretti C, Frajese G, Isidori A, Fabbri A. Leptin and androgens in male obesity: evidence for leptin contribution to reduced androgen levels. J Clin Endocrinol Metab. 1999;84:3673–80.

Jaffe TM, Kim ED, Hoekstra TH, Lipshultz LI. Sperm pellet analysis: a technique to detect the presence of sperm in men considered to have azoospermia by routine semen analysis. J Urol. 1998;159:1548–50.

Jarow JP, Chen H, Rosner TW, Trentacoste S, Zirkin BR. Assessment of the androgen environment within the human testis: minimally invasive method to obtain intratesticular fluid. J Androl. 2001;22:640–5.

Kamischke A, Gromoll J, Simoni M, Behre HM, Nieschlag E. Transmission of a Y chromosomal deletion involving the deleted in azoospermia (DAZ) and chromodomain (CDY1) genes from father to son through intracytoplasmic sperm injection: case report. Hum Reprod. 1999;14: 2320–2.

Kato Y, Shiraishi K, Matsuyama H. Expression of testicular androgen receptor in non-obstructive azoospermia and its change after hormonal therapy. Andrologia. 2014;2(5):734–40. doi:10.11 11/j.2047-2927.2014.00240.

Keel BA. Within- and between-subject variation in semen parameters in infertile men and normal semen donors. Fertil Steril. 2006;85:128–34.

Keenan DM, Veldhuis JD. Divergent gonadotropin-gonadal dose-responsive coupling in healthy young and aging men. Am J Physiol. 2004;286:R381–9.

Kent-First MG, Kol S, Muallem A, Ofir R, Manor D, Blazer S, First N, Itskovitz-Eldor J. The incidence and possible relevance of Y-linked microdeletions in babies born after intracytoplasmic sperm injection and their infertile fathers. Mol Hum Reprod. 1996;2:943–50.

Kleiman SE, Almog R, Yogev L, Hauser R, Lehavi O, Paz G, Yavetz H, Botchan A. Screening for partial AZFa microdeletions in the Y chromosome of infertile men: is it of clinical relevance? Fertil Steril. 2012;98:43–7.

Kleiman SE, Yogev L, Lehavi O, Hauser R, Botchan A, Paz G, Yavetz H, Gamzu R. The likelihood of finding mature sperm cells in men with AZFb or AZFb-c deletions: six new cases and a review of the literature (1994–2010). Fertil Steril. 2011;95:2005–12.

Krausz C, Hoefsloot L, Simoni M, Tüttelmann F. EAA/EMQN best practice guidelines for molecular diagnosis of Y-chromosomal microdeletions: state-of-the-art 2013. Andrology. 2014;2:5–19.

Krausz C, Quintana-Murci L, Barbaux S, Siffroi JP, Rouba H, Delafontaine D, Souleyreau-Therville N, Arvis G, Antoine JM, Erdei E, Taar JP, Tar A, Jeandidier E, Plessis G, Bourgeron T, Dadoune JP, Fellous M, McElreavey K. A high frequency of Y chromosome deletions in males with nonidiopathic infertility. J Clin Endocrinol Metab. 1999;84:3606–12.

Krausz C, Quintana-Murci L, McElreavey K. Prognostic value of Y deletion analysis: what is the clinical prognostic value of Y chromosome microdeletion analysis? Hum Reprod. 2000;15:1431–4.

Kumar R. Medical management of non-obstructive azoospermia. Clinics (Sao Paulo). 2013;68 Suppl 1:75–9.

Kumar M, Kumar K, Jain S, Hassan T, Dada R. Novel insights into the genetic and epigenetic paternal contribution to the human embryo. Clinics (Sao Paulo). 2013;68 Suppl 1:5–14.

Leão RB, Esteves SC. Gonadotropin therapy in assisted reproduction: an evolutionary perspective from biologics to biotech. Clinics (Sao Paulo). 2014;69:279–93.

Longepied G, Saut N, Aknin-Seifer I, Levy R, Frances AM, Metzler-Guillemain C, Guichaoua MR, Mitchell MJ. Complete deletion of the AZFb interval from the Y chromosome in an oligozoospermic man. Hum Reprod. 2010;25:2655–63.

Matthiesson KL, MnLachlan RI, O'Donnell L, Frydenberg M, Robertson DM, Stanton PG, Meachem SJ. The relative roles of follicle-stimulating hormone and luteinizing hormone in maintaining spermatogonial maturation and spermiation in normal men. J Clin Endocrinol Metab. 2006;91:3962–9.

McLachlan RI, O'Donnell L, Meachem SJ, Stanton PG, de Kretser DM, Pratis K, Robertson DM. Identification of specific sites of hormonal regulation in spermatogenesis in rats, monkeys, and man. Recent Prog Horm Res. 2002;57:149–79.

Meseguer M, Santiso R, Garrido N, Gil-Salom M, Remohí J, Fernandez JL. Sperm DNA fragmentation levels in testicular sperm samples from azoospermic males as assessed by the sperm chromatin dispersion test. Fertil Steril. 2009;92:1638–45.

Mitra A, Dada R, Kumar R, Gupta NP, Kucheria K, Gupta SK. Y chromosome microdeletions in azoospermic patients with Klinefelter's syndrome. Asian J Androl. 2006;8:81–8.

Miyaoka R, Esteves SC. A critical appraisal on the role of varicocele in male infertility. Adv Urol. 2012;2012:597495.

Mulhall JP, Reijo R, Alagappan R, Brown L, Page D, Carson R, Oates RD. Azoospermic men with deletion of the DAZ gene cluster are capable of completing spermatogenesis: fertilization, normal embryonic development and pregnancy occur when retrieved testicular spermatozoa are used for intracytoplasmic sperm injection. Hum Reprod. 1997;12:50–8.

Navarro-Costa P, Plancha CE, Gonçalves J. Genetic dissection of the AZF regions of the human Y chromosome: thriller or filler for male (in)fertility? J Biomed Biotechnol. 2010;2010:936569.

Oates RD, Silber S, Brown LG, Page DC. Clinical characterization of 42 oligospermic or azoospermic men with microdeletion of the AZFc region of the Y chromosome, and of 18 children conceived via ICSI. Hum Reprod. 2002;17:2813–24.

Okada H, Dobashi M, Yamazaki T, Hara I, Fujisawa M, Arakawa S, Kamidono S. Conventional versus microdissection testicular sperm extraction for nonobstructive azoospermia. J Urol. 2002;168:1063–7.

O'Shaughnessy PJ, Verhoeven G, De Gendt K, Monteiro A, Abel MH. Direct action through the Sertoli cells is essential for androgen stimulation of spermatogenesis. Endocrinology. 2010;15:2343–8.

Ozkavukcu S, Ibis E, Kizil S, Isbacar S, Aydos K. A laboratory modification to testicular sperm preparation technique improves spermatogenic cell yield. Asian J Androl. 2014;16(6):852–7. doi:10.4103/1008-682X.132468.

Palermo GD, Schlegel PN, Hariprashad JJ, Ergün B, Mielnik A, Veeck LL, Rosenwaks Z. Fertilization and pregnancy outcome with intracytoplasmic sperm injection for azoospermic men. Hum Reprod. 1999;14:741–8.

Patsalis PC, Sismani C, Quintana-Murci L, Taleb-Bekkouche F, Krausz C, McElreavey K. Effects of transmission of Y chromosome AZFc deletions. Lancet. 2000;360:1222–4.

Pavlovich CP, King P, Goldstein M, Schlegel PN. Evidence of a treatable endocrinopathy in infertile men. J Urol. 2001;165:837–41.

Peterlin B, Kunej T, Sinkovec J, Gligorievska N, Zorn B. Screening for Y chromosome microdeletions in 226 Slovenian subfertile men. Hum Reprod. 2002;17:17–24.

Popal W, Nagy ZP. Laboratory processing and intracytoplasmic sperm injection using epididymal and testicular spermatozoa: what can be done to improve outcomes? Clinics (Sao Paulo). 2013;68 Suppl 1:125–30.

Quigley CA, de Bellis A, Marschke KB, El-Awady MK, Wilson EM, French FS. Androgen receptor defects: historical, clinical and molecular perspectives. Endocr Rev. 1995;16:271–321.

Rajpert-De Meyts E, Ottesen AM, Garn ID, Aksglaede L, Juul A. Deletions of the Y chromosome are associated with sex chromosome aneuploidy but not with Klinefelter syndrome. Acta Paed. 2011;100:900–2.

Raman JD, Schlegel PN. Testicular sperm extraction with intracytoplasmic sperm injection is successful for the treatment of nonobstructive azoospermia associated with cryptorchidism. J Urol. 2003;170:1287–90.

Ramasamy R, Ricci JA, Palermo GD, Gosden LV, Rosenwaks Z, Schlegel PN. Successful fertility treatment for Klinefelter's syndrome. J Urol. 2009;182:1108–13.

Ramasamy R, Stahl PJ, Schlegel PN. Medical therapy for spermatogenic failure. Asian J Androl. 2012;14:57–60.

Ramasamy R, Yagan N, Schlegel PN. Structural and functional changes to the testis after conventional versus microdissection testicular sperm extraction. Urology. 2005;65:1190–4.

Reifsnyder JE, Ramasamy R, Husseini J, Schlegel PN. Role of optimizing testosterone before microdissection testicular sperm extraction in men with nonobstructive azoospermia. J Urol. 2012;188:532–6.

Repping S, Skaletsky H, Lange J, Silber S, Van Der Veen F, Oates RD, Page DC, Rozen S. Recombination between palindromes P5 and P1 on the human Y chromosome causes massive deletions and spermatogenic failure. Am J Hum Genet. 2002;71:906–22.

Sato T, Katagiri K, Gohbara A, Inoue K, Ogonuki N, Ogura A, Kubota Y, Ogawa T. In vitro production of functional sperm in cultured neonatal mouse testes. Nature. 2011;471:504–7.

Schiff JD, Palermo GD, Veeck LL, Goldstein M, Rosenwaks Z, Schlegel PN. Success of testicular sperm extraction [corrected] and intracytoplasmic sperm injection in men with Klinefelter syndrome. J Clin Endocrinol Metab. 2005;90(6263). Erratum in: J Clin Endocrinol Metab, 2006. 91:4027.

Shinjo E, Shiraishi K, Matsuyama H. The effect of human chorionic gonadotropin-based hormonal therapy on intratesticular testosterone levels and spermatogonial DNA synthesis in men with non-obstructive azoospermia. Andrology. 2013;1:929–35.

Schlegel PN, Kaufmann J. Role of varicocelectomy in men with nonobstructive azoospermia. Fertil Steril. 2004;81:1585–8.

Schlegel PN, Su LM. Physiological consequences of testicular sperm extraction. Hum Reprod. 1997;12:1688–92.

Schlegel PN. Testicular sperm extraction: microdissection improves sperm yield with minimal tissue excision. Hum Reprod. 1999;14:131–5.

Siffroi JP, Le Bourhis C, Krausz C, Barbaux S, Quintana-Murci L, Kanafani S, Rouba H, Bujan L, Bourrouillou G, Seifer I, Boucher D, Fellous M, McElreavey K, Dadoune JP. Sex chromosome mosaicism in males carrying Y chromosome long arm deletions. Hum Reprod. 2000;15:2559–62.

Silber SJ. Microsurgical TESE and the distribution of spermatogenesis in non-obstructive azoospermia. Hum Reprod. 2000;15:2278–84.

Simoni M, Tuttelmann F, Gromoll J, Nieschlag E. Clinical consequences of microdeletions of the Y chromosome: the extended Munster experience. Reprod Biomed Online. 2008;16:289–303.

Soares AR, Costa P, Silva J, Sousa M, Barros A, Fernandes S. AZFb microdeletions and oligozoospermia–which mechanisms? Fertil Steril. 2012;97:858–63.

Shiraishi K, Ohmi C, Shimabukuro T, Matsuyama H. Human chorionic gonadotrophin treatment prior to microdissection testicular sperm extraction in non-obstructive azoospermia. Hum Reprod. 2012;27:331–9.

Sokol RZ, Swerdloff RS. Endocrine evaluation. In: Lipshultz LI, Howards SS, editors. Infertility in the male. 3rd ed. New York: Churchill Livingstone; 1997. p. 210–8.

Spratt DI, Carr DB, Merriam GR, Scully RE, Rao PN, Crowley Jr WF. The spectrum of abnormal patterns of gonadotropin-releasing hormone secretion in men with idiopathic hypogonadotropic hypogonadism: clinical and laboratory correlations. J Clin Endocrinol Metab. 1987;64:283–91.

Stahl PJ, Masson P, Mielnik A, Marean MB, Schlegel PN, Paduch DA. A decade of experience emphasizes that testing for Y microdeletions is essential in American men with azoospermia and severe oligozoospermia. Fertil Steril. 2010;94:1753–6.

Strain G, Zumoff B, Rosner W, Pi-Sunyer X. The relationship between serum levels of insulin and sex hormone-binding globulin in men: the effect of weight loss. J Clin Endocrinol Metab. 1994;9:1173–6.

Sussman EM, Chudnovsky A, Niederberger CS. Hormonal evaluation of the infertile male: has it evolved? Urol Clin North Am. 2008;35:147–55.

Tchernof A, Despres JP, Belanger A, Dupont A, Prud'homme D, Moorjani S, et al. Reduced testosterone and adrenal C19 steroid levels in obese men. Metabolism. 1995;44:513–9.

Tournaye H, Verheyen G, Nagy P, Ubaldi F, Goossens A, Silber S, Van Steirteghem AC, Devroey P. Are there any predictive factors for successful testicular sperm recovery in azoospermic patients? Hum Reprod. 1997;12:80–6.

Tsujimura A. Microdissection testicular sperm extraction: prediction, outcome, and complications. Int J Urol. 2007;14:883–9.

Tyler-Smith C, Krausz C. The will-o'-the-wisp of genetics hunting for the azoospermia factor gene. N Engl J Med. 2009;360:925–7.

van Golde RJ, Wetzels AM, de Graaf R, Tuerlings JH, Braat DD, Kremer JA. Decreased fertilization rate and embryo quality after ICSI in oligozoospermic men with microdeletions in the azoospermia factor c region of the Y chromosome. Hum Reprod. 2001;16:289–92.

Vernaeve V, Bonduelle M, Tournaye H, Camus M, Van Steirteghem A, Devroey P. Pregnancy outcome and neonatal data of children born after ICSI using testicular sperm in obstructive and non-obstructive azoospermia. Hum Reprod. 2003;18:2093–7.

Verza Jr S, Esteves SC. Sperm defect severity rather than sperm source is associated with lower fertilization rates after intracytoplasmic sperm injection. Int Braz J Urol. 2008;34:49–56.

Verza Jr S, Esteves SC. Microsurgical versus conventional single-biopsy testicular sperm extraction in nonobstructive azoospermia: a prospective controlled study. Fertil Steril. 2011; 96(Suppl):S53. (abstract).

Vloeberghs V, Verheyen G, Tournaye H. Intracytoplasmic spermatid injection and in vitro maturation: fact or fiction? Clinics (Sao Paulo). 2013;68 Suppl 1:151–6.

Vogt PH, Bender U. Human Y chromosome microdeletion analysis by PCR multiplex protocols identifying only clinically relevant. AZF microdeletions. Methods Mol Biol. 2013;927:187–204.

Vozdova M, Heracek J, Sobotka V, Rubes J. Testicular sperm aneuploidy in non-obstructive azoospermic patients. Hum Reprod. 2012;27:2233–9.

Weedin JW, Khera M, Lipshultz LI. Varicocele repair in patients with nonobstructive azoospermia: a meta-analysis. J Urol. 2010;183:2309–15.

Wistuba J, Luetjens CM, Stukenborg JB, Poplinski A, Werler S, Dittmann M, Damm OS, Hamalainen T, Simoni M, Gromoll J. Male 421, XX^{Y}mice as a model for Klinefelter syndrome: hyperactivation of Leydig cells. Endocrinology. 2010;151:2898–910.

World Health Organization. WHO manual for the standardised investigation and diagnosis of the infertile male. Cambridge: Cambridge University Press; 2000.

Management of Infertility in Klinefelter Syndrome

8

Ranjith Ramasamy and Affan Zafar

8.1 Introduction

Klinefelter syndrome (KS) is the most common genetic cause of primary hypogonadism in males. Chromosome analysis of most individuals with KS shows a chromosome pattern of 47,XXY; the extra X chromosome causes the clinical and pathological manifestations of the disorder. About 20 % of KS individuals have a different sex chromosome aneuploidy, 48,XXXY, for example, or are genetic mosaics, and only some of their cells have a Klinefelter karyotype (Tuttelmann and Gromoll 2010; Maiburg et al. 2012). The phenotype of mosaic individuals is mild and depends on the percentage of cells which have the Klinefelter karyotype; most individuals are never diagnosed with the syndrome (Fruhmesser and Kotzot 2011). The hallmarks of the syndrome include small testes, gynecomastia, elevated gonadotropins, and azoospermia (Klinefelter et al. 1942). Less than 10 % of KS males are diagnosed before puberty; the most common presentation is an adult who experiences infertility (Bojesen et al. 2003). The prevalence of KS is about 1 in 600 males, corresponding to approximately 544,000 people in the United States and making it the most common sex chromosome abnormality (Nielsen and Wohlert 1990). The prevalence has increased in recent years for unknown reasons. It is known that the increase cannot be attributed to improved technology alone because the prevalence of other anomalous sex chromosome disorders has not increased similarly (Morris et al. 2008). The management of KS has a significant impact on the healthcare system; treatment of hypogonadism can cost over $1000 per year for hormone replacement in addition to expensive diagnostic tests and biopsies (Maggi et al. 2007).

R. Ramasamy, MD (✉)
Baylor College of Medicine, 1150 Northwest 14th Street 309, Miami, FL 33136, USA
e-mail: ranjithrama@gmail.com

A. Zafar, BS
Department of Urology, University of Miami, Miami, FL, USA

K. Gunasekaran, N. Pandiyan (eds.), *Male Infertility*,
DOI 10.1007/978-81-322-3604-7_8

Comorbidities, such as cardiovascular problems, also require management and increase the financial burden on patients.

Healthcare practitioners do not accurately diagnose KS adolescents. One study screened newborns in Denmark for KS and found that the condition is much more common than previously thought. The actual diagnosis of KS is made in only about 25 % of cases when compared to the prevalence of the condition found in this study (Groth et al. 2013). This statistic has sparked a debate over screening of newborns for the syndrome. Experts in favor of screening argue that early diagnosis would allow appropriate management of the comorbidities and early planning for fertility options for the adult years. Additionally, since currently only 25 % of KS individuals are diagnosed, screening would expand care to the remaining 75 % of patients. Those against newborn screening comment that early interventions for KS have not been studied well enough and may not be cost effective. According to the World Health Organization (WHO) public health screening principles, general screening should be implemented for a disease if it poses an important health problem, has a latent early symptomatic stage, and a well-understood natural history and if diagnostic and treatment modalities are available, if a suitable diagnostic test is available, and if that test is cost effective (Wilson and Jungner 1968). Two tests are available for newborn screening of KS. The Barr body analysis has fallen out of favor and is rarely used; however, it is a relatively inexpensive potential option. It is 82 % sensitive and 95 % specific for detecting a Klinefelter chromosome abnormality (Kamischke et al. 2003). Implementing this older test for newborn screening would drastically improve physicians' ability to screen for KS. Karyotyping is now the test of choice for KS because of its 100 % sensitivity and specificity; however, it is more time consuming and expensive (Hager et al. 2012). KS is a relatively common disorder; much is known about the disease process; accurate and cheap tests exist, and evidence is starting to build in favor of early management, as will be discussed later in the chapter. In addition, in the United States screening is performed in newborns for many genetic disorders that are much less common than KS. An example is phenylketonuria (PKU), which has an incidence of 1 in 10,000 (Williams et al. 2008). Since KS meets the WHO principles, screening for KS should be strongly considered by physicians and healthcare policy makers. It is imperative that clinicians be knowledgeable about Klinefelter syndrome, especially those who specialize in adolescent and reproductive medicine.

8.2 Disease Progression of Klinefelter Syndrome

Typically, a KS patient is a 25-year-old male with a tall stature, long legs, short trunk, small testes, gynecomastia, and little facial/body hair who complains of symptoms of androgen deficiency and infertility. It is important to keep in mind that not every patient has all of these characteristics and sometimes the phenotype can be indistinguishable from an individual with a normal karyotype. It is difficult to distinguish a Klinefelter patient from any other boy on the basis of appearance alone, and most pass through puberty with only mild symptoms. Children with KS have normal levels of follicle-stimulating hormone (FSH), luteinizing hormone

Table 8.1 Pubertal stage-related serum gonadotropin and gonadal steroid concentrations in boys with a 47,XXY karyotype compared to control siblings

Pubertal stage	Subjects	*n*	FSH (μg/dl)	LH (μg/dl)	T (ng/dl)	E2 (ng/dl)
PH_1	47,XXY	40	8.0 (3.6–23.0)	2.5 (1.3–6.7)	14 (<10–135)	1.0 (<1.0–6.5)
	Controls	14	9.2 (2.7–30.0)	2.5 (1.5–5.1)	11 (<10–145)	1.0 (<1.0–2.0)
PH_2	47,XXY	6	42.5 (15.0–150)*	5.4 (1.1–19.0)	69 (<10–115)	2.2 (<1.0–4.6)**
	Controls	9	11.0 (6.1–16.0)	2.5 (2.1–4.8)	15 (<10–110)	1.0 (<1.0–2.2)
PH_{3-5}	47,XXY	18	150 (44.5–264)***	24.0 (7.0–63.0)***	367 (92–566)	3.2 (<1.0–7.4)
	Controls	8	22.5 (10.0–35.0)	5.7 (2.5–8.4)	316 (31–462)	3.0 (1.9–5.6)

Adapted from Salbenblatt et al. (1985)

Values are median with the range in parentheses. To reduce sampling frequency bias, no more than one specimen was included from each subject per year. Pubertal stage was assigned according to pubic hair development. Differences between 47,XXY subjects and control siblings were calculated with a two-tailed Mann-Whitney test and are significant where indicated with *p=0.003, **p<0.05, and ***p <0.001

Table 8.2 Sertoli and Leydig cell dysfunction during puberty in males with KS (Wikstrom et al. 2007)

	Control adolescent	KS adolescent
AMH	Intermediate production	Decreased
Androgen receptors on Sertoli cells	Normal	Decreased
Leydig cells	Few, normal testosterone production	Hyperplasia, low testosterone production

(LH), testosterone, and estradiol before puberty, and germ cells are seen in the testes by histology. The average age at puberty is the same as that of other individuals.

There are several differences between individuals with KS and the general population with regard to the progression of puberty. In males with KS, serum levels of FSH, LH, testosterone, and estradiol are significantly higher and at an earlier age than in normal controls (Table 8.1). The testes stop growing in mid-puberty in males with KS and do not ever reach normal size (Salbenblatt et al. 1985). Germ cells during puberty differentiate to the spermatogonium stage only; virtually no mature spermatozoa are present in the testes. By the end of puberty, few or no germ cells remain. Only a few seminiferous tubules with complete spermatogenesis can be seen, and most tubules are fibrosed with hyalinization. Degeneration of testicular function and eventual androgen deficiency are seen at a cellular and biochemical level as well. As puberty progresses in a KS male, there is evidence of Sertoli and Leydig cell dysfunction. Sertoli cell malfunction is marked by decreased production of anti-Mullerian hormone (AMH, regulates sex hormone production) and decreased androgen receptors on the Sertoli cell when compared with normal controls. Leydig cell dysfunction is marked by hyperplasia of the cells and inadequate testosterone production; in contrast, controls have fewer Leydig cells and normal levels of testosterone (Table 8.2). (Wikstrom et al. 2007).

Due to the gonadal dysfunction that occurs during puberty, individuals with KS have several manifestations of androgen deficiency. The testes are small and firm, about 4 mL in males with KS as compared to 20 mL in eugonadal males (Corona et al. 2010). Male-pattern body hair is sparse. Sexual problems include lack of libido and erectile dysfunction, which affect 70 % of KS males over the age of 25. Infertility is another sexual problem and is the most common reason for presentation and eventual diagnosis of KS. Of affected males, 90 % are shown to be azoospermic on semen analysis, and no sperm are found on examination of the centrifuged semen sediment. The remaining 10 % have oligoasthenoteratozoospermia, meaning few sperm exist on semen analysis, and some or all spermatozoa have abnormal motility and morphology (Bojesen et al. 2011).

Briefly, Klinefelter syndrome and androgen deficiency have other manifestations that affect an individual's overall health. The imbalance of estrogen and low testosterone give rise to various problems. KS patients typically develop some degree of gynecomastia and have a slightly increased risk of male breast cancer. They also have an increased propensity to form blood clots and varicose veins and are at higher risk of musculoskeletal pain, osteoporosis, and hip fractures. Central obesity, diabetes mellitus type 2, and the metabolic syndrome become concerning as men with KS begin to age (Kamischke et al. 2003). Typical neurological and psychosocial features are also associated with the syndrome. A higher risk of epilepsy exists, and patients often have cognitive difficulties, legasthenia (inability to formulate words from letters), learning problems, and trouble socializing.

The life expectancy is 11.5 years less than that of the general male population (Bojesen et al. 2011). Although testosterone deficiency would seem to be the major player, early death cannot be attributed to this alone (Nieschlag et al. 1993). Early diagnosis of KS is important so that interventions can be initiated to mitigate the risks posed by the comorbid conditions (Swerdlow et al. 2005; Nieschlag 2013). This chapter seeks to explore management options for fertility and overall health in males with KS, from adolescence to adulthood.

8.3 Management of the KS Adolescent

In earlier years, patients with KS were thought to have lifelong infertility. Due to advances in technology, it is now well established that these individuals can have isolated foci of spermatogenesis in the testis, and when sperm are extracted and injected into an egg, KS patients can conceive a biological child (Aksglaede and Juul 2013). Management now focuses on preserving fertility, but there is debate about how best to accomplish this goal as there have been no good controlled studies of adolescent males with KS. *The choice boils down to one of three options: expectantly manage until the patient reaches adulthood and desires fertility, initiate medical treatment in adolescence and defer invasive biopsy until fertility is desired, or biopsy in adolescence with cryopreservation of sperm for future use.*

Once the clinical features of KS are observed in an adolescent and the diagnosis is confirmed by karyotype, the question to be answered is whether the hypogonadism is symptomatic. The symptoms of low testosterone include fatigue, difficulty gaining muscle mass, trouble concentrating, and delayed secondary sex characteristics. A serum total testosterone level should be measured, and if it is less than 300 ng/dL on a morning blood draw, the diagnosis of male hypogonadism can be made, and the patient can begin testosterone supplementation therapy. The immediate goals for testosterone therapy are to promote secondary sex characteristics and stimulate linear growth, bone development, and muscle bulk. Long-term goals include possible augmentation of the disease process so that the cardiovascular, metabolic, and psychosocial features are less severe. Research has been published which recommends hormone therapy in adolescents with KS; however, there have been no controlled studies to determine the effect of testosterone supplementation on the progression of puberty (Bojesen and Gravholt 2007, Rogol and Tartaglia 2010). The method of application and dose of testosterone should be discussed with the patient, combining the clinician's expertise and patient preference. Testosterone supplementation has side effects, as does any medication, and these should be discussed with the patient; however, the potential benefit of initiating early therapy seems to outweigh the risk of adverse effects. The particular side effect of exogenous testosterone administration of concern in a patient with KS is inhibition of already low testicular function, specifically spermatogenesis. Some cite this as an argument against administering testosterone therapy, since the effect on fertility is important to consider in this disorder (de Souza and Hallak 2011). In fact, a history of testosterone therapy is associated with a decreased sperm retrieval rate during microdissection testicular sperm extraction (TESE) in the general male population (Schiff et al. 2005, Ramasamy et al. 2009). However, men without KS who received human chorionic gonadotropin (hCG) in addition to testosterone therapy had no difference in semen parameters between their initial semen samples and samples obtained after 1 year of therapy (Hsieh et al. 2013). HCG is a luteinizing hormone (LH) analog and stimulates endogenous testosterone production and other testicular functions (Coviello et al. 2005). The drug is generally well tolerated and has few side effects. The drawbacks of using hCG are that it is expensive and it requires injections in addition to administration of testosterone. Thus, for an adolescent with KS and symptomatic hypogonadism, it is best to initiate testosterone supplementation therapy and hCG to prevent the comorbidities of the disorder while preserving testicular function. Clomiphene and anastrazole are other adjuncts to testosterone supplementation for preserving fertility and endogenous testicular function, but they have not been thoroughly studied for this specific use (Moskovic et al. 2012, Burnett-Bowie et al. 2008). Some experts still argue against initiating any therapy before fertility is desired, thus additional clinical trials are required to determine the best management plan for adolescent patients with KS.

Cryopreservation should be considered in this population only when mature and viable sperm are found on an ejaculated specimen. Obtaining mature sperm or germ cells by TESE followed by cryopreservation is not recommended for the adolescent with KS for several reasons. Since sperm retrieval rates are relatively high in KS adults, at least equal to those of men with other causes of nonobstructive azoospermia, there is no advantage in performing the procedure on an adolescent, especially since he may be unsure of desiring fertility in the future (Vernaeve et al. 2004). Moreover, the procedure could have a negative impact on testicular function. In a

KS patient, the chance of finding viable germ cells in normal seminiferous tubules is low, and multiple biopsies would likely be required. After any TESE, serum testosterone levels decrease and do not reach preprocedure levels even a year later (Okada et al. 2004). In addition, the seminiferous tubule volume decreases in the testicular parenchyma around the biopsy site, and the number of germ cells per tubule decreases (Tash and Schlegel 2001).

Experimental options are on the horizon for adolescent males with KS who desire to preserve fertility. Preservation of spermatogonial stem cells (SSC) is one such option. Although only experimental at this point, transplantation of SSC into a fibrosed adult KS testis for in vitro maturation may become a therapeutic option in the future.

In summary, the adolescent KS patient with symptoms of hypogonadism and a serum testosterone level less than 300 ng/dL should receive testosterone supplementation therapy with concurrent hCG. Further management should be delayed until the patient desires fertility (Fig. 8.1). *Further controlled studies are needed in this population to optimize the management of the syndrome.*

8.4 Management of Fertility in KS Adults

The management of adults with KS is more straightforward because it is centered on achieving fertility and has numerous studies to guide management. The treatment focuses on optimizing testicular function, obtaining sperm via biopsy, and utilizing intracytoplasmic sperm injection (ICSI) to obtain a pregnancy. ICSI involves injection of a single sperm into the cytoplasm of the oocyte. Afterward, the oocyte is placed in cell culture and checked for signs of fertilization. If fertilization is successful, it is implanted into the female's uterus.

In an adult KS patient desiring fertility, testosterone supplementation therapy should be suspended, and a serum testosterone level should be measured after 6 months. Men with levels less than 300 ng/dL should be treated with anastrazole for 2–3 months because patients with KS have low testosterone levels and are associated with a low testosterone-to-estradiol ratio (Mehta et al. 2012). Anastrazole is an aromatase inhibitor that increases the testosterone-to-estradiol ratio and also increases sperm concentration and motility (Raman and Schlegel 2002). Men who do not respond to anastrazole therapy with a normal testosterone level after 1 month should also be treated with hCG injections. HCG is analogous to luteinizing hormone which improves intratesticular testosterone levels and semen quality parameters (Hussein et al. 2013, Schill et al. 1982, Miyagawa et al. 2005).

After medical treatment, or if the serum testosterone is normal, microdissection TESE should be performed. Sperm is retrieved in 68 % of attempts in males with KS, a rate which is comparable to or better than the success rate in non-KS men with nonobstructive azoospermia. Studies show that normal baseline testosterone is predictive of a successful TESE; 86 % of attempts were successful in this subgroup. In patients whose testosterone level normalized after 2 months of medical therapy,

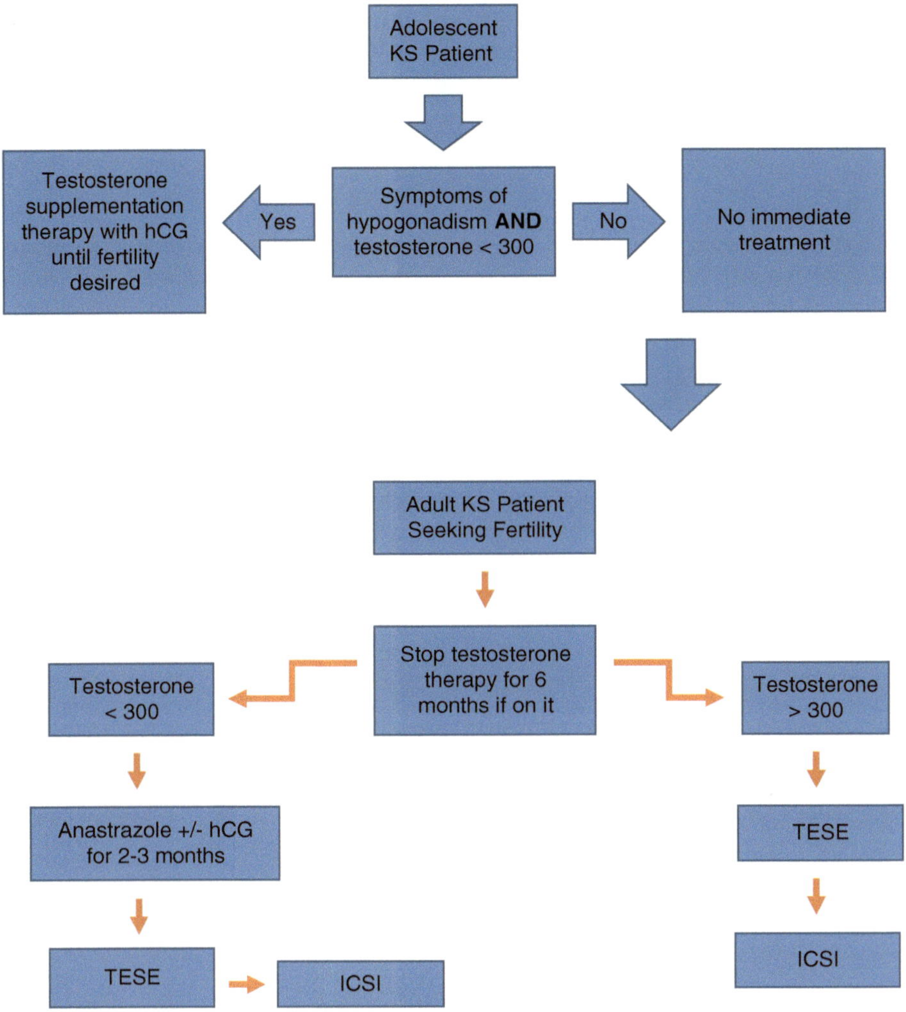

Fig. 8.1 Management of infertility in KS

77 % of attempts were successful. A low testosterone level after medical therapy was the least favorable; sperm was obtained in only 55 % of TESE attempts (Ramasamy et al. 2009).

With the sperm obtained from micro-TESE, the couple can proceed to intracytoplasmic sperm injection (ICSI). ICSI is well established as a fertility option for many types of male-factor infertility issues including nonmosaic KS (Palermo et al. 1998). In those men who successfully undergo sperm retrieval, 57 % are able to obtain a clinical pregnancy by utilizing ICSI and 45 % of those pregnancies progress to live births (Ramasamy et al. 2009). After TESE, resumption of testosterone supplementation therapy should be considered.

In summary, for an adult KS patient seeking to father a child, testosterone therapy should be suspended for 6 months. Then, if the testosterone level is less than 300 ng/dL, the patient should receive medical therapy with anastrazole ± hCG for 2–3 months. Afterward, or if the testosterone level is normal, a micro-TESE followed by ICSI should be performed (Fig. 8.1).

Conclusion

The best management of KS in adolescents is still not established and requires further study. For patients receiving testosterone therapy, hormone levels should be checked regularly in order to optimize the dose of testosterone. Referral to a medical geneticist is warranted for discussion about the disorder. When parenthood is desired and after ICSI has been performed, a preimplantation genetic diagnosis should be offered to ensure the embryo which will be implanted does not have a Klinefelter karyotype. This procedure involves biopsy for genetic testing of a part of the embryo that is unnecessary, such as a polar body. Regular primary care follow-up should be ensured so patients can be screened and treated for the chronic comorbidities associated with KS. In addition to the infertility management, referral to a psychiatrist, psychologist, and social counselor should be considered to address the cognitive, learning, and psychosocial issues associated with Klinefelter syndrome.

References

Aksglaede L, Juul A. Testicular function and fertility in men with Klinefelter syndrome: a review. Eur J Endocrinol/Eur Fed Endocrine Soc. 2013;168(4):R67–76. doi:10.1530/eje-12-0934.

Bojesen A, Gravholt CH. Klinefelter syndrome in clinical practice. Nat Clin Pract Urol. 2007;4(4):192–204. doi:10.1038/ncpuro0775.

Bojesen A, Juul S, Gravholt CH. Prenatal and postnatal prevalence of Klinefelter syndrome: a national registry study. J Clin Endocrinol Metab. 2003;88(2):622–6. doi:10.1210/jc.2002-021491.

Bojesen A, Stochholm K, Juul S, Gravholt CH. Socioeconomic trajectories affect mortality in Klinefelter syndrome. J Clin Endocrinol Metab. 2011;96(7):2098–104. doi:10.1210/jc.2011-0367.

Burnett-Bowie SA, Roupenian KC, Dere ME, Lee H, Leder BZ. Effects of aromatase inhibition in hypogonadal older men: a randomized, double-blind, placebo-controlled trial. Clin Endocrinol (Oxf). 2008;70(1):116–23. doi:10.1111/j.1365-2265.2008.03327.x.

Corona G, Petrone L, Paggi F, Lotti F, Boddi V, Fisher A, Vignozzi L, Balercia G, Sforza A, Forti G, Mannucci E, Maggi M. Sexual dysfunction in subjects with Klinefelter's syndrome. Int J Androl. 2010;33(4):574–80. doi:10.1111/j.1365-2605.2009.00986.x.

Coviello AD, Matsumoto AM, Bremner WJ, Herbst KL, Amory JK, Anawalt BD, Sutton PR, Wright WW, Brown TR, Yan X, Zirkin BR, Jarow JP. Low-dose human chorionic gonadotropin maintains intratesticular testosterone in normal men with testosterone-induced gonadotropin suppression. J Clin Endocrinol Metab. 2005;90(5):2595–602. doi:10.1210/jc.2004-0802.

de Souza GL, Hallak J. Anabolic steroids and male infertility: a comprehensive review. BJU Int. 2011;108(11):1860–5. doi:10.1111/j.1464-410X.2011.10131.x.

Fruhmesser A, Kotzot D. Chromosomal variants in klinefelter syndrome. Sex Dev Genet Mol Biol Evol Endocrinol Embryol Pathol Sex Determination Differ. 2011;5(3):109–23. doi:10.1159/000327324.

Groth KA, Skakkebaek A, Host C, Gravholt CH, Bojesen A. Clinical review: Klinefelter syndrome–a clinical update. J Clin Endocrinol Metab. 2013;98(1):20–30. doi:10.1210/jc.2012-2382.

Hager K, Jennings K, Hosono S, Howell S, Gruen JR, Rivkees SA, Tartaglia NR, Rinder HM. Molecular diagnostic testing for Klinefelter syndrome and other male sex chromosome aneuploidies. Int J Pediatr Endocrinol. 2012;2012(1):8. doi:10.1186/1687-9856-2012-8.

Hsieh TC, Pastuszak AW, Hwang K, Lipshultz LI. Concomitant intramuscular human chorionic gonadotropin preserves spermatogenesis in men undergoing testosterone replacement therapy. J Urol. 2013;189(2):647–50. doi:10.1016/j.juro.2012.09.043.

Hussein A, Ozgok Y, Ross L, Rao P, Niederberger C. Optimization of spermatogenesis-regulating hormones in patients with non-obstructive azoospermia and its impact on sperm retrieval: a multicentre study. BJU Int. 2013;111(3 Pt B):E110–4. doi:10.1111/j.1464-410X.2012.11485.x.

Kamischke A, Baumgardt A, Horst J, Nieschlag E. Clinical and diagnostic features of patients with suspected Klinefelter syndrome. J Androl. 2003;24(1):41–8.

Klinefelter H, Reifenstein E, Albright F. Syndrome characterized by gynecomastia aspermatogenesis without a-Leydigism and increased excretion of follicle-stimulating hormone. J Clin Endocrinol Metabol. 1942;2:615–24.

Maggi M, Schulman C, Quinton R, Langham S, Uhl-Hochgraeber K. The burden of testosterone deficiency syndrome in adult men: economic and quality-of-life impact. J Sex Med. 2007;4(4 Pt 1):1056–69. doi:10.1111/j.1743-6109.2007.00531.x.

Maiburg M, Repping S, Giltay J. The genetic origin of Klinefelter syndrome and its effect on spermatogenesis. Fertil Steril. 2012;98(2):253–60. doi:10.1016/j.fertnstert.2012.06.019.

Mehta A, Malek-Jones M, Bolyakov A, Mielnik A, Schlegel PN, Paduch DA. Methylation-specific PCR allows for fast diagnosis of X chromosome disomy and reveals skewed inactivation of the X chromosome in men with Klinefelter syndrome. J Androl. 2012;33(5):955–62. doi:10.2164/jandrol.111.016030.

Miyagawa Y, Tsujimura A, Matsumiya K, Takao T, Tohda A, Koga M, Takeyama M, Fujioka H, Takada S, Koide T, Okuyama A. Outcome of gonadotropin therapy for male hypogonadotropic hypogonadism at university affiliated male infertility centers: a 30-year retrospective study. J Urol. 2005;173(6):2072–5. doi:10.1097/01.ju.0000158133.09197.f4.

Morris JK, Alberman E, Scott C, Jacobs P. Is the prevalence of Klinefelter syndrome increasing? Eur J Hum Genet: EJHG. 2008;16(2):163–70. doi:10.1038/sj.ejhg.5201956.

Moskovic DJ, Katz DJ, Akhavan A, Park K, Mulhall JP. Clomiphene citrate is safe and effective for long-term management of hypogonadism. BJU Int. 2012;110(10):1524–8. doi:10.1111/j.1464-410X.2012.10968.x.

Nielsen J, Wohlert M. Sex chromosome abnormalities found among 34,910 newborn children: results from a 13-year incidence study in Arhus, Denmark. Birth Defects Orig Artic Ser. 1990;26(4):209–23.

Nieschlag E. Klinefelter syndrome: the commonest form of hypogonadism, but often overlooked or untreated. Dtsch Arztebl Int. 2013;110(20):347–53. doi:10.3238/arztebl.2013.0347.

Nieschlag E, Nieschlag S, Behre HM. Lifespan and testosterone. Nature. 1993;366(6452):215. doi:10.1038/366215a0.

Okada H, Shirakawa T, Ishikawa T, Goda K, Fujisawa M, Kamidono S. Serum testosterone levels in patients with nonmosaic Klinefelter syndrome after testicular sperm extraction for intracytoplasmic sperm injection. Fertil Steril. 2004;82(1):237–8. doi:10.1016/j.fertnstert.2003.11.047.

Palermo GD, Schlegel PN, Sills ES, Veeck LL, Zaninovic N, Menendez S, Rosenwaks Z. Births after intracytoplasmic injection of sperm obtained by testicular extraction from men with nonmosaic Klinefelter's syndrome. N Engl J Med. 1998;338(9):588–90. doi:10.1056/nejm199802263380905.

Raman JD, Schlegel PN. Aromatase inhibitors for male infertility. J Urol. 2002;167(2 Pt 1):624–9.

Ramasamy R, Ricci JA, Palermo GD, Gosden LV, Rosenwaks Z, Schlegel PN. Successful fertility treatment for Klinefelter's syndrome. J Urol. 2009;182(3):1108–13. doi:10.1016/j.juro.2009.05.019.

Rogol AD, Tartaglia N. Considerations for androgen therapy in children and adolescents with Klinefelter syndrome (47, XXY). Pediatr Endocrinol Rev PER. 2010;8 Suppl 1:145–50.

Salbenblatt JA, Bender BG, Puck MH, Robinson A, Faiman C, Winter JS. Pituitary-gonadal function in Klinefelter syndrome before and during puberty. Pediatr Res. 1985;19(1):82–6. doi:10.1203/00006450-198501000-00022.

Schiff JD, Palermo GD, Veeck LL, Goldstein M, Rosenwaks Z, Schlegel PN. Success of testicular sperm extraction [corrected] and intracytoplasmic sperm injection in men with Klinefelter syndrome. J Clin Endocrinol Metab. 2005;90(11):6263–7. doi:10.1210/jc.2004-2322.

Schill WB, Jungst D, Unterburger P, Braun S. Combined hMG/hCG treatment in subfertile men with idiopathic normogonadotrophic oligozoospermia. Int J Androl. 1982;5(5):467–77.

Swerdlow AJ, Higgins CD, Schoemaker MJ, Wright AF, Jacobs PA. Mortality in patients with Klinefelter syndrome in Britain: a cohort study. J Clin Endocrinol Metab. 2005;90(12):6516–22. doi:10.1210/jc.2005-1077.

Tash JA, Schlegel PN. Histologic effects of testicular sperm extraction on the testicle in men with nonobstructive azoospermia. Urology. 2001;57(2):334–7.

Tuttelmann F, Gromoll J. Novel genetic aspects of Klinefelter's syndrome. Mol Hum Reprod. 2010;16(6):386–95. doi:10.1093/molehr/gaq019.

Vernaeve V, Staessen C, Verheyen G, Steirteghem AV, Devroey P, Tournaye H. Can biological or clinical parameters predict testicular sperm recovering in 47, XXY Klinefelter's syndrome patients? Hum Reprod. 2004;19(5):1135–9.

Wikstrom AM, Hoei-Hansen CE, Dunkel L, Rajpert-De Meyts E. Immunoexpression of androgen receptor and nine markers of maturation in the testes of adolescent boys with Klinefelter syndrome: evidence for degeneration of germ cells at the onset of meiosis. J Clin Endocrinol Metab. 2007;92(2):714–9. doi:10.1210/jc.2006-1892.

Williams RA, Mamotte CDS, Burnett JR. Phenylketonuria: an inborn error of phenylalanine metabolism. Clin Biochem Rev. 2008;29(1):31–41.

Wilson JMG, Jungner G. Principles and practice of screening for disease. Geneva: World Health Organization; 1968.

Varicocele

9

Karthik Gunasekaran

9.1 Introduction

The pampiniform plexus is a venous network that drains blood from the testis. A varicocele is an abnormal dilatation of the pampiniform plexus and usually occurs on the left side. The incidence of varicocele is almost as high as 15 % in the general population afflicting up to 35 % of men with primary infertility and 81 % of men with secondary infertility. Although other studies have found an equal incidence of varicocele among both primary and secondary infertility, this discrepancy remains to be explored (Jarow et al. 1996; Gorelick and Goldstein 1993; Saypol 1981). A recent Cochrane review suggested that varicocele is the most frequent physical abnormality found in subfertile men (Kroese et al. 2012). The varicocele has always been a controversial topic and highly debated among specialists in the field. The effect of varicocele on semen parameters, its association with infertility, and its effect on pregnancy rates have been avidly debated. Subfertile men show a higher incidence of varicocele prompting researchers to believe that the varicocele is a cause of infertility (WHO 1992). Further, repair of varicocele has seemingly documented some beneficial effects (Newton et al. 1980). However, critics are skeptical as the effects of varicocele repair are inconsistent across studies.

The aim of this chapter is to throw light on the current concepts on the etiology of varicocele, its pathophysiology, its association with infertility, and choice of treatment and finally to look at the cost–benefit analysis in treating it. This hopefully would translate into guiding the physicians in giving a well-informed choice to the patient.

K. Gunasekaran, MBBS, MS, FIAGES, FIMSA, FECSM
The Metromale Clinic: Super Specialty Clinic for Male Sexual Health and Fertility, No. 1, Crescent Park Street, T. Nagar, Landmark: Near BR Mathsya, Chennai, India
e-mail: gunasek@gmail.com

K. Gunasekaran, N. Pandiyan (eds.), *Male Infertility*,
DOI 10.1007/978-81-322-3604-7_9

9.2 Anatomy and Etiology

Though a varicocele is more common on the left, bilateralism seems to be on the rise with recent data suggesting over 30–80 % of varicocele being bilateral (Gat and Bachar 2004). When an isolated right-sided varicocele is identified, it warrants further investigation to rule out a retroperitoneal anomaly, although it could also be a normal anatomical variant. Why are varicoceles more common on the left side? The left internal spermatic vein follows a perpendicular course that is approximately 8–10 cm longer than the right before it enters the left renal vein. This results in increased hydrostatic pressure in the left internal spermatic vein. Also, the left internal spermatic vein because of its perpendicular insertion allows the direct transmission of renal vein pressure to the left internal spermatic vein. The right spermatic vein enters the inferior vena cava at an angle, thus preventing direct pressure transmissions from occurring (Siegel et al. 2006). Furthermore, the left internal spermatic vein lacks functional valves that can lead to regression of blood. There could be a partial obstruction of the left internal spermatic vein because of the compression of the left renal vein between the aorta and upper mesenteric artery (nutcracker syndrome) (Naugton et al. 2001).

9.3 Etiopathogenesis of Varicocele

The etiology of varicocele is multifactorial; similarly the pathophysiology too involves multiple mechanisms. Increased scrotal temperature, high intratesticular pressures, reflux of toxic metabolites, hypoxia and reactive oxygen species, and effect on hormones have all been suggested as possible mechanisms (Fuzisawa et al. 1989; Comhaire 1991). The increased temperature of the scrotum results from reflux of warm blood from the abdominal cavity. This may be a result of the damage or absence of valves in both the internal spermatic vein and cremasteric or external spermatic veins (Goldstein and Eid 1989). The venous tone of the spermatic plexus increases resulting in high hydrostatic pressures.

One study demonstrated that the pressures were actually 19.7 mmHg higher than when compared to the control groups (Shafik and Bedeir 1980). This increased venous pressure can compromise arterial pressure which is required to maintain homeostasis of intratesticular pressure. In the lab looking at fragments from the spermatic vein has revealed alterations in the longitudinal muscle layers, in addition to a decrease in the number of nerve elements and vasa vasorum present in the vessel wall. However, we do not know whether the decrease in the vasa vasorum is a change that suggests causation due to the varicocele or whether this is simply a reactive change of no clinical significance. Nevertheless, these findings suggest a defective contractile mechanism of blood transport through the venous plexus (Tilki et al. 2007). Dysfunction may result by means of chronic vasoconstriction of the spermatic epithelium caused by an increased concentration of toxic metabolites from the adrenal gland (Naugton et al. 2001). Oxidative stress which results from excessive reactive oxygen species (ROS) is increasingly being recognized as a major factor in infertility Said et al. 2005, 1; Agarwal et al. 1994; De Lamirande and Gagnon 1992).

The human body possesses a minimum quantity of ROS for regulating normal sperm function; however, in about 25–40 % of infertile men, the semen contains an excessive amount Marmar 2001; Padron et al. 1997). ROS are needed for regulating normal sperm functions such as sperm capacitation, the acrosome reaction, and sperm–oocyte fusion (De Lamirande and Gagnon 1992; Marmar 2001; Padron et al. 1997).

Elevated ROS and diminished antioxidant capacity have been associated with varicocele (Hendin et al. 1999). However, since both fertile and infertile men show similar findings, it is unclear whether ROS is a cause or consequence. Oxidative stress has also been associated with increased DNA fragmentation in patients with varicocele (Smith et al. 2006). Altered production of steroids in the testis is also a proposed mechanism of varicocele affecting fertility. Some early reports suggested decreased testosterone levels in men with varicocele, whereas others suggested that this was not the cause (Hudson et al. 1983; Swerdloff and Walsh 1975).

9.4 Varicocele and Semen Parameters

The jury has still not given a verdict on the effect that varicocele has on semen parameters and its subsequent effect on male infertility. Semen parameters can either be normal, or there can be different findings like oligozoospermia, asthenozoospermia, teratozoospermia, or a combination of findings. Some studies suggest a gradual deterioration of seminal parameters in the presence of varicocele, ultimately leading to azoospermia (Papadimas and Mantalenakis 1983). Other studies reveal that semen parameters may not be affected at all as there is no significant difference between infertile men and men in the general population with or without varicocele (Redmon et al. 2002). Interestingly, a large-scale study by the WHO showed significantly lower sperm concentration in infertile men with varicocele compared to men with idiopathic infertility, but did not give any evidence regarding the impact of varicocele on sperm motility and morphology (WHO 1992). Strictly speaking a cause–effect relationship between the presence of varicocele and its impact on semen parameters remains unproven. Another plausibility explanation is that varicocele may be an incidental finding in men with idiopathic infertility and men with isolated seminal plasma abnormalities.

9.5 Diagnosis of Varicocele

9.5.1 Physical Examination

A physical exam consisting of inspection and palpation still remains the best method to diagnose a varicocele. Large varicoceles are easily visible and on palpation they give “a bag of worms feel” as described by Dublin. Dublin et al. also graded varicocele based on size. Easily visible varicoceles are grade 3 or large, grade 2 or medium refers to varicoceles that are palpable without a Valsalva, and grade 1 or small refers to varicoceles that are palpable only with Valsalva (Dublin and Amelar 1977).

The grading may be of clinical importance as Steckel and colleagues observed that men with larger varicocele had poorer semen parameters preoperatively and showed an improvement in semen parameters after their repair compared to the repair of small- or medium-sized varicocele (Steckel et al. 1993). It may be important to observe decompression of varicocele in the supine position after examination in the standing position. A varicocele that does decompress after lying down may signify other pathology like a cord lipoma or a hernia.

9.5.2 Doppler Testing

Reflux seen with a Valsalva maneuver can point to a varicocele. Recording the signal and visualizing the images help clinch a diagnosis. Arterial and venous flow should not be confused together. A persistent and reproducible venous rush is to be looked for. A pencil probe Doppler can be used in most cases (Greenberg et al. 1977).

9.5.3 Ultrasound

Ultrasound is being increasingly combined with Doppler for the diagnosis of varicocele. Color Doppler ultrasound had a sensitivity of 93 % and specificity of 85 % when compared to physical examination. It is especially useful in diagnosing a not so easily palpable varicocele (Chiou et al. 1997). Whether subclinical varicocele, picked up only by color Doppler ultrasound, warrants any intervention is a subject of intense debate (Petros 1991).

9.5.4 Venography

Venography is used more as a treatment option than as a diagnostic procedure. It is very sensitive, but not that specific (Ahlberg et al. 1996). It is performed using the Seldinger technique via the right femoral or right internal jugular vein (Sigman and Jarrow 2002). Given the invasive nature of the procedure, routine use is not recommended. However, it has been used as the procedure of choice for detecting persistent varicocele post-surgery (Seyferth et al. 1981).

9.6 Indications for Varicocelectomy

9.6.1 Symptoms of a Varicocele

Large varicoceles are usually symptomatic. Scrotal pain may be an important symptom. Other causes of scrotal pain need to be ruled out before any intervention. Different surgical approaches have been tried with varying results (Karademir 2005; Yeniyol et al. 2003; Chawla et al. 2005).

9.7 Varicocele and Its Effect on Fertility

Varicocele and its effect on semen parameters have been a subject of intense debate. Varicocele can affect sperm concentration, count, and motility. Some studies suggest that varicocele may affect spermatogenesis, regardless of fertility status. Sperm counts in both fertile and infertile men with varicocele were lower compared to controls, but the fertile group showed higher sperm counts (Nagao et al. 1986). The lower concentration and motility reported according to researchers could be attributed to germ cell apoptosis, to increased concentration of reactive oxygen species, or to the presence of antisperm antibodies (Yeniyol et al. 2003). According to MacLeod and colleagues, varicocele induces what is known as a stress pattern on sperm morphology in over 90 % of his infertile patients (MacLeod 1965). Others opined that the stress pattern may not be pathognomonic of a varicocele (Saypol 1981). It is currently difficult to come to any conclusion regarding the effect of varicocele on semen parameters.

9.8 Varicocele in Azoospermia

The complete absence of sperm in the ejaculate in a neat and centrifuged sample is azoospermia. The incidence ranges from 1–15 % of all subfertile men (Jarow et al. 1989; Pagani et al. 2002). The prevalence of varicocele in men with azoospermia is 5–10 % (Matthews et al. 1998; Kim et al. 1999). As early as 1955, Tuloch reported spermatogenesis in a patient treated with varicocele. Motile sperm appeared in the ejaculate of 21–55 % of men following varicocele repair (Lee et al. 2007). This suggests that varicocele repair may obviate the need for assisted reproduction techniques. However, one should also remember that these effects may only be temporary, as in a recent study, more than 50 % men relapsed back to azoospermia in 1 year (Pasqualotto et al. 2006). The varicocele correction or the mere appearance of sperm in the ejaculate post-surgery alone cannot predict whether a natural conception would occur. Also one should be aware of the etiology of azoospermia before initiating treatment. Y-chromosome micro-deletions and karyotype abnormalities are clinically significant findings in men with azoospermia. About 16.6 % of azoospermia men have Y-chromosome micro-deletions or karyotype anomalies (Kleiman et al. 1999). A few studies have addressed the effects of varicocele repair in infertile men presenting with coexisting genetic abnormalities. In a study of varicocele repair in men with infertility and Y-chromosome micro-deletions vs. no deletions, the men with no deletion ($n = 4$) were found to have an improvement in their semen parameters, while men in the deletion group ($n = 5$) did not exhibit any improvement (Dada et al. 2007). Importantly, one must understand that, most of these studies are based on small case series, much larger randomized controlled trials may solve the debate on whether varicocele surgery can be offered to select subgroups of men with azoospermia. Currently there is low-quality evidence to suggest that varicocele surgery may be no better than expectant management (Biyani et al. 2009).

9.9 Varicocele and ICSI

A common question troubling infertility specialists who treat patients with low sperm counts and coexistent varicocele is whether to surgically correct the varicocele or to offer ICSI directly. The points in favor of a varicocele repair would be that if the procedure is successful, then there would be a paradigm shift in the concept of *ICSI for all patients presenting with male infertility (*ASRM 2004). On an additional note, if the couple has a good prognosis of a future natural pregnancy, a varicocele repair would be cost-effective (Penson et al. 2002).

9.10 Treatment of Varicocele

9.10.1 Antegrade Sclerotherapy

Tauber described sclerotherapy for varicoceles as early as 1988 (Tauber and Johnson 1994). High scrotal incision is made and the cord is hooked out. The large spermatic vein is injected with contrast medium. It is then injected with sclerosing agent mixed with air. Zucchi et al. compared sclerotherapy to surgery and showed that results were comparable (Zucchi et al. 2005).

9.10.2 Percutaneous Occlusion

The procedure is usually performed on an outpatient basis with IV sedation. Various techniques like balloon or coils can be employed to achieve occlusion of the internal spermatic vein. Though a surgical procedure can be avoided, still the effect of radiation lingers and patients are concerned about this. There is also a risk of recurrence and balloon migration. Success rates for venous occlusion are less than that of surgery (Pryor and Howards 1987).

9.11 Surgical Strategies

9.11.1 Retroperitoneal Approach

The idea is to ligate the internal spermatic vein retroperitoneally. It is hypothesized that at this level the number of veins that needs *ligation is less and hence recurrence is less* (Cockett et al. 1984). This is also known as the modified Palomo *technique. Palomo in his original description ligated the artery along with the internal spermatic vein* (Palomo 1969). In the modified Palomo technique, the artery is spared (Wright and Goldstein 1994). A known pitfall to this technique is that there is no scope for ligation of the cremasteric vessels which can cause recurrence (Coolsaet 1980).

9.11.2 Laparoscopic Varicocelectomy

This technique is very similar to the modified Palomo technique with the exception of a laparoscopic entry with carbon *dioxide insufflation. Hydrocele appears to be a common complication associated with varicocele. Some surgeons do a bunch ligation of the artery, vein, and lymphatics in the laparoscopic approach. Contrary to popular belief, ligation of the testicular artery does not result in testicular atrophy, and a single group proved lower recurrence rates with the en masse technique (*Kass and Marcol 1992). However, Goldstein and colleagues had lower success rates when the testicular artery was divided (Wright and Goldstein 1994).

9.11.3 Inguinal Approach

This technique aims to tackle the internal spermatic vessels in the inguinal canal. The vessels here are more visible because of the size, and an important advantage is that the external cremasteric vessels may be ligated here (Ivanissevich 1960). A Doppler probe may be utilized to identify and spare the artery along with an operating microscope (Goldstein et al. 1992). Some authors advocate the delivery of the testicle through the inguinal wound to ligate all the testicular venous channels (Goldstein et al. 1992). However, this claim has been refuted by others (Ramaswamy and Shlegel 2006).

9.11.4 Subinguinal Approach

The main advantage of this technique is that the inguinal canal is not breached. As the external oblique is not cut, there is less pain and also the chances of injuring the ilioinguinal nerve are less (Marmar and Kim 1994). The external cremasteric vessels can be ligated at this level. The main disadvantage is that this is a more taxing technique due to the fact that the internal spermatic veins are more branched at that level. A microscope may come in handy when this technique is employed due to the smaller size of the vessels here.

Conclusion

Varicocele and its effect on fertility always have been and will continue to be a subject of intense debate in the years to come. Our limited understanding of the *pathophysiology of varicocele and response to treatment continues to evolve over time. Evidence suggests that there could be a significant improvement in sperm concentration and motility in carefully selected patients albeit without any evidence to suggest improvement in spontaneous pregnancy rates. For now, subclinical varicocele is best left alone. Microsurgery through the subinguinal route may be the mainstay of treatment.*

References

Agarwal A, Ikemoto I, Loughlin KR. Relationship of sperm parameters with levels of reactive oxygen species in semen specimens. J Urol. 1994;152:107–10.

Ahlberg NE, Bartley O, Chidekel N, Fritjoffson A. Phlebography in Varicocelescroti. Acta Radiol Diagn (Stockh). 1996;4:517–28.

Biyani CS, Cartledge J, Janetschek G. Varicocele. BMJ Clin Evid. 2009;2009.

Chawla A, Kulkarni G, Kamal K, Zini A. Microsurgical Varicocelectomy for recurrent or persistent varicoceles associated with orchalgia. Urology. 2005;66:1072–4.

Chiou RK, Anderson JC, Wobig RK, et al. Color Doppler ultrasound criteria to diagnose varicoceles: correlation of a new scoring system with physical examination. Urology. 1997;50:953–6.

Cockett AT, Takihara H, Consentino MJ. The varicocele. Fertil Steril. 1984;41:5–11.

Comhaire F. The pathogenesis of epididymo-testicular dysfunction in varicocele: factors other than temperature. Adv Exp Med Biol. 1991;286:281–7.

Coolsaet BL. The varicocele syndrome: venography determining the optimal level of surgical management. J Urol. 1980;124:833–9.

Dada R, Kumar R, Shamsi MB, Sidhu T, Mitra A, Singh S, et al. Azoospermia factor deletions in varicocele cases with severe oligozoospermia. Indian J Med Sci. 2007;61(9):505–10. http://dx.doi.org/10.4103/0019-5359.34519.

De Lamirande E, Gagnon C. Reactive oxygen species and human spermatozoa. II. Depletion of adenosine triphosphate plays an important role in the inhibition of sperm motility. J Androl. 1992;13:379–86.

Dublin L, Amelar RD. The Varicocele and infertility. In: Amelar RD, Dublin L, Walsh PC, editors. Male infertility. Philadelphia: Saunders; 1977. p. 57–68.

Fuzisawa M, Yoshida S, Kojima K, Kamidono S. Biochemical changes in testicular varicocele. Archs Androl. 1989;22:149–59.

Gat Y, Bachar GN, Zuckerman Z, et al. Varicocele: a bilateral disease. Fertil Steril. 2004;81(2):424–9.

Goldstein M, Eid JF. Elevation of intratesticular and scrotal skin surface temperature in men with varicocele. J Urol. 1989;142:7.

Goldstein M, Gibert BR, Dicker AP, dwosh J, Gnecco C. Microsurgical inguinal varicocelectomy with delivery of the testis: an artery and lymphatic sparing technique. J Urol. 1992;148:1808–11.

Gorelick JI, Goldstein M. Loss of fertility in men with Varicocele. Fertil Steril. 1993;59(3):613–6.

Greenberg SH, Lipshultz LI, Morganroth J, Wein AJ. The use of Doppler stethoscope in the evaluation of varicoceles. J Urol. 1977;117:296–8.

Hendin BN, Kolettis PN, Sharma RK, Thomas AJ, Agarwal A. Varicocele is associated with elevated spermatozoal reactive oxygen species production and diminished seminal plasma antioxidant capacity. J Urol. 1999;161:1831–4.

Hudson RW, PEREZ-Marrero RA, Crawford VA, Mc Kay D. Seminal plasma testosterone and dihydrotestosterone levels in males with varicoceles. Int J Androl. 1983;6:135–42.

Ivanissevich O. Left Varicocele due to reflux: experience with 4.470 cases in forty-two years. J Int Coll Surg. 1960;34:742–5.

Jarow JP, Espeland MA, Lipshultz LI. Evaluation of the azoospermic patient. J Urol. 1989;142:62–5.

Jarow JP, Coburn M, Sigman M. Incidence of varicoceles in men with primary and secondary infertility. Urology. 1996;47(1):73–6.

Karademir K, Senkul T, Baykal K, et al. Evaluation of the role of Varicocelectomy including external spermatic vein ligation in patients with scrotal pain. Int J Urol. 2005;12:484–8.

Kass EJ, Marcol B. Results of varicocele surgery in adolescents: a comparison of techniques. J Urol. 1992;148:694–6.

Kim ED, Leibman BB, Grinblat DM, Lipshultz LI. Varicocele repair improves semen parameters in azoospermic men with spermatogenic failure. J Urol. 1999;162(3 Pt 1):737.

Kleiman SE, Yogev L, Gamzu R, Hauser R, Botchan A, Lessing JB, et al. Genetic evaluation of infertile men. Hum Reprod. 1999;14(1):33–8. http://dx.doi.org/10.1093/humrep/14.1.33.

Kroese AC, de Lange NM, Collins JA, Evers JL. Surgery or embolization for varicocele in subfertile men. Cochrane Database Syst Rev 2012;10:CD000479. doi:10.1002/14651858.CD000479.pub5

Lee JS, Park HJ, Seo JT. What is the indication of varicocelectomy in men with non obstructive azoospermia? Urology. 2007;69:352–5.

MacLeod J. Seminal cytology in the presence of Varicocele. Fertil Steril. 1965;16:735–57.

Marmar JL. The pathophysiology of varicoceles in the light of current molecular and genetic information. Hum Reprod Update. 2001;7:461–72.

Marmar JL, Kim Y. Subinguinal microsurgical varicocelectomy: a technical critique and statistical analysis of semen and pregnancy data. J Urol. 1994;152:1127–32.

Matthews GJ, Matthews ED, Goldstein M. Induction of spermatogenesis and achievement of pregnancy after microsurgical varicocelectomy in men with azoospermia and severe oligoasthenospermia. Fertil Steril. 1998;70:71–5.

Nagao RR, Plymate SR, Berger RE, Perin EB, Paulsen CA. Comparison of gonadal function between fertile and infertile men with Varicoceles. Fertil Steril. 1986;46:930–3.

Naugton DK, Nangia AK, Agarwal A. Varicocele and male infertility: part II. Pathophysiology of varicoceles in male infertility. Hum Reprod Update. 2001;7:473–81.

Newton R, Schinfeld JS, Schiff I. The effect of varicocelectomy on sperm count, motility and conception rate. Fertil Steril. 1980;34:250–4.

Padron OF, Brackett NL, Sharma RK, Lynne CM, Thomas Jr AJ, Agarwal A. Seminal reactive oxygen species and sperm motility and morphology in men with spinal cord injury. Fertil Steril. 1997;67:1115–20.

Pagani R, Brugh 3rd VM, Lamb DJ. Y chromosome genes and male infertility. Urol Clin North Am. 2002;29:745–53.

Palomo A. Radical cure of varicocele by a new technique: preliminary report. J Urol. 1969;61:604–7.

Papadimas J, Mantalenakis S. Hormonal profile in infertile men. Arch Androl. 1983;11:73–80.

Pasqualotto FF, Sobreiro BP, Hallak J, Pasqualotto EB, Lucon AM. Induction of spermatogenesis in azoospermic men after varicocelectomy repair: an update. Fertil Steril. 2006;85:635–9.

Penson DF, Paltiel AD, Krumholz HM, Palter S. The cost-effectiveness of treatment for varicocele related infertility. J Urol. 2002;168:2490–4.

Petros JA, Andriole GL, Middleton WD, Picus DA. Correlation of testicular color Doppler ultrasonography, physical examination and venography in the detection of left varicoceles in men with infertility. J Urol. 1991;145(4):785–8.

Pryor JL, Howards SS. Varicocele. Urol Clin North Am. 1987;14:449–513.

Ramaswamy R, Shlegel PN. Microsurgical inguinal varicocelectomy with and without testicular delivery. Urology. 2006;68:1323–6.

Redmon JB, Carey P, Pryor JL. Varicocele – the most common cause of male factor infertility? Hum Reprod Update. 2002;8:53–8.

Said TM, Agarwal A, Sharma RK, Thomas Jr AJ, Sikka SC. Impact of sperm morphology on DNA damage caused by oxidative stress induced by beta-nicotinamide adenine dinucleotide phosphate. Fertil Steril. 2005;83(1):95–103.

Saypol DC. Varicocele. J Androl. 1981;2:61–71.

Seyferth W, Jecht E, Zeitler E. Percutaneous sclerotherapy of varicoceles. Radiology. 1981;139:335–40.

Shafik A, Bedeir GA. Venous tension patterns in cord veins in normal and varicocele individuals. J Urol. 1980;123:383–5.

Siegel Y, Gat Y, Bacher GN, Gornish M. A proposed anatomic typing of the right internal spermatic vein: importance for percutaneous sclerotherapy of varicocele. Cardiovasc Intervent Radiol. 2006;29(2):192–7.

Sigman M, Jarrow JP. Male infertility. In: Walsh PC, Retik AB, Vaughan ED, Wein AJ, editors. Campbells urology, vol. 2. 8th ed. Philadelphia: Saunders; 2002. p. 1475–515.

Smith R, Kaune H, Parodi d, et al. Increased sperm DNA damage in patients with varicocele: relationship with seminal oxidative stress. Hum Reprod. 2006;21:986–93.
Steckel J, Dicker AP, Goldstein M. Relationship between Varicocele size and response to Varicocelectomy. J Urol. 1993;149:769–71.
Swerdloff RS, Walsh PC. Pituitary and Gonadal Hormones in patients with varicocele. Fertil Steril. 1975;26:1006–12.
Tauber R, Johnson N. Antegrade scrotal sclerotherapy for the treatment of varicocele: technique and late results. J Urol. 1994;151:386–90.
The Male Infertility Best Practice Policy Committee of the American Urological Association and The Practice Committee of the American Society for Reproductive Medicine. Report on varicocele and infertility. Fertil Steril. 2004;82 Suppl 1:S142–5.
Tilki D, Kilic E, Tauber R, Pfeiffer D, Stief CG, Tauber R, et al. The complex structure of the smooth muscle layer of spermatic veins and its potential role in the development of varicocele testis. Eur Urol. 2007;51:1402–9; discussion 10.
WHO. The influence of varicoceles on parameters in a large group of men presenting to infertility clinics. Fertil Steril. 1992;57:1289–93.
World Health Organization. The influence of varicocele on parameters of fertility in a large group of men presenting to infertility clinics. Fertil Steril. 1992;57:1289–93.
Wright EJ, Goldstein M. Ligation of the testicular artery during micro surgical varicocelectomy: incidence and implications. Abstract presented at the 89th Annual meeting of the American Urological association. Monterey; 1994.
Yeniyol CO, Tuna A, Yener H, Zeyrek N, Tilki A. High ligation to treat pain in Varicocele. Int Urol Nephrol. 2003;35(1):65–8.
Zucchi A, et al. Treatment of varicocele: randomized prospective study on open surgery versus Tauber antegrade sclerotherapy. J Androl. 2005;26:328–32.

Sperm DNA Damage: Causes and Laboratory Detection

10

Satish Kumar Adiga and Guruprasad Kalthur

10.1 Introduction

Infertility is a major health issue globally which is defined as "the inability of a sexually active couple having unprotected sexual intercourse to achieve pregnancy within one year." Prevalence of infertility in the general population is estimated to be around 15–20 %, and in India alone there are more than 20 million infertile couples (Poongothai et al. 2009). Approximately 50 % of the infertility is due to male factor, which makes up 15 % of all couples. Decrease in semen quality and concomitant increase in the incidence of male infertility (Adiga et al. 2008; Feki et al. 2009; Joffe 2010) all over the world have drawn attention to the medical and scientific communities to focus on understanding the pathophysiology as well as on correcting the problem. Though the exact cause for the decline in semen quality is unclear, environmental factors, change in lifestyle, and pathological conditions like testicular cancer, cryptorchidism, varicocele, etc. show a strong correlation (Carlsen et al. 1992, 1993; Li et al. 2011; Jørgensen et al. 2012).

Semen analysis is the cornerstone of male infertility evaluation. Though it is an excellent tool to assess the testicular function, its ability to predict the fertilizing ability of the spermatozoa is not clear. Though the conventional parameters such as sperm concentration, motility, and morphology are higher in normal fertile men, there exists some degree of overlap between fertile and infertile men with respect to semen parameters, especially in the idiopathic group (Aitken et al. 1984). Approximately 15 % of the infertile men are said to have normal spermiogram (Guzick et al. 1998). Therefore, more emphasis is given on correlating the genetic integrity of the spermatozoa with fertility potential.

S.K. Adiga, PhD (✉) • G. Kalthur, PhD
Division of Clinical Embryology, Kasturba Medical College,
Manipal University, Manipal 576 104, India
e-mail: satish.adiga@manipal.edu

K. Gunasekaran, N. Pandiyan (eds.), *Male Infertility*,
DOI 10.1007/978-81-322-3604-7_10

10.2 Structure of Sperm DNA

A human spermatozoon has unique characteristics with respect to its structure and function. Specifically, the nucleus has a stable, highly condensed, and compact organization of chromatin which probably ensures that the genetic material of the paternal origin is protected from the harsh environments. High degree of compaction observed in sperm chromatin is provided by the presence of protamines which contributes to approximately 85–90 % of the nuclear protein in spermatozoa. Protamines replace the histones during spermiogenesis process which are highly basic due to the presence of basic amino acids such as arginine in high percentage. This confers a very strong affinity toward the nucleic acids compared to the histones. In addition, the disulfhydryl linkage between SH groups of two cysteine residues which are placed far apart in their native conformation further helps in compaction of the nuclear material. Due to these reasons, it is quite resistant to nucleases unlike in somatic cells (Sotolongo et al. 2003).

10.3 Etiology of Sperm DNA Damage

The origin of sperm DNA damage is complex and a diverse phenomenon. Various possible causes of sperm DNA damage are listed below:

(a) *Chromatin remodeling*: The sperm chromatin is highly packed compared to somatic cell nucleus. McPherson and Longo (1993) postulated that the extensive modification of chromatin during spermiogenesis requires temporary nicks in sperm DNA. Endogenous nuclease such as topoisomerase II may help in generating and then ligating nicks to facilitate protamination by relieving torsional stress (McPherson and Longo, 1993). However, these endogenous nicks may persist in mature spermatozoa suggesting an incomplete maturation process and abnormal chromatin organization (Manicardi et al. 1995).

(b) *Membrane organization*: The membrane of the human spermatozoa is rich in polyunsaturated fatty acids (PUFAs) which are the major sites of lipid peroxidation which generates reactive oxygen species (ROS). In addition, spermatozoa have minimal cytoplasm and hence lack the support of cytoplasmic antioxidant enzymes as well as molecules to tackle the free radicals. Therefore, although spermatozoa have a very compact chromatin organization, they are highly susceptible to free radical-induced DNA damage.

(c) *Poor antioxidant defense*: Seminal plasma is rich in enzymatic and nonenzymatic antioxidants which work together to counteract with ROS. The major antioxidant enzymes present in seminal plasma are superoxide dismutase (SOD), catalase (CAT), and glutathione peroxidase (GPX). Besides these enzymes, the seminal plasma is rich in low-molecular-weight compounds such as glutathione, pantothenic acid, carnitine, coenzyme Q, vitamin E, vitamin C, selenium, and zinc (Walczak-Jedrzejowska et al. 2013). Decrease in the level of either of them can decrease the total antioxidant capacity of the seminal plasma. A large number of studies have observed that the infertile men have low level of antioxidants in their seminal plasma (Smith et al. 1996; Sanocka et al. 1996; Lewis et al. 1997) which also correlates well with high level of oxidative stress (Agarwal et al. 2004; Zini et al. 2009; Aitken et al. 2010) and DNA damage (Cohen-Bacrie et al. 2009).

(d) *Apoptosis*: Spermatogenesis is a complex process which involves mitotic and meiotic events in highly proliferating germ cell compartment after attaining puberty. An intricate relation with Sertoli cell during the entire process is very crucial for the production of genetically normal spermatozoa. The abnormal germ cells, similar to all other histone-containing cells, are eliminated by apoptosis. However, it is not clear whether the protamine-containing spermatozoa are eliminated by apoptosis or not (Aitken et al. 2013). Once the spermatozoon leaves the lumen of seminiferous tubule, it is not in contact with Sertoli cells. The harsh conditions to which spermatozoa are exposed during their transport and storage in male reproductive tract may induce sperm DNA damage without apoptosis.

(e) *Infections and pathological conditions*: Various pathological conditions and genital tract infections in men have been associated with sperm DNA damage. Men with recurrent genitourinary infection such as paraplegics are noted to have high level of DNA damage (Brackett et al. 2008). Increased leukocyte concentration and DNA damage are observed in the ejaculates of men with genital tract infection or inflammation. Systemic infections with HIV, hepatitis B and C, leprosy, malaria, etc. have been associated with increased DNA damage which is thought to be due to elevated oxidative stress or the chromatin modification induced by proinflammatory cytokines during spermiogenesis process. Similarly, conditions like cryptorchidism, varicocele, and testicular cancer are usually associated with high percentage of spermatozoa with DNA damage in the ejaculate. Commonly used chemotherapeutic agents like cyclophosphamide and cis-platinum are known to induce DNA damage in spermatozoa (Das et al. 2002).

(f) *In vitro conditions*: Spermatozoa experience various types of stress during their manipulation in vitro which culminates in loss of DNA integrity. Rigorous pipetting, centrifugation, exposure to light, and cryopreservation process can lead to oxidative stress-induced DNA damage (Iwasaki and Gagnon 1992; Shekarriz et al. 1995; Watson 2000). In addition, the removal of seminal plasma rich in antioxidants during processing of ejaculate for assisted reproductive technologies (ARTs) can further increase the oxidative stress (Potts et al. 2000). Presence of leukocytes, round cells, and immature spermatozoa in the sperm pellet are the possible source of ROS during the in vitro incubation of spermatozoa.

10.4 Types of DNA Damage in Spermatozoa

Usually spermatozoa carry both single- and double-strand DNA breaks. In addition, damaged sperm chromatin is known to contain base adducts like 8-OHdG and ethenonucleosides such as 1,N6-ethenoadenosine and 1,N6-ethenoguanosine (Badouard et al. 2008). Recent evidences suggest that spermatozoa contain numerous cross-linking with DNA–DNA or DNA–protein cross-linking which are significantly greater than in the dispersed interphase nuclei of somatic cells (Qiu et al. 1995).

10.4.1 Methods to Assess Sperm DNA Damage

Comet Assay Also known as single-cell gel electrophoresis (SCGE), it is a popular electrophoretic method used to assess the DNA integrity. Under electrophoretic conditions, the broken DNA strands migrate to anode. The broken DNA strands are visualized using fluorescent dye which binds to DNA. The spermatozoa with DNA damage will have a head composed of intact DNA and tail containing broken DNA fragments, attaining typical comet shape. The amount of DNA present in the tail and tail length indicates the extent of DNA damage (Fig. 10.1). The DNA damage assessment can be made by using software or by manual scoring. Even though with this test both single- and double-strand breaks can be assessed, it is a time-consuming method, and the threshold level is not defined for clinical application.

Sperm Chromatin Structure Assay (SCSA) This is a flow-cytometric method which is based on the susceptibility of the sperm chromatin to undergo partial denaturation in situ under acidic conditions. Spermatozoa with damaged chromatin denature when exposed to acidic conditions, while those with normal chromatin remain stable (Evenson et al. 1980). After exposure of spermatozoa to acidic conditions, spermatozoa are stained with acridine orange (AO), a metachromatic fluorescent dye.

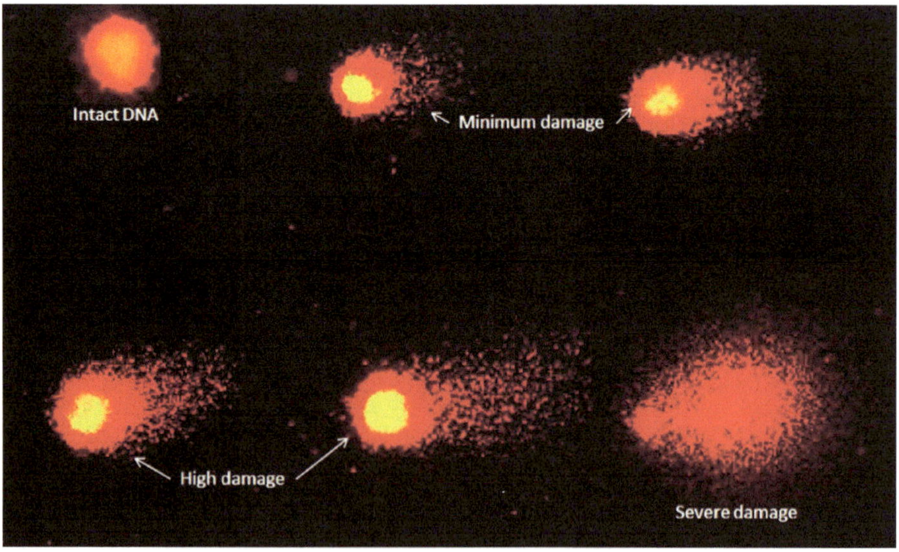

Fig 10.1 Comet assay: human spermatozoa stained with ethidium bromide and observed under fluorescent microscope (400× magnification)

When it intercalates with double-stranded DNA, it fluoresces green and fluoresces red when bound to single-stranded DNA. The extent of DNA denaturation following acid treatment is determined by measuring the metachromatic shift from green fluorescence to red fluorescence. Usually five to ten thousand cells are analyzed and assessed using a specific software. Though the method is highly reproducible and quite rapid, it is an expensive method.

Acridine Orange Test (AOT) This test is the simplified version of SCSA which uses fluorescent microscope to assess the metachromatic shift in the fluorescence by acridine orange (Tejada et al. 1984). It fluoresces green when bound to double-stranded DNA (excitation maximum at 502 nm and an emission maximum at 525 nm) and fluoresces red when bound to single-stranded DNA or RNA (excitation maximum 460 nm and an emission maximum 650 nm). For the assay, spermatozoa are exposed to mild acid treatment and stained with AO. Spermatozoa with intact DNA fluoresce green, and sperm with DNA damage fluoresces red or orange (Fig. 10.2). It is relatively a simple, rapid, and cheap method. The major disadvantages of this method are heterogeneous staining of the slide, rapid quenching, development of series of intermediate colors depending on the extent of chromatin denaturation, and large degree of inter- and intra-observer variations. Therefore, this method is considered to have low sensitivity and specificity to detect sperm DNA damage.

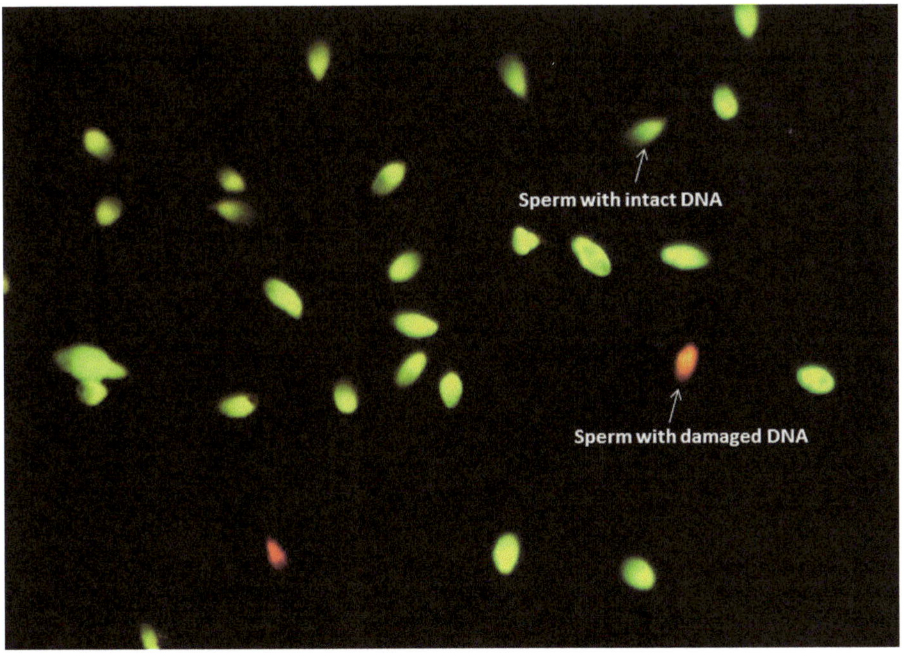

Fig. 10.2 Acridine orange test: human spermatozoa stained with acridine orange and observed under fluorescent microscope (400× magnification)

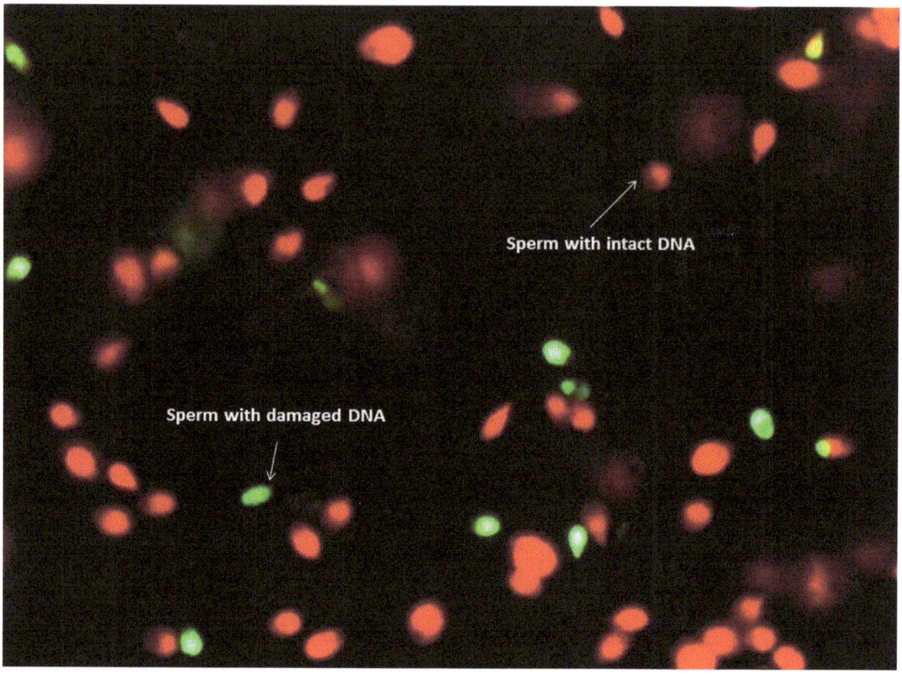

Fig. 10.3 TUNEL assay: human spermatozoa counterstained with propidium iodide (PI) and observed under fluorescent microscope using FITC filter (400× magnification)

Terminal Deoxynucleotidyl Transferase (TdT)-Mediated 2′-Deoxyuridine 5′-Triphosphate Nick-End Labeling (TUNEL) Assay This assay detects the DNA breaks directly without changing the chromatin structure unlike in comet assay or sperm chromatin structure assay. The assay is based on the ability of the terminal deoxynucleotidyl transferase (TdT) to label the 3′-OH end of broken DNA strand with nucleotides (5-bromo-2′-deoxyuridine 5′-triphosphate nucleotide) usually tagged with a fluorochrome (Fig. 10.3) or a chromogen which can be visualized by observing under fluorescent or light microscope, respectively. The advantage of light microscopic method is that the signal obtained is permanent unlike in fluorescent microscopic method. Since it is a kit-based method, the results are reproducible. However, the kits are usually expensive with differences in working protocol, and the threshold level is not defined for clinical application.

Sperm Chromatin Dispersion (SCD) Test This test is based on the principle that mild acidic denaturation of sperm DNA and lysis of protamines will create a halo of chromatin loops around the sperm head when DNA is intact and small or no halo around the sperm head when DNA is fragmented (Fig. 10.4). It is a relatively simple and inexpensive method to detect sperm DNA integrity which was first described by Fernández et al. (2003). However, it does not give information on the extent of DNA damage in spermatozoa, and there are a limited number of studies to support its clinical application.

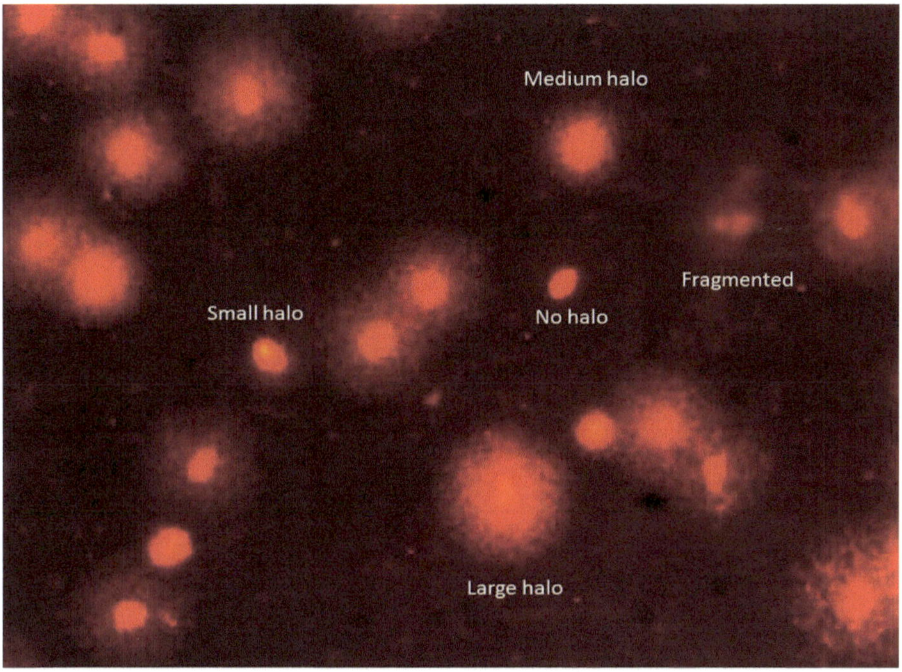

Fig. 10.4 Sperm chromatin dispersion test: human spermatozoa stained with ethidium bromide and observed under fluorescent microscope (400× magnification)

Aniline Blue Staining This is a very simple light microscopic method which is based on the difference in chromatin packing of spermatozoa. It gives an indirect measure of protamine–histone ratio in spermatozoa. Aniline blue is an acidic dye which has a greater permeability/affinity for histones in the sperm nucleus. Increased aniline blue staining of sperm indicates loose chromatin packing. The blue-stained spermatozoa are considered as immature, and pinkish sperm are mature (Fig. 10.5). Even though it is a rapid and cheap method, heterogeneous staining pattern limits its clinical application.

Toluidine Blue Staining Toluidine blue is a nuclear dye used for metachromatic and orthochromatic staining of chromatin that stains phosphate residues of the sperm DNA with loosely packed chromatin and fragmented ends. When the stain attaches with lysine-rich regions of histone, it produces a violet-bluish intense coloration, whereas a pale-blue color is produced by interactions with protamines in the chromatin. The sample can be analyzed using an ordinary microscope, but intermediate coloration increases inter-user variability.

Chromomycin A3 (CMA3) Staining This method is a simple fluorescence microscopic method which gives information on the degree of protamination and chromatin packing in spermatozoa. CMA3 specifically binds to GC (guanine–cytosine)-rich sequences in DNA. GC-rich region is also the site where protamines bind with DNA. The higher the CMA3 staining, the lower will be the protamine level and the

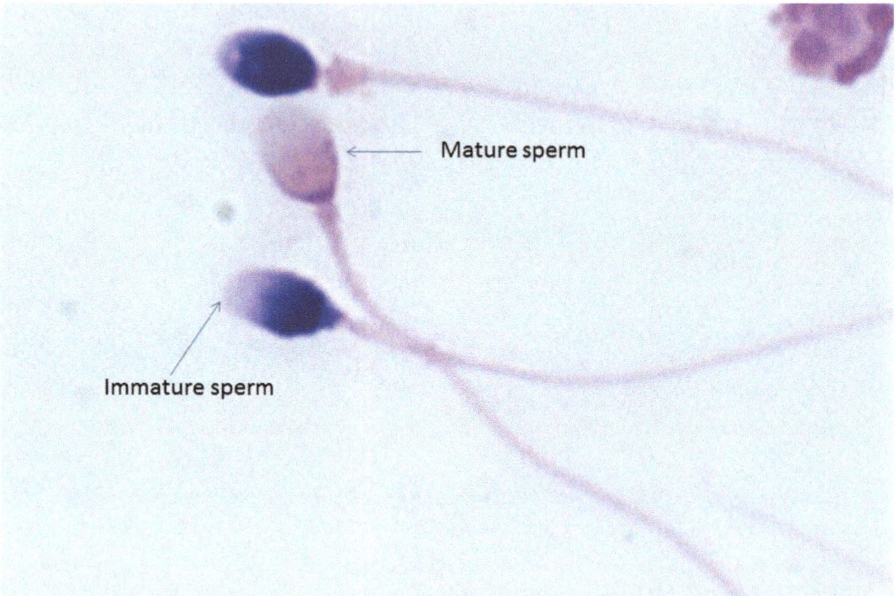

Fig. 10.5 Aniline blue staining: human spermatozoa stained with aniline blue dye and observed under light microscope (1000× magnification)

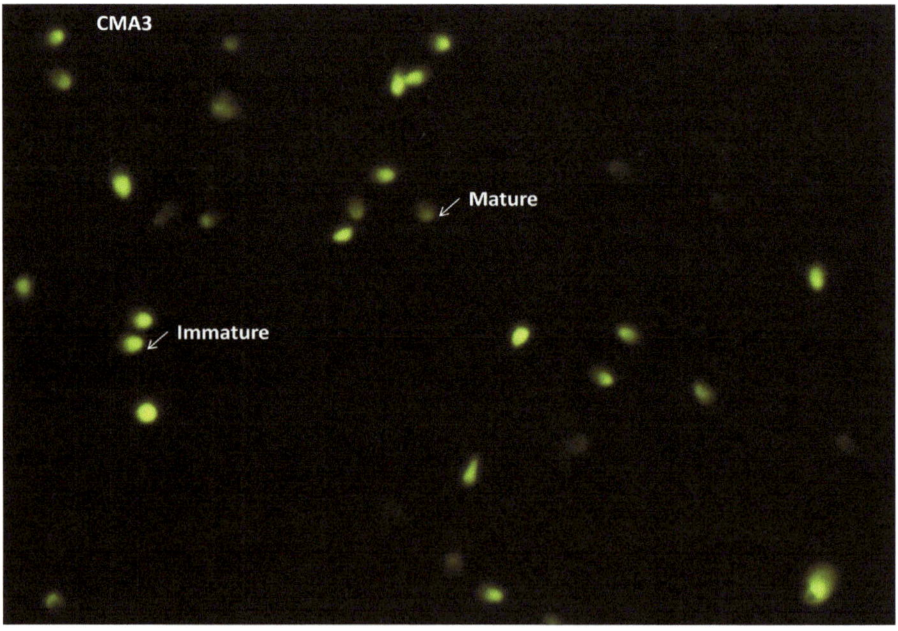

Fig. 10.6 Chromomycin A3 staining: human spermatozoa stained with chromomycin A3 and observed under fluorescent microscope (400× magnification)

poorer will be the chromatin packing in spermatozoa (Fig. 10.6). The spermatozoa with bright yellow are considered as immature, while with dull yellow are considered as mature. Due to rapid quenching of fluorescence and high inter- and intra-observer variation, this method has low clinical application.

8-OH Deoxyguanosine (8-OHdG) Estimation This is a chromatographic method which detects the level of ROS-induced by-product, 8-OHdG level in sperm DNA. The assay requires HPLC (high-performance liquid chromatography) which involves DNA extraction, enzymatic digestion of DNA, elution through HPLC column, and finally analysis of 8-OHdG. The method is very expensive and depends upon the DNA yield.

10.5 Clinical Management of Sperm DNA Damage

With considerable evidence of association of sperm DNA damage and male infertility, more research emphasis is given on enhancing the DNA integrity both in vivo and ex vivo. Treating of male infertility patients with antioxidant molecules to reduce the oxidative stress has become the most sensible approach (Fraga et al. 1991; Zini et al. 2005). Similarly, supplementation of culture medium with antioxidants, vitamins, and metals during in vitro processing of semen sample has shown drastic improvement in sperm functional competence (Kalthur et al. 2012; Talevi et al. 2013; Fanaei et al. 2014) suggesting its promising role during the preparation of spermatozoa for ART which could improve the outcome.

References

Adiga SK, Jayaraman V, Kalthur G, Upadhya D, Kumar P. Declining semen quality among south Indian infertile men: a retrospective study. J Hum Reprod Sci. 2008;1:15–8.

Agarwal A, Nallella KP, Allamaneni SS, Said TM. Role of antioxidants in treatment of male infertility: an overview of the literature. Reprod Biomed Online. 2004;8:616–27.

Aitken RI, Best FS, Warner F, Templeton A. A prospective study of the relationship between semen quality and fertility in cases of unexplained infertility. J Androl. 1984;5:297–303.

Aitken RJ, De Iuliis GN, Finnie JM, Hedges A, McLachlan RI. Analysis of the relationships between oxidative stress, DNA damage and sperm vitality in a patient population: development of diagnostic criteria. Hum Reprod. 2010;25:2415–26.

Aitken RJ, Bronson R, Smith TB, De Iuliis GN. The source and significance of DNA damage in human spermatozoa; a commentary on diagnostic strategies and straw man fallacies. Mol Hum Reprod. 2013;19:475–85.

Badouard C, Ménézo Y, Panteix G, Ravanat JL, Douki T, Cadet J, Favier A. Determination of new types of DNA lesions in human sperm. Zygote. 2008;16:9–13.

Brackett NL, Ibrahim E, Grotas JA, Aballa TC, Lynne CM. Higher sperm DNA damage in semen from men with spinal cord injuries compared to controls. J Androl. 2008;29:93–9.

Carlsen E, Giwercman A, Keiding N, Skakkebaek NE. Evidence for decreasing quality of semen during past 50 years. BMJ. 1992;305:609–13.

Carlsen E, Giwercman A, Skakkabaek NE, Keiding N. Decreasing quality of semen. BMJ. 1993; 306:461.

Cohen-Bacrie P, Belloc S, Ménézo YJ, Clement P, Hamidi J, Benkhalifa M. Correlation between DNA damage and sperm parameters: a prospective study of 1,633 patients. Fertil Steril. 2009;91:1801–5.

Das UB, Mallick M, Debnath JM, Ghosh D. Protective effect of ascorbic acid on cyclophosphamide-induced testicular gametogenic and androgenic disorders in male rats. Asian J Androl. 2002;4:201–7.

Evenson DP, Darzynkiewicz Z, Melamed MR. Relation of mammalian sperm chromatin heterogeneity to fertility. Science. 1980;210:1131–3.

Fanaei H, Khayat S, Halvaei I, Ramezani V, Azizi Y, Kasaeian A, Mardaneh J, Parvizi MR, Akrami M. Effects of ascorbic acid on sperm motility, viability, acrosome reaction and DNA integrity in teratozoospermic samples. Iran J Reprod Med. 2014;12:103–10.

Feki NC, Abid N, Rebai A, Sellami A, Ayed BB, Guermazi M, Bahloul A, Rebai T, Ammar LK. Semen quality decline among men in infertile relationships: experience over 12 years in the South of Tunisia. J Androl. 2009;5:541–7.

Fernández JL, Muriel L, Rivero MT, Goyanes V, Vazquez R, Alvarez JG. The sperm chromatin dispersion test: a simple method for the determination of sperm DNA fragmentation. J Androl. 2003;24:59–66.

Fraga CG, Motchnik PA, Shigenaga MK, Helbock HJ, Jacob RA, Ames BN. Ascorbic acid protects against endogenous oxidative DNA damage in human sperm. Proc Natl Acad Sci U S A. 1991;88:11003–6.

Guzick DS, Sullivan MW, Adamson GD, Cedars MI, Falk RJ, Peterson EP, Steinkampf MP. Efficacy of treatment for unexplained infertility. Fertil Steril. 1998;70:207–13.

Iwasaki A, Gagnon C. Formation of reactive oxygen species in spermatozoa of infertile patients. Fertil Steril. 1992;57:409–16.

Joffe M. Semen quality analysis and the idea of normal fertility. Asian J Androl. 2010;12:79–82.

Jørgensen N, Joensen UN, Jensen TK, Jensen MB, Almstrup K, Olesen IA, Juul A, Andersson AM, Carlsen E, Petersen JH, Toppari J, Skakkebæk NE. Human semen quality in the new millennium: a prospective cross-sectional population-based study of 4867 men. BMJ Open. 2012;2:e000990.

Kalthur G, Salian SR, Keyvanifard F, Sreedharan S, Thomas JS, Kumar P, Adiga SK. Supplementation of biotin to sperm preparation medium increases the motility and longevity in cryopreserved human spermatozoa. J Assist Reprod Genet. 2012;29(7):631–5.

Lewis SE, Sterling ES, Young IS, Thompson W. Comparison of individual antioxidants of sperm and seminal plasma in fertile and infertile men. Fertil Steril. 1997;67:142–7.

Li Y, Lin H, Li Y, Cao J. Association between socio-psycho-behavioral factors and male semen quality: systematic review and meta-analyses. Fertil Steril. 2011;95:116–23.

Manicardi GC, Bianchi PG, Pantano S, Azzoni P, Bizzaro D, Bianchi U, Sakkas D. Presence of endogenous nicks in DNA of ejaculated human spermatozoa and its relationship to chromomycin A3 accessibility. Biol Reprod. 1995;52:864–7.

McPherson S, Longo FJ. Chromatin structure-function alterations during mammalian spermatogenesis: DNA nicking and repair in elongating spermatids. Eur J Histochem. 1993;37:109–28.

Poongothai J, Gopenath TS, Manonayaki S. Genetics of human male infertility. Singapore Med J. 2009;50:336–47.

Potts RJ, Notarianni LJ, Jefferies TM. Seminal plasma reduces exogenous oxidative damage to human sperm, determined by the measurement of DNA strand breaks and lipid peroxidation. Mutat Res. 2000;447:249–56.

Qiu J, Hales BF, Robaire B. Damage to rat spermatozoal DNA after chronic cyclophosphamide exposure. Biol Reprod. 1995;53:1465–73.

Sanocka D, Miesel R, Jedrzejczak P, Kurpisz MK. Oxidative stress and male infertility. J Androl. 1996;17:449–54.

Shekarriz M, Thomas Jr AJ, Agarwal A. Incidence and level of seminal reactive oxygen species in normal men. Urology. 1995;45:103–7.

Smith R, Vantman D, Ponce J, Escobar J, Lissi E. Total antioxidant capacity of human seminal plasma. Hum Reprod. 1996;11:1655–60.

Sotolongo B, Lino E, Ward WS. Ability of hamster spermatozoa to digest their own DNA. Biol Reprod. 2003;69:2029–35.

Talevi R, Barbato V, Fiorentino I, Braun S, Longobardi S, Gualtieri R. Protective effects of in vitro treatment with zinc, d-aspartate and coenzyme q10 on human sperm motility, lipid peroxidation and DNA fragmentation. Reprod Biol Endocrinol. 2013;11:81. doi:10.1186/1477-7827-11-81.

Tejada RI, Mitchell JC, Norman A, Marik JJ, Friedman S. A test for the practical evaluation of male fertility by acridine orange (AO) fluorescence. Fertil Steril. 1984;42:87–91.

Walczak-Jedrzejowska R, Wolski JK, Slowikowska-Hilczer J. The role of oxidative stress and antioxidants in male fertility. Cent Euro J Urol. 2013;66:60–7.

Watson PF. The causes of reduced fertility with cryopreserved semen. Anim Reprod Sci. 2000;60–61:481–92.

Zini A, Blumenfeld A, Libman J, Willis J. Beneficial effect of microsurgical varicocelectomy on human sperm DNA integrity. Hum Reprod. 2005;20:1018–21.

Zini A, San Gabriel M, Baazeem A. Antioxidants and sperm DNA damage: a clinical perspective. J Assist Reprod Genet. 2009;26:427–32.

Sexually Transmitted Infections and Impact on Male Fertility

11

Gulfam Ahmad, Stefan S. du Plessis, and Ashok Agarwal

11.1 Introduction

Microorganisms residing in the male or female genital tracts cause sexually transmitted infections (STIs) and are generally transmitted through unprotected intercourse or other sexual acts. The increasing prevalence of STIs as a whole, and curable STIs in particular, has become a global challenge. A total of 498.9 million cases of curable STIs were reported by the World Health Organization (WHO) in 2008 compared to 448.3 million in 2005 indicating an 11.3 % increase in the incidence rate (Fig. 11.1) (WHO 2008).

Studies focusing on human infertility have been more comprehensive with regard to the female's contribution to compromised fertility, with a lesser degree of focus on the male partner's role. STIs can impact the reproductive process at varying stages, ranging from the division, differentiation, and development of germ cells to viability and ultimate survival of the newborn (Baecher-Lind 2009). Infection in the male urogenital system can prove to be problematic, with the localization of microorganisms residing in the upper genital tract causing contamination of the semen sample (Fourie et al. 2011). It is troubling to note that since certain STIs can also present asymptomatically, the male partner can remain undiagnosed and subsequently untreated.

G. Ahmad, PhD
Department of Physiology and Cell Biology, University of Health Sciences, Lahore 54600, Pakistan

S.S. du Plessis, PhD
Division of Medical Physiology, Stellenbosch University, Tygerberg 7505, Western Cape, South Africa

A. Agarwal, PhD, HCLD (✉)
American Center for Reproductive Medicine, Cleveland Clinic, Mail Code X-11 10681 Carnegie Avenue, Cleveland, OH 44195, USA
e-mail: agarwaa@ccf.org

K. Gunasekaran, N. Pandiyan (eds.), *Male Infertility*,
DOI 10.1007/978-81-322-3604-7_11

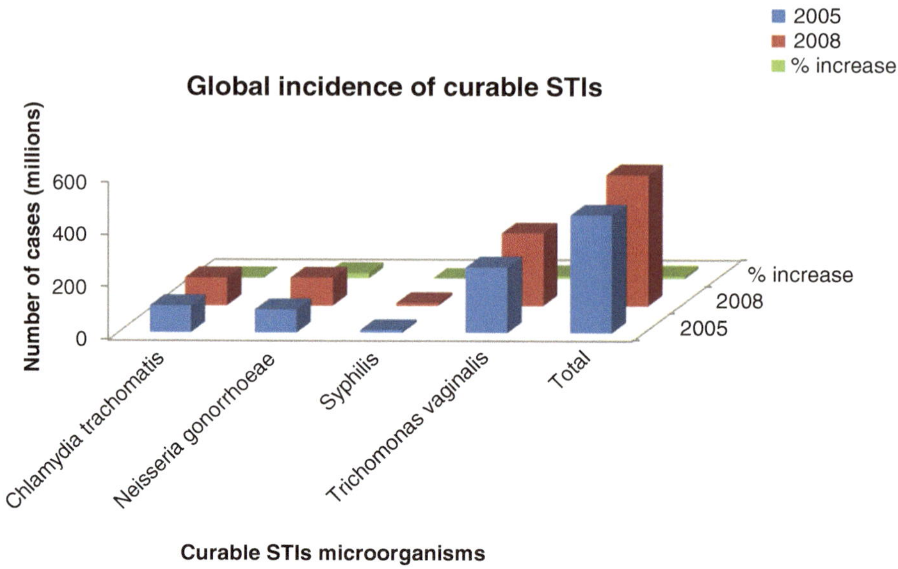

Fig. 11.1 Global incidence of curable STIs (millions) (WHO 2008)

Previously, studies focused on the influence of STIs on male fertility status have shown the impact of infection on sperm parameters as well as the resultant inflammation in the testicles (orchitis), epididymis (epididymitis), and urethra (urethritis) which can ultimately result in spermatogenetic arrest (Parekattil and Agarwal 2012). An additional factor that can impact on the male fertility status is the high concentration of white blood cells (WBCs) that can be found in semen samples from STI-positive subjects (Flint 2012). This condition is termed leukocytospermia and is defined by WHO as the presence of $>1 \times 10^6$ WBC/ml of semen (WHO 2010). The etiology of these infections and their relevance to male infertility vary geographically and generally include bacterial, viral, and protozoan origin (Fig. 11.2). The rest of the chapter will focus on the etiology of common STIs, and their impact on male fertility will be discussed in relevant sections.

11.2 Bacterial Infection in Semen

11.2.1 *Chlamydia trachomatis*

This bacterial infection is the most common among curable STIs in the United States, Europe, and Eastern Mediterranean as highlighted by the WHO (2008). Therefore, this bacterium has received the most attention from earlier studies regarding infertility. Infected males can suffer from asymptomatic infection of the urethra, epididymis, and prostate. This infection can result into urethritis which can

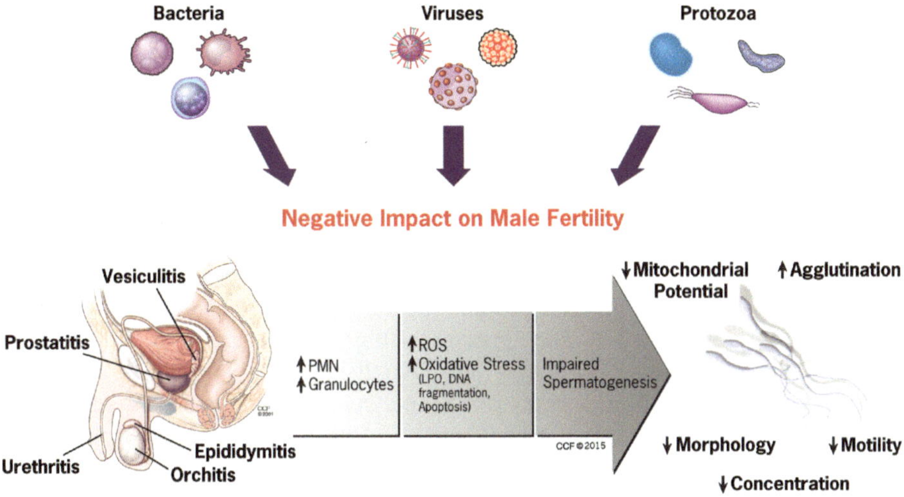

Fig. 11.2 Common pathogens of STIs and impact on male fertility

become even more symptomatic in males compared to females (Parekattil and Agarwal 2012).

Looking strictly at sperm parameters with regard to C. *trachomatis* infection, results are variable. One study reported no change in sperm viability, morphology, and the percentage of motile spermatozoa (Kokab et al. 2012), while another showed no change in any of the sperm parameters (Vigil et al. 2002). However, some studies have reported a reduction in the percentage of progressively motile spermatozoa (Brookings et al. 2013; Kokab et al. 2012; Gallegos et al. 2008; Gdoura et al. 2001) as well as a decline in sperm viability and increase in abnormal morphology (Brookings et al. 2013; Cengiz et al. 1997) from semen samples positive for *C. trachomatis*. A recent study on the effects of C. *trachomatis* infection on male fertility status showed a decrease in sperm concentration (Rybar et al. 2012). Another study investigating chronic prostatitis as a result of *C. trachomatis* infection also showed lowered sperm concentrations, reduced motility, and increased morphological abnormalities (Mazzoli et al. 2010). When investigating semen from asymptomatic male patients, it has been found that the presence of deoxyribonucleic acid (DNA) of *C. trachomatis* in the semen was associated with reduced sperm concentration (Bezold et al. 2007).

Limited in vivo studies have investigated the effect of C. *trachomatis* on the male fertility status and have reported conflicting results. When utilizing a zona-free hamster oocyte penetration assay to analyze the acrosome reaction of male partners infected with *C. trachomatis*, results showed that semen quality and spermatozoa function were unaffected by the presence of the *bacterium* (Vigil et al. 2002). In contrast to the results of the above research, another study reported conflicting results by showing a decrease in acrosome activity in men suffering from *C. trachomatis* (Jungwirth et al. 2003; Eley et al. 2005)

The inconsistency in the results between different studies could be attributed to several reasons and can be influenced by the duration of infection and time of semen analysis. Regarding *C. trachomatis*, the timing of semen analysis following bacterial contact in the reproductive tract, methods of detections in the upper genital tract, and possible relevance of differential diagnosis would have an impact on the sperm parameters (Eley et al. 2005).

Several theories regarding the mechanisms behind the resultant compromised fertility in men suffering from chlamydial infection are inconsistent. When the infection reaches the epithelial cells, the initial response is the generation of interleukin-1 (IL-1), resulting in the stimulation of polymorphonuclear WBCs which subsequently secretes IL-8. The abnormally high concentration of WBCs in the semen sample induces leukocytospermia (Flint 2012). This in turn leads to the generation of reactive oxygen species (ROS) and subsequently oxidative stress (OS) which can affect sperm parameters (Comhaire 1999). Due to scanty cytoplasm in spermatozoa and low antioxidant activity, the spermatozoa are highly susceptible to OS and sperm membrane damage due to lipid peroxidation (Smith 2013). This can impair the acrosomal reaction and subsequently has a negative impact on male fertility (Monavari et al. 2013). The link between *C. trachomatis* and the generation of ROS is conceivable due to the presence of lipopolysaccharides on its surface (Matthews 1951; Hosseinzadeh and Pacey 2003). This compound is able to bind to the CD14 receptor situated on the spermatozoa membrane (Harris et al. 2001). Studies suggest that lipopolysaccharides induce excessive ROS production by spermatozoa; this is confirmed by the decreases seen in sperm motility and concentration in endotoxin-treated samples (Lee and Lee 2013; Urata et al. 2001).

An additional theory regarding the relationship between chlamydial infection and male infertility is the development of antisperm antibodies. The bacterium induces invasion of lymphocytes, macrophages, plasma cells, and eosinophils in response to the infection. The release of cytokines then stimulates the inflammatory cascade, invoking a humoral cell response of secretory IgA and circulatory IgM and IgG antibodies (Lee and Lee 2013). In infertile men, *C. trachomatis* antibodies, IgG and IgA, were shown to be *associated* with a negative impact on semen characteristics and pregnancy outcome (Idahl et al. 2010). Problems arise, when chlamydia IgG or IgA antibodies in semen do not reflect the bacterial presence in the genital tract because some routine antibody analysis are done by specific antibody detection tests instead of cultures, and can provide conflicting results (Parekattil and Agarwal 2012). Sometimes, a negative relation between chlamydial antibodies (IgA and IgG) and semen characteristics is difficult to establish (Eggert-Kruse et al. 1996).

Direct detection tests would be more effective in isolation of the bacteria and to understand its impact on sperm parameters for successful fertilization. During the event of capacitation, tyrosine phosphorylation of sperm proteins was observed to be associated with spermatozoa capacitation in vitro. Thus, *C. trachomatis* attachment to target cells could involve contact with host signal transduction pathways (Hosseinzadeh et al. 2000). Further, genitourinary infection of *C. trachomatis* has been found to be associated with an increase in sperm DNA fragmentation (Gallegos et al. 2008). Semen analysis positive for *C. trachomatis* revealed a significant loss of sperm mitochondrial potential and nonsignificant increase in sperm DNA fragmentation compared to *C. trachomatis*-negative semen samples (Sellami et al. 2014).

11.2.2 *Neisseria gonorrhoeae*

N. gonorrhoeae is a Gram-negative bacterium which infects both men and women. Based on the WHO estimates (2005), each year more than 82 million individuals are infected by this pathogen across the world. Despite its common prevalence, *N. gonorrhoeae* is least studied compared to other STI-causing microorganisms in relation to male infertility. It affects the male urethra, causing urethritis, and has also been found to interact with spermatozoa through its lipooligosaccharides. Gonococcal lipooligosaccharides are immunochemically similar to human glycosphingolipid antigens, which favor the gonococci to evade the host immune response during infection. The importance of the similarity was observed when there was an increased frequency of this structure in gonorrhea-positive males (Schneider et al. 1991). Gonococci attach to the spermatozoa by asialoglycoprotein receptor (ASGP-R) present on sperm and are subsequently transmitted to the female partner (Harvey et al. 2000). Prevalence of *N. gonorrhoeae*, as detected by the presence of its DNA in semen, has been found to be higher in infertile men (6.5 %) compared to fertile men (0 %) (Abusarah et al. 2013).

N. gonorrhoeae contributes to urethritis (Lee and Lee 2013) and chronic infections and, if left untreated, can cause complications in the epididymis. Additionally, epididymitis can largely affect the sperm concentration leading to oligospermia and azoospermia in cases of bilateral epididymitis or vas deferens occlusion (Ndowa and Lusti-Narasimhan 2012). The link between *N. gonorrhoeae* infection and male fertility is further supported by a cohort modeling Swedish study reporting a decline in secondary subfertility with the eradication of gonorrhea (Akre et al. 1999).

11.2.3 *Mycoplasmas*

Two genital mycoplasmas, *Mycoplasma hominis* and *Mycoplasma genitalium*, are found in both male and female reproductive tracts (Gimenes et al. 2014). Although in men mycoplasmas were isolated about a decade ago, their exact role in the development of male infertility is still under debate (Maeda et al. 2004; Al-Sweih et al. 2012). Different studies have reported varying prevalence rates of mycoplasma infection based on the laboratory detection method of bacteria. When urine samples of patients with persistent or recurrent urethritis were examined, 41 % of the population was positive for *M. genitalia* (Wikstrom and Jensen 2006). In Tunisian infertile men, *M. genitalium* DNA was detected in 4.8 % of semen samples, while the detection for *M. hominis* DNA was 9.6 %. The prevalence of *M. genitalium* DNA was significantly higher in azoospermic semen samples compared to non-azoospermic. However, no association of *M. genitalium* and *M. hominis* was found attributing to the abnormal semen characteristics (concentration, motility, morphology, viability, volume, and leukocyte count) (Gdoura et al. 2008). Although the relation of mycoplasmas with male infertility is not clearly documented, attachment of *M. genitalium* to spermatozoa was observed. This attachment is of significant importance not only in transmitting the infection to the female partner but also in causing sperm agglutination, thereby rendering them immotile and ultimately resulting in male infertility (Svenstrup et al. 2003; Pellati et al. 2008). In another study, negative effects of *M. hominis* infection on semen viscosity, volume, sperm morphology, motility, and concentration have been documented (Zinzendorf et al. 2008). In vitro incubation of mycoplasmas with semen has shown significant reduction in sperm motility and morphology and increase in the higher rates of the acrosome reaction and capacitation. This means mycoplasma species can negatively impair the fertilizing capacity of spermatozoa (Rose and Scott 1994).

11.2.4 *Ureaplasmas*

Ureaplasmas (*Ureaplasma urealyticum and Ureaplasma parvum*) reside in the male urethra where they contaminate the semen at the time of ejaculation (Zeighami et al. 2009). The incidence of *U. urealyticum* infection in infertile men is variable, ranging from 5 to 42 % (Abusarah et al. 2013). A total of 18.3 % infertile Tunisian men were found positive for ureaplasmas, of which, the percentage of men infected with *U. urealyticum* was higher (15.4 %) compared to *U. parvum* (2.9 %) (Gdoura et al. 2001). In another study 27.6 % infertile men were found positive for *U. urealyticum* (Zinzendorf et al. 2008). The data on effects of ureaplasmas on semen parameters are conflicting. Some studies found no relation between the *U. urealyticum* infection and the quality of sperm parameters (Andrade-Rocha 2003), while others documented low sperm motility, reduced concentration, and morphology (Zeighami et al. 2009; Zinzendorf et al. 2008). Furthermore, in an animal study where rats were experimentally infected with *U. urealyticum*, remarkable change in spermatogenesis was observed. When these rats were allowed to mate, in 33 % of the cases, post-mating plug was not observed, while in the rest of the cases who mated successfully, offspring were significantly smaller compared to uninfected or control rats (Xu et al. 1997). In a later study, in vitro experiments on co-incubation of human and ram sperm with *U. urealyticum* revealed a dose-dependent decrease in viability and motility in human spermatozoa and only motility in ram spermatozoa compared to controls. The same study found time- and dose-dependent DNA damage both in human and ram spermatozoa, which suggests that ureaplasmas can affect quantitative (motility, concentration) as well as qualitative (DNA, morphology) sperm parameters (Reichart et al. 2000). Damage to quality of spermatozoa can have serious effects on the fertility of the couple as reduced pregnancy rates have been reported after embryo transfer in *U. urealyticum*-infected groups compared to normal (Montagut et al. 1991). Care must be taken while using ureaplasma-infected semen samples for assisted reproductive technology (ART) as semen washing procedures may not always remove the pathogens completely from the spermatozoa (Knox et al. 2003).

11.2.5 *Treponema pallidum*

T. pallidum is most commonly acquired through close sexual contact and results in syphilis. Despite the curable nature of the disease, it remains a big challenge, infecting around 12 million people worldwide every year (Rodriguez-Cerdeira and Silami-Lopes 2012). This pathogen gets significant attention due to its link with HIV (human immunodeficiency virus) transmission (Spielmann et al. 2010). Although nothing much is documented on the role of *T. pallidum* and male infertility, complications of the disease can have a negative impact on fertility. One proposed indication regards the inflammation of the epididymis which can cause epididymal obstruction. In tertiary syphilis, gummatous lesions cause destruction of local tissue. If lesions occur in the testicles, the infection may have an impact on testicular function and therefore infertility. Effects of this pathogen are even more severe and drastic on pregnancy and the infant with evidence of 50 % abortions and stillbirths and more than 10 % infant mortality (Brookings et al. 2013). Therefore, during ART procedures it is imperative that both partners are screened for the pathogen and should be treated accordingly.

11.3 Semen and Viral Infection

11.3.1 Human Immunodeficiency Virus (HIV)

HIV is a lentivirus belonging to the subgroup of retrovirus that causes acquired immune deficiency syndrome (AIDS). The two types of this virus are known as HIV-1 and HIV-2. Despite similarities between both types of HIV, they differ in pathogenicity, infectivity, and prevalence. HIV-1 transmission is easy and rapid resulting in vast majority of infections worldwide (Weiss 1993; Gimenes et al. 2014). Common routes of HIV-1 transmission include blood, breast milk, and vaginal as well as seminal fluid. There have been some studies validating the viral impact on male infertility. The concept of how viral infections could weaken the male genital function is by direct invasion of the male genital tract cells or indirect inflammatory or immunological responses. Semen parameters of men with asymptomatic disease can be in normal range (van Leeuwen et al. 2008); nevertheless, with disease progression it can negatively affect sperm motility, morphology (Bujan et al. 2007; Pavili et al. 2010), and concentration (Crittenden et al. 1992; Nicopoullos et al. 2004).

This virus is also known to cause secondary hypogonadism resulting in low testosterone levels. Reduced concentration of the androgen would have an impact on spermatogenesis reducing the sperm count (Crum-Cianflone et al. 2007). The viral infection resides in the germ cells of the testes, and an extended duration of infection is associated with germ cell loss (Shevchuk et al. 1999). In one study, a positive correlation between CD4+ count and sperm concentration as well as motility together with a negative correlation with normal sperm morphology has been documented as reviewed by Brookings et al. (2013).

With the introduction of highly active antiretroviral therapy (HAART) for HIV-positive patients, survival rate and life expectancy have tremendously improved (Sabin 2013). HAART has given a new direction of investigation because changes in semen of HIV-positive men currently found are largely attributed to this therapy (Kehl et al. 2011). In addition to the changes in semen as discussed earlier, sperm mitochondrial toxicity and high aneuploidy have also been reported in HIV-positive men (Pavili et al. 2010). When spermatozoa from healthy men were incubated in vitro with different concentrations of HAART agents, decreases in sperm motility and mitochondrial potential and an increase in acrosome reaction were observed at higher doses of saquinavir (a protease inhibitor used in HAART) (Ahmad et al. 2011).

ART are the best options for HIV-positive men who wish to father a child. The use of HAART decreases the viral load in semen; further sperm washing procedures have improved the utility of semen from HIV-positive men in intrauterine insemination or in vitro fertilization (IVF). Washed spermatozoa from HIV-positive men have been used in assisted reproduction and have resulted in successful live births without HIV transmission to mother or the child (Nicopoullos et al. 2004).

11.3.2 Human Papillomavirus

HPV is considered the most common sexually transmitted viral disease among young men and women. Out of 100 identified genotypes, 40–50 are found to infect the genital tract. High-risk genotypes 16, 18, 31, and 45 are associated with malignancy of the squamous cells localized in the genital tract and anus (Medicine 2013). Identification of HPV through polymerase chain reaction (PCR) and fluorescence in situ hybridization (FISH) in semen cultures revealed reduced sperm motility (Foresta et al. 2010) and sperm concentration (Bezold et al. 2007). In contrast, a study of 308 HPV-positive males showed that the infection does not correlate with an impact on the sperm parameters (Schillaci et al. 2013). In addition, the gene-targeting region of HPV in sperm reports no change in hyperactivation of spermatozoa, which proposes preservation of the fertilizing capacity of spermatozoa (Lee et al. 2002). In view of published data, a clear link between HPV and male infertility remains inconclusive (Fr 2008). Nevertheless, a significant increase in the abortion rate was observed in couples where the semen sample of the male was positive for viral DNA. Similarly, a recent study reported a significant increase in pregnancy loss after IVF in couples where semen samples were positive for viral DNA (Perino et al. 2011). Therefore, HPV infection should be dealt with seriously in all couples seeking fertility treatment.

11.3.3 Herpes Simplex Virus

Herpes simplex virus contains two genital virus strains: HSV-1 and HSV-2. HSV-1 is commonly involved in oral and occasionally in genital infections, but HSV-2 is the most common etiology of genital herpes (Wald et al. 2000). Prevalence of both HSV strains is quite variable ranging from 2 to 50% as detected in semen of asymptomatic men, but no association to change in sperm parameters or male infertility was established (Neofytou et al. 2009). In contrast, reduced sperm motility and concentration was attributed to the presence of HSV DNA detected through nested PCR in 49.5 % of semen samples from infertile men compared to controls (Kapranos et al. 2003). Further, decline in sperm concentration, higher rates of apoptosis, and disrupted spermatogenesis were observed in patients infected with HSV.

An animal study utilized transgenic mice as subjects to investigate the molecular impact of HSV on spermatogenesis. The expression of the pathogen's thymidine kinase in the testis correlated with sperm structural abnormalities and defects in spermatogenesis (Braun et al. 1990). This was substantiated in 2009, when results confirmed the correlation of the thymidine kinase activity to the loss of germ cells in the testes (Cai et al. 2009). Apparently, the published data accord the negative effects of HSV on sperm parameters and male fertility.

11.3.4 Human Cytomegalovirus

Human cytomegalovirus (HCMV) has been isolated from different body secretions including blood, urine, milk, cervical and vaginal secretions, and semen (Eggert-Kruse et al. 2009; Roback et al. 2001). Sexual transmission does not appear to be the common route of HCMV infection; however, if the accessory glands are infected with the virus, it can be discharged into the male reproductive tract and can encounter the spermatozoa easily (Eggert-Kruse et al. 2009). Although presence of HCMV in semen is debated, some studies have confirmed its presence in seminal fluid (Bezold et al. 2007; Levy et al. 1997). The relevance of this virus or the detection of its DNA in semen and its impact on semen parameters are uncertain. A fairly large body of evidence has shown no relation between the infection and change in semen characteristics (Bezold et al. 2007; Neofytou et al. 2009; Eggert-Kruse et al. 2009, Pallier et al. 2002).

11.3.5 Hepatitis B Virus

Hepatitis B virus (HBV) is present in semen and other bodily fluids of infected people. HBV is sometimes considered even more challenging than HIV due to its ability to cross the blood-testis barrier and its penetration into the sperm genome (Garolla et al. 2013). Viral load in semen of infected men seeking assisted reproductive treatments has been quantified by real-time PCR (Qian et al. 2005). Integration of HBV into sperm chromosomes was confirmed by FISH in carrier men (Huang et al. 2003). The integration of virus into the sperm genome can cause mutagenic and hereditary effects that are serious threats in vertical transmission.

Several studies have reported alterations in sperm parameters in HBV-infected semen samples including decrease in sperm concentration, motility, and morphology (Lorusso et al. 2010; Vicari et al. 2006; Zhou et al. 2011). Others have reported increased germ cell apoptosis (Kang et al. 2012; Moretti et al. 2008) and spermatozoa aneuploidy (Huang et al. 2003; Kang et al. 2012; Moretti et al. 2008) in response to HBV infection.

Infertility treatment of HBV-infected patients is a great concern for health professionals. When zona-free hamster eggs were injected with human spermatozoa infected with the HBV DNA plasmid, HBV gene expression was noted in the embryo (Ali et al. 2006). Furthermore, a reduction in IVF success rates has been reported in HBV-infected couples (Zhou et al. 2011). The vertical transmission of the virus demands extreme care since even ART cannot exclude the risk of viral transmission to the offspring.

11.3.6 Hepatitis C Virus

Sexual transmission of hepatitis C virus (HCV) is not common, and very low viral loads in semen of infected patients have been detected. Only 5 % vertical and sexual transmission of HCV has been documented by some authors (Durazzo et al. 2006), while some cohort studies report even less (0–0.6 %) infection rates per year in seronegative counter partners (Piazza et al. 1997; Vandelli et al. 2004; Tahan et al. 2005). According to the Center for Disease Control and Prevention (CDC, USA), sexual transmission of HCV is rare CDC guidelines (2010). Though HCV RNA has been detected in seminal plasma of infected men, in one particular study, no changes in seminal parameters were attributed to the presence of viral RNA (Bourlet et al. 2009). In contrast, other studies have reported negative effects of HCV infection on semen parameters. For example, reductions in sperm motility, morphology, and sperm count have been reported in infected samples (Durazzo et al. 2006; Lorusso et al. 2010; Hofny et al. 2011; La Vignera et al. 2012). Additionally, sperm aneuploidy, alterations in sperm mitochondrial potential, and DNA fragmentation were observed in HCV-positive samples (La Vignera et al. 2012).

The transmission of HCV during ART procedure is not well reported. However, the virus has been identified in follicular fluid in women infected with HCV (Papaxanthos-Roche et al. 2004). Thus far, follow-up studies on couples, where at least one partner was HCV positive, have reported no infected births (Savasi et al. 2013; Bourlet et al. 2009). Although the transmission of HCV is low, extreme care must be taken while handling infected samples. Density gradient centrifugation (DGC) and sperm swim-up methods are the recommended procedures for sperm preparation to be used in ART (Savasi et al. 2013; Bourlet et al. 2009).

11.4 Semen and Protozoa Infection

11.4.1 *Trichomonas vaginalis*

Current statistics suggest that the infection of trichomoniasis is more prevalent among women affecting more than 160 million people worldwide (WHO 2005). The prevalence and virulence of the pathogen are well studied in women compared to men. The reason for this ignorance of its impact on male infertility may be due to its asymptomatic nature in men. This pathogen was detected in 72 % of the asymptomatic male population (Flint 2012). This high percentage of asymptomatic cases can be due to the cytotoxic role of prostatic zinc toward protozoan pathogenesis (Harp and Chowdhury 2011) which can mask the symptoms of the infection. However, untreated trichomoniasis can result in urethritis, epididymitis, and prostatitis as well as detrimental impact on the female partner, which can result in pelvic inflammatory disease, cervicitis, urethritis, vaginitis, and preterm delivery (Flint 2012).

T. vaginalis was found more common in infertile men compared to fertile men. Further, a decrease in sperm count was also reported in infected semen samples. Significant reductions in sperm motility, morphology, and viability were reported in a large number of asymptomatic male subjects (Gopalkrishnan and Kumar 1990). The change in sperm parameters in infected samples is an indication of *T. vaginalis*' association to male fertility, but further research is required.

Conclusions

For male patients positive for STIs, there are established laboratory practices that can be implemented in an in vitro setting to minimize the risk of transmission of infectious agent to the mother or progeny. Density gradient centrifugation (DGC) and direct swim-up are the two known techniques associated with sperm washing which allows for the removal of infectious agents from the semen sample. Though highly efficient, sperm washing mediums can result in minute quantities of the viral DNA remaining (Kuji et al. 2008). This problem can be resolved by the addition of serine proteases and a "novel tube insert" in the process of DGC. Serine proteases can significantly reduce the virus number attached to the sperm, notably with HIV-1 (Loskutoff et al. 2005; Blevins et al. 2008). The usage of DGC improves the sperm yield from highly viscous samples and prevents the formation of sperm antibodies, a benefit for male HIV-positive patients who wish to undergo IVF (Fourie et al. 2012). The viral STI that exhibits difficulty in removal for IVF is HPV. This can be improved by the addition of heparinase-III to the washing media, and it has shown significant reduction of HPV DNA in infected samples (Garolla et al. 2012).

Implementation of STI screening in males could offer a long-term advantage for the male patient, while early detection could allow for the avoidance of healthcare costs and decreased coinfection with other STIs such as HIV (Domes et al. 2012; Chesson et al. 2013). When analysis can be approached from a proteomic and molecular level, there can be an improvement of detection and management for the patient. Since prevention is the best cure, utmost attention must be given when dealing with such STIs to prevent their spread. Proper vaccination must be ensured in cases where required and available like HBV. Protected intercourse is essential in cases where seminal transmission of the virus or bacteria is common, i.e., HBV or HIV.

References

Abusarah EA, Awwad ZM, Charvalos E, Shehabi AA. Molecular detection of potential sexually transmitted pathogens in semen and urine specimens of infertile and fertile males. Diagn Microbiol Infect Dis. 2013;77:283–6.

Ahmad G, Moinard N, Jouanolou V, Daudin M, Gandia P, Bujan L. In vitro assessment of the adverse effects of antiretroviral drugs on the human male gamete. Toxicol In Vitro. 2011;25:485–91.

Akre O, Cnattingius S, Bergstrom R, Kvist U, Trichopoulos D, Ekbom A. Human fertility does not decline: evidence from Sweden. Fertil Steril. 1999;71:1066–9.

Ali BA, Huang TH, Salem HH, Xie QD. Expression of hepatitis B virus genes in early embryonic cells originated from hamster ova and human spermatozoa transfected with the complete viral genome. Asian J Androl. 2006;8:273–9.

Al-Sweih NA, Al-Fadli AH, Omu AE, Rotimi VO. Prevalence of Chlamydia trachomatis, Mycoplasma hominis, Mycoplasma genitalium, and Ureaplasma urealyticum infections and seminal quality in infertile and fertile men in Kuwait. J Androl. 2012;33:1323–9.

Andrade-Rocha FT. Ureaplasma urealyticum and Mycoplasma hominis in men attending for routine semen analysis. Prevalence, incidence by age and clinical settings, influence on sperm characteristics, relationship with the leukocyte count and clinical value. Urol Int. 2003;71: 377–81.

Baecher-Lind LE, Miller WC, Wilcox AJ. Infectious disease and reproductive health: a review. Obstet Gynecol Surv. 2009;65:53–65.

Bezold G, Politch JA, Kiviat NB, Kuypers JM, Wolff H, Anderson DJ. Prevalence of sexually transmissible pathogens in semen from asymptomatic male infertility patients with and without leukocytospermia. Fertil Steril. 2007;87:1087–97.

Blevins BA, D. L. R. M., Loskutoff NM. Technical note: effect of density gradient centrifugation with trypsin on the in vivo fertilising capability of bovine spermatozoa. Reproduction, Fertility, And Development 2008;20:784–8.

Bourlet T, Lornage J, Maertens A, Garret AS, Saoudin H, Tardy JC, Jimenez C, Guerin JF, Pozzetto B, Levy R. Prospective evaluation of the threat related to the use of seminal fractions from hepatitis C virus-infected men in assisted reproductive techniques. Hum Reprod. 2009;24: 530–5.

Braun RE, Lo D, Pinkert CA, Widera G, Flavell RA, Palmiter RD, Brinster RL. Infertility in male transgenic mice: disruption of sperm development by HSV-tk expression in postmeiotic germ cells. Biol Reprod. 1990;43:684–93.

Brookings C, Goldmeier D, Sadeghi-Nejad H. Sexually transmitted infections and sexual function in relation to male infertility. Korean J Urol. 2013;54:149–56.

Bujan L, Hollander L, Coudert M, Gilling-Smith C, Vucetich A, Guibert J, Vernazza P, Ohl J, Weigel M, Englert Y, Semprini AE. Safety and efficacy of sperm washing in HIV-1-serodiscordant couples where the male is infected: results from the European CREAThE network. Aids. 2007;21:1909–14.

Cai LY, Kato T, Nakayama M, Susa T, Murakami S, Izumi S, Kato Y. HSV type 1 tymidine kinase protein accumulation in round spermatids induces male infertility by spermatogenesis disruption and apoptotic loss of germ cells. Reprod Toxicol. 2009;27:14–21.

CDC. Http://Www.Cdc.Gov/Std/Treatment/2010/

Cengiz T, Aydoganli L, Baykam M, Mungan NA, Tuncbilek E, Dincer M, Yakupoglu K, Akalin Z. Chlamydial infections and male infertility. Int Urol Nephrol. 1997;29:687–93.

Chesson HW, Bernstein KT, Gift TL, Marcus JL, Pipkin S, Kent CK. The cost-effectiveness of screening men who have sex with men for rectal chlamydial and gonococcal infection to prevent HIV infection. Sex Transm Dis. 2013;40:366–71.

Comhaire FEA. Mechanisms and effects of male genital tract infection on sperm quality and fertilization potential: the andrologist's viewpoint. Hum Reprod Update. 1999;5:393–5.

Crittenden JA, Handelsman DJ, Stewart GJ. Semen analysis in human immunodeficiency virus infection. Fertil Steril. 1992;57:1294–9.

Crum-Cianflone NF, Bavaro M, Hale B, Amling C, Truett A, Brandt C, Pope B, Futek K, Medina S, Wallace MR. Erectile dysfunction and hypogonadism among men with HIV. Aids Patient Care Stds. 2007;21:9–19.

Domes T, Lo KC, Grober ED, Mullen JB, Mazzulli T, Jarvi K. The utility and cost of Chlamydia trachomatis and Neisseria gonorrhoeae screening of a male infertility population. Fertil Steril. 2012;97:299–305.

Durazzo M, Premoli A, Di Bisceglie C, Bertagna A, Faga E, Biroli G, Manieri C, Bo S, Pagano G. Alterations of seminal and hormonal parameters: an extrahepatic manifestation of HCV infection? World J Gastroenterol. 2006;12:3073–6.

Eggert-Kruse W, Buhlinger-Gopfarth N, Rohr G, Probst S, Aufenanger J, Naher H, Runnebaum B. Antibodies to Chlamydia trachomatis in semen and relationship with parameters of male infertility. Hum Reprod. 1996;11:1408–17.

Eggert-Kruse W, Reuland M, Johannsen W, Strowitzki T, Schlehofer JR. Cytomegalovirus (CMV) infection–related to male and/or female infertility factors? Fertil Steril. 2009;91:67–82.

Eley A, Pacey AA, Galdiero M, Galdiero M, Galdiero F. Can Chlamydia trachomatis directly damage your sperm? Lancet Infect Dis. 2005;5:53–7.

Flint M. Gamete proteomic profile of male patients suffering from STIs. PhD Protocol, University of Stellenbosch; 2012. https://scholar.sun.ac.za/handle/10019.1/98639

Flint M, Du Plessis SS. Trichomonas Vaginalis in Sub-Saharan Africa: occurrence and diagnostic approaches for the male partner. Stellenbosch University; Medical Technology SA. 2013;27:26–28.

Foresta C, Pizzol D, Moretti A, Barzon L, Palù G, Garolla A. Clinical and prognostic significance of human papillomavirus DNA in the sperm or exfoliated cells of infertile patients and subjects with risk factors. Fertil Steril. 2010;94:1723–7.

Fourie J, Loskutoff N, Huyser C. Elimination of bacteria from human semen during sperm preparation using density gradient centrifugation with a novel tube insert. Andrologia. 2011;44:513–7.

Fourie J, Loskutoff N, Huyser C. Treatment of human sperm with serine protease during density gradient centrifugation. J Assist Reprod Genet. 2012;29:1273–9.

Fr O. Sexually transmitted infections: impact on male fertility. Andrologia. 2008;40:72–5.

Gallegos G, Ramos B, Santiso R, Goyanes V, Gosálvez J, Fernández JL. Sperm DNA fragmentation in infertile men with genitourinary infection by Chlamydia trachomatis and Mycoplasma. Fertil Steril. 2008;90:328–34.

Garolla A, Lenzi A, Palù G, Pizzol D, Bertoldo A, De Toni L, Foresta C. Human papillomavirus sperm infection and assisted reproduction: a dangerous hazard with a possible safe solution. Hum Reprod. 2012;27:967–73.

Garolla A, Pizzol D, Bertoldo A, Menegazzo M, Barzon L, Foresta C. Sperm viral infection and male infertility: focus on HBV, HCV, HIV, HPV, HSV, HCMV, and AAV. J Reprod Immunol. 2013;100:20–9.

Gdoura R, Keskes-Ammar L, Bouzid F, Eb F, Hammami A, Orfila J. Chlamydia trachomatis and male infertility in Tunisia. Eur J Contracept Reprod Health Care. 2001;6:102–7.

Gdoura R, Kchaou W, Ammar-Keskes L, Chakroun N, Sellemi A, Znazen A, Rebai T, Hammami A. Assessment of Chlamydia trachomatis, Ureaplasma urealyticum, Ureaplasma parvum, Mycoplasma hominis, and Mycoplasma genitalium in semen and first void urine specimens of asymptomatic male partners of infertile couples. J Androl. 2008;29:198–206.

Gimenes F, Souza RP, Bento JC, Teixeira JJ, Maria-Engler SS, Bonini MG, Consolaro ME. Male infertility: a public health issue caused by sexually transmitted pathogens. Nat Rev Urol. 2014;11:672–87.

Gopalkrishnan K, Hinduja IN, Kumar TC. Semen characteristics of asymptomatic males affected by Trichomonas vaginalis. J In Vitro Fertil Embryo Trans Ivf. 1990;7:165–7.

Harp DF, Chowdhury I. Trichomoniasis: evaluation to execution. Eur J Obstet Gynecol Reprod Biol. 2011;157:3–9.

Harris CL, Vigar MA, Rey Nores JE, Horejsi V, Labeta MO, Morgan BP. The lipopolysaccharide co-receptor CD14 is present and functional in seminal plasma and expressed on spermatozoa. Immunology. 2001;104:317–23.

Harvey HA, Porat N, Campbell CA, Jennings M, Gibson BW, Phillips NJ, Apicella MA, Blake MS. Gonococcal lipooligosaccharide is a ligand for the asialoglycoprotein receptor on human sperm. Mol Microbiol. 2000;36:1059–70.

Hofny ER, Ali ME, Taha EA, Nafeh HM, Sayed DS, Abdel-Azeem HG, Abdou EF, Kamal GM, Mostafa T. Semen and hormonal parameters in men with chronic hepatitis C infection. Fertil Steril. 2011;95:2557–9.

Hosseinzadeh S, Brewis IA, Pacey AA, Moore HDM, Eley A. Coincubationn of Human Spermatozoa Chlamydia trachomatis in votro causes increased tyrosine phosphorylation of sperm proteins. Infect Immun. 2000;68:4872–6.

Hosseinzadeh S, Pacey AA, Eley A. Chlamydia Trachomatis-induced death of human spermatozoa is cause primarily by Lipopolysaccharide. J Med Microbiol. 2003;52:193–200.

Huang JM, Huang TH, Qiu HY, Fang XW, Zhuang TG, Liu HX, Wang YH, Deng LZ, Qiu JW. Effects of hepatitis B virus infection on human sperm chromosomes. World J Gastroenterol. 2003;9:736–40.

Idahl A, Lundin E, Elgh F, Jurstrand M, Moller JK, Marklund I, Lindgren P, Ottander U. Chlamydia trachomatis, Mycoplasma genitalium, Neisseria gonorrhoeae, human papillomavirus, and polyomavirus are not detectable in human tissue with epithelial ovarian cancer, borderline tumor, or benign conditions. Am J Obstet Gynecol. 2010;1:71.E1–6.

Jungwirth A, Straberger A, Esterbauer B, Fink K, Schmeller N. Acrosome reaction in Chlamydia-positive and negative patients. Andrologia. 2003;35:314–6.

Kang X, Xie Q, Zhou X, Li F, Huang J, Liu D, Huang T. Effects of hepatitis B virus S protein exposure on sperm membrane integrity and functions. Plos One. 2012;7:E33471.

Kapranos N, Petrakou E, Anastasiadou C, Kotronias D. Detection of herpes simplex virus, cytomegalovirus, and Epstein-Barr virus in the semen of men attending an infertility clinic. Fertil Steril. 2003;79 Suppl 3:1566–70.

Kehl S, Weigel M, Muller D, Gentili M, Hornemann A, Sutterlin M. HIV-infection and modern antiretroviral therapy impair sperm quality. Arch Gynecol Obstet. 2011;284:229–33.

Knox CL, Allan JA, Allan JM, Edirisinghe WR, Stenzel D, Lawrence FA, Purdie DM, Timms P. Ureaplasma parvum and Ureaplasma urealyticum are detected in semen after washing before assisted reproductive technology procedures. Fertil Steril. 2003;80:921–9.

Kokab A, Akhondi MM, Sadeghi MR, Modarresi MH, Aarabi M, Jennings R, Pacey AA, Eley A. Raised inflammatory markers in semen from men with asymptomatic chlamydia infection. J Androl. 2012;31:114–20.

Kuji N, Yoshii T, Hamatani T, Hanabusa H, Yoshimura Y, Kato S. Buoyan density and sedimentation dynamics of HIV-1 in two density-gradient media for semen processing. Fertil Steril. 2008;90:1983–7.

La Vignera S, Condorelli RA, Vicari E, D'agata R, Calogero AE. Sperm DNA damage in patients with chronic viral C hepatitis. Eur J Intern Med. 2012;23:E19–24.

Lee S, Lee KS. Chlamydia and male lower urinary tract diseases. Korean J Urol. 2013;54:73–7.

Lee CA, Huang CT, King A, Chan PJ. Differential effects of human papollomavirus DNA types on p53 tumor-suppressor gene apoptosis in sperm. Gynecol Oncol. 2002;85:511–6.

Levy R, Najioullah F, Keppi B, Thouvenot D, Bosshard S, Lornage J, Lina B, Guerin JF, Aymard M. Detection of cytomegalovirus in semen from a population of men seeking infertility evaluation. Fertil Steril. 1997;68:820–5.

Lorusso F, Palmisano M, Chironna M, Vacca M, Masciandaro P, Bassi E, Selvaggi Luigi L, Depalo R. Impact of chronic viral diseases on semen parameters. Andrologia. 2010;42:121–6.

Loskutoff NM, Huyser C, Singh R, Thornhill AR, Morris L, Webber L. Use orf a novel washing method combining multiple density gradients and trypsin for removing human immunodeficiency virus-1 and hepatitis C virus from semen. Fertil Steril. 2005;84:1001–10.

Maeda S, Deguchi T, Ishiko H, Matsumoto T, Naito S, Kumon H, Tsukamoto T, Onodera S, Kamidono S. Detection of Mycoplasma genitalium, Mycoplasma hominis, Ureaplasma parvum (biovar 1) and Ureaplasma urealyticum (biovar 2) in patients with non-gonococcal urethritis using polymerase chain reaction-microtiter plate hybridization. Int J Urol. 2004;11: 750–4.

Matthews CS, Buxton CL. Bacteriology of the cervix in cases of infertility. Fertil Steril. 1951;2: 45–52.

Mazzoli S, Cai T, Addonisio P, Bechi A, Mondaini N, Bartoletti R. Chlamydia trachomatis infection is related to poor semen quality in young prostatitis. Eur Urol. 2010;57:708–14.

Medicine, P. C. O. A. S. F. R. Recommendations for reducing the risk of viral transmission during fertility treatment with the use of autologous gametes: a committee opinion. Fertil Steril. 2013;99:340–6.

Monavari S, Vaziri MS, Khalili M, Shamsi-Shahrabadi M, Keyvani H, Mollaei H, Fazlalipour M. Asymptomatic seminal infection of herpes simplex virus: impact on male infertility. J Biomed Res. 2013;27:56–61.

Montagut JM, Lepretre S, Degoy J, Rousseau M. Ureaplasma in semen and IVF. Hum Reprod. 1991;6:727–9.

Moretti E, Federico MG, Giannerini V, Collodel G. Sperm ultrastructure and meiotic segregation in a group of patients with chronic hepatitis B and C. Andrologia. 2008;40:286–91.

Ndowa F, Lusti-Narasimhan M. The threat of untreatable gonorrhoea: implications and consequences for reproductive and sexual morbidity. Reprod Health Matters. 2012;20:76–82.

Neofytou E, Sourvinos G, Asmarianaki M, Spandidos DA, Makrigiannakis A. Prevalence of human herpes virus types 1–7 in the semen of men attending an infertility clinic and correlation with semen parameters. Fertil Steril. 2009;91:2487–94.

Nicopoullos JD, Almeida PA, Ramsay JW, Gilling-Smith C. The effect of human immunodeficiency virus on sperm parameters and the outcome of intrauterine insemination following sperm washing. Hum Reprod. 2004;19:2289–97.

Pallier C, Tebourbi L, Chopineau-Proust S, Schoevaert D, Nordmann P, Testart J, Courtot AM. Herpesvirus, cytomegalovirus, human sperm and assisted fertilization. Hum Reprod. 2002;17(5):1281–7.

Papaxanthos-Roche A, Trimoulet P, Commenges-Ducos M, Hocke C, Fleury HJ, Mayer G. PCR-detected hepatitis C virus RNA associated with human zona-intact oocytes collected from infected women for ART. Hum Reprod. 2004;19:1170–5.

Parekattil S, Agarwal A. Infection in infertility. In: Parekattil S, Agarwal A, editors. Male infertility: contemporary clinical approaches. New York: Springer Science + Business Media; 2012.

Pavili L, Daudin M, Moinard N, Walschaerts M, Cuzin L, Massip P, Pasquier C, Bujan L. Decrease of mitochondrial DNA level in sperm from patients infected with human immunodeficiency virus-1 linked to nucleoside analogue reverse transcriptase inhibitor. Fertil Steril. 2010;94:2151–6.

Pellati D, Mylonakis I, Bertoloni G, Fiore C, Andrisani A, Ambrosini G, Armanini D. Genital tract infections and infertility. Eur J Obstet Gynecol Reprod Biol. 2008;140:3–11.

Perino A, Giovannelli L, Schillaci R, Ruvolo G, Fiorentino FP, Alimondi P, Cefalù E, Ammatuna P. Human papillomavirus infection in couples undergoing in vitro fertilization procedures: impact on reproductive outcomes. Fertil Steril. 2011;95:1845–48.

Piazza M, Sagliocca L, Tosone G, Guadagnino V, Stazi MA, Orlando R, Borgia G, Rosa D, Abrignani S, Palumbo F, Manzin A, Clementi M. Sexual transmission of the hepatitis C virus and efficacy of prophylaxis with intramuscular immune serum globulin. Arch Intern Med. 1997;157:1537–44.

Qian WP, Tan YQ, Chen Y, Peng Y, Li Z, Lu GX, Lin MC, Kung HF, He ML, Shing LK. Rapid quantification of semen hepatitis B virus DNA by real-time polymerase chain reaction. World J Gastroenterol. 2005;11:5385–9.

Reichart M, Kahane I, Bartoov B. In vivo and in vitro impairment of human and ram sperm nuclear chromatin integrity by sexually transmitted Ureaplasma urealyticum infection. Biol Reprod. 2000;63:1041–8.

Roback JD, Hillyer CD, Drew WL, Laycock ME, Luka J, Mocarski ES, Slobedman B, Smith JW, Soderberg-Naucler C, Todd DS, Woxenius S, Busch MP. Multicenter evaluation of PCR methods for detecting CMV DNA in blood donors. Transfusion. 2001;41:1249–57.

Rodriguez-Cerdeira C, Silami-Lopes VG. Congenital syphilis in the 21st century. Actas Dermosifiliogr. 2012;103:679–93.

Rose BI, Scott B. Sperm motility, morphology, hyperactivation, and ionophore-induced acrosome reactions after overnight incubation with mycoplasmas. Fertil Steril. 1994;61:341–8.

Rybar R, Prinosilova P, Kopecka V, Hlavicova J, Veznik Z, Zajicova A, Rubes J. The effect of bacterial contamination of semen on sperm chromatin integrity and standard semen parameters in men from infertile couples. Andrologia. 2012;44:410–8.

Sabin CA. Do people with HIV infection have a normal life expectancy in the era of combination antiretroviral therapy? BMC Medicine. 2013;11:251.

Savasi V, Oneta M, Parrilla B, Cetin I. Should HCV discordant couples with a seropositive male partner be treated with assisted reproduction techniques (ART)? Eur J Obstet Gynecol Reprod Biol. 2013;167:181–4.

Schillaci R, Capra G, Bellavia C, Ruvolo G, Scazzone C, Venezia R, Perino A. Detection of oncogenic human papillomavirus genotypes on spermatozoa from male partners of infertile couples. Fertil Steril. 2013;100:1236–40.

Schneider H, Griffiss JM, Boslego JW, Hitchcock PJ, Zahos KM, Apicella MA. Expression of paragloboside-like lipooligosaccharides may be necessary component of gonococcal pathogenesis in men. J Exp Med. 1991;174:1601–5.

Sellami H, Znazen A, Sellami A, Mnif H, Louati N, Zarrouk SB, Keskes L, Rebai T, Gdoura R, Hammami A. Molecular detection of Chlamydia trachomatis and other sexually transmitted bacteria in semen of male partners of infertile couples in Tunisia: the effect on semen parameters and spermatozoa apoptosis markers. Plos One. 2014;9:E98903.

Shevchuk Mm PJ, Khalife G, Armenakas NA, Fracchia JA. Changing testicular histology in AIDS: its implication for sexual transmission of HIV. Urology. 1999;53:203–8.

Smith T. Male infertility. In: Walsh TJ, Smith JF, editors. General urology. 18th ed. New York: Mcgraw Hill; 2013.

Spielmann N, Munstermann D, Hagedorn HJ, An Der Heiden M, Houareau C, Gunsenheimer-Bartmeyer B, Kucherer C, Keeren K, Hamouda O, Marcus U. Time trends of syphilis and HSV-2 co-infection among men who have sex with men in the German HIV-1 seroconverter cohort from 1996–2007. Sex Transm Infect. 2010;86:331–6.

Svenstrup HF, Fedder J, Abraham-Peskir J, Birkelund S, Christiansen G. Mycoplasma genitalium attaches to human spermatozoa. Hum Reprod. 2003;18:2103–9.

Tahan V, Karaca C, Yildirim B, Bozbas A, Ozaras R, Demir K, Avsar E, Mert A, Besisik F, Kaymakoglu S, Senturk H, Cakaloglu Y, Kalayci C, Okten A, Tozun N. Sexual transmission of HCV between spouses. Am J Gastroenterol. 2005;100:821–4.

Urata K, Narahara H, Tanaka Y, Egashira T, Takayama F, Miyakawa I. Effect of endotoxin-induced reactive oxygen species on sperm motility. Fertil Steril. 2001;76:163–6.

Van Leeuwen E, Wit FW, Prins JM, Reiss P, Van Der Veen F, Repping S. Semen quality remains stable during 96 weeks of untreated human immunodeficiency virus-1 infection. Fertil Steril. 2008;90:636–41.

Vandelli C, Renzo F, Romano L, Tisminetzky S, De Palma M, Stroffolini T, Ventura E, Zanetti A. Lack of evidence of sexual transmission of hepatitis C among monogamous couples: results of a 10-year prospective follow-up study. Am J Gastroenterol. 2004;99:855–9.

Vicari E, Arcoria D, Di Mauro C, Noto R, Noto Z, La Vignera S. Sperm output in patients with primary infertility and hepatitis B or C virus; negative influence of HBV infection during concomitant varicocele. Minerva Med. 2006;97:65–77.

Vigil P, Morales P, Tapia A, Riquelme R, Salgado AM. Chlamydia trachomatis infection in male partners of infertile couples: incidence and sperm function. Andrologia. 2002;34:155–61.

Wald A, Zeh J, Selke S, Warren T, Ryncarz AJ, Ashley R, Krieger JN, Corey L. Reactivation of genital herpes simplex virus type 2 infection in asymptomatic seropositive persons. N Engl J Med. 2000;342:844–50.

Weiss RA. How does HIV cause AIDS? Science. 1993;260:1273–9.

WHO. 2008. Http://Apps.Who.Int/Iris/Bitstream/10665/75181/1/9789241503839_Eng.Pdf.

WHO Estimates. 2005. Http://Www.Who.Int/Whosis/Mme_2005.Pdf.

Wikstrom A, Jensen JS. Mycoplasma genitalium: a common cause of persistent urethritis among men treated with doxycycline. Sex Transm Infect. 2006;82:276–9.

World Health Organization, Department of Reproductive Health and Research. WHO laboratory manual for the examination and processing of human semen. 5th ed. Cambridge university Press; 2010.

Xu C, Sun GF, Zhu YF, Wang YF. The correlation of Ureaplasma urealyticum infection with infertility. Andrologia. 1997;29:219–26.

Zeighami H, Peerayeh SN, Yazdi RS, Sorouri R. Prevalence of Ureaplasma urealyticum and Ureaplasma parvum in semen of infertile and healthy men. Int J Std Aids. 2009;20:387–90.

Zhou XP, Hu XL, Zhu YM, Qu F, Sun SJ, Qian YL. Comparison of semen quality and outcome of assisted reproductive techniques in Chinese men with and without hepatitis B. Asian J Androl. 2011;13:465–9.

Zinzendorf NY, Kouassi-Agbessi BT, Lathro JS, Don C, Kouadio L, Loukou YG. Ureaplasma Urealyticum or Mycoplasma Hominis infections and semen quality of infertile men in Abidjan. J Reprod Contracept. 2008;19(2):65–72.

Ionizing Radiation and Male Fertility

12

Gulfam Ahmad and Ashok Agarwal

12.1 Introduction

Exposure to ionizing radiation (IR) is becoming more common in the medical field for disease diagnoses and cancer treatment. In addition to patients undergoing treatment, IR exposure also poses a big threat to health professionals. The majority of medical investigations require radiographic testing to diagnose the disease followed by treatment, which in case of cancer patients may also require radiotherapy. Although all living creatures are at the risk of damage in response to ionizing radiation, the mammalian testes are much more sensitive to ionizing radiation. In man and in majority of animals, the testes lie outside the body and are susceptible to radiation damage (Abuelhija et al. 2013). Damage to the testes is directly proportional to the dose and time of exposure to artificial radiation or treatment. Evidence exists for sperm count reduction after treatment with low-dose testis irradiation. Moderate- to high-dose irradiation can lead to prolonged drastic decline in sperm count or even azoospermia (Abuelhija et al. 2013). The human testes appear to be more sensitive, and the recovery of spermatogenesis after radiotherapy is significantly delayed compared to most other rodents (Meistrich and Samuels 1985). This delay suggests that during the treatment period, spermatogonial stem cells become arrested at a point of their differentiation; however, the underlying mechanism of the spermatogenesis arrest and subsequent recovery in human is not known.

G. Ahmad, PhD
Department of Physiology and Cell Biology, University of Health Sciences, Lahore 54600, Pakistan

A. Agarwal, PhD, HCLD (✉)
American Center for Reproductive Medicine, Cleveland Clinic, Mail Code X-11, 10681 Carnegie Avenue, Cleveland, OH 44195, USA
e-mail: agarwaa@ccf.org

K. Gunasekaran, N. Pandiyan (eds.), *Male Infertility*,
DOI 10.1007/978-81-322-3604-7_12

This raises an important question about the post-treatment fertility of the patients and also the consequences of IR exposure on the reproductive health in medical professionals.

This chapter aims to focus on the impact of ionizing radiation on male fertility. Following a brief overview of ionizing radiation, this review will discuss selected research published on ionizing radiation, with a greater emphasis on radiotherapy and male fertility.

12.2 Ionizing Radiation

Ionizing radiation occurs in the form of an atomic or subatomic particle or an electromagnetic wave with very high kinetic energy, which has an ability to ionize the nucleus of a substance. It is believed that radioactive decay is the major reason for ionizing radiation. Electrons, protons, or neutrons are released during this process; therefore, theoretically any molecule can produce IR. However, the rate of decay differs for each molecule and can be controlled with advanced technologies. Microwaves, infrared rays, radio waves, radiant heat waves, and ultraviolet rays are generally not considered as IR. However, persistent exposure to any of the above can result into the similar effects as induced by IR (Lancranjan et al. 1975).

12.3 Sources

Classic sources of radiation which are of main concern to human beings include natural and artificial sources. Among natural sources, gamma rays from the decay products of uranium, radon gas decay products in the atmosphere, naturally occurring radionuclides, and cosmic rays from the outer space are common. A living being has daily exposure to the natural IR as they are present throughout the natural world. For example, radioactive radon gas is present in the atmosphere, and the Earth itself produces gamma rays from the decay of uranium. On an average, a person is exposed to 2.1 mSv natural radiation annually (du Plessis et al. 2014). Personnel whose work involves dealing with the general public such as teachers, physicians, and health professionals should be equipped with the basic knowledge of such radiation exposure to guide the rest of the population.

Sources of artificial radiations include radionuclides present in eating and drinking materials, X-rays used in medical diagnostic procedures, and gamma rays produced as by-products in the nuclear industry and products formed during atmospheric nuclear testing (du Plessis et al. 2014). Artificial radiation exposure can cause detrimental effects on the health of living beings. Common risk factors which can cause cancer in human beings and the impact on male fertility are summarized in Fig. 12.1. The subsequent discussion will focus on the impact of ionizing radiations on male fertility.

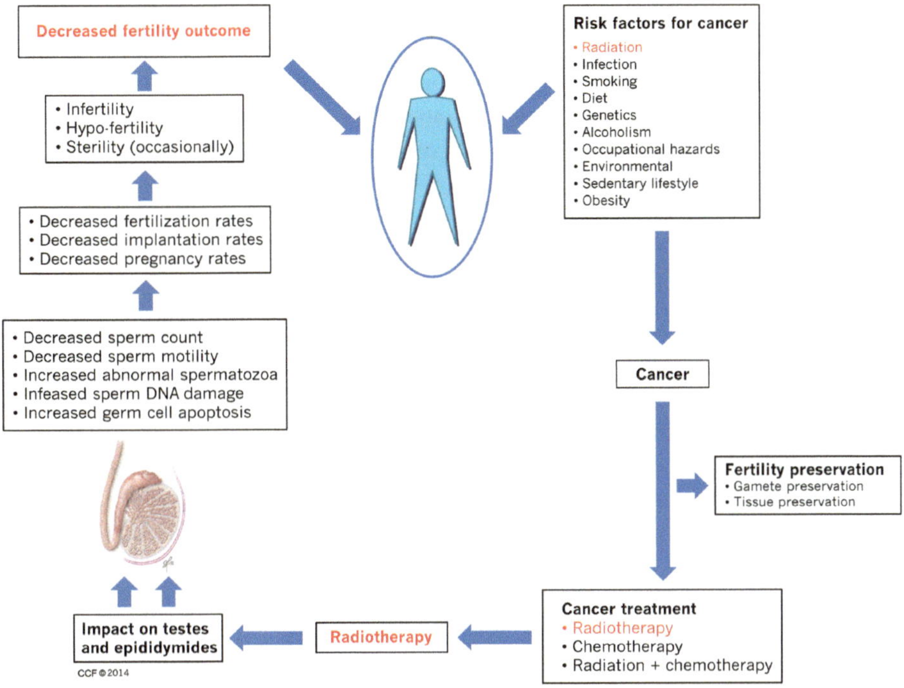

Fig. 12.1 Risk factors for cancer and impact of radiation therapy on male fertility

12.4 Radiation and Spermatogenesis

12.4.1 Animal Studies

12.4.1.1 Rodent Model

Studies conducted on different rodent models have shown that radiation have direct and dose-dependent mutagenic effects on the germ cells. High doses lead to drastically lethal effects, chromosomal aneuploidy, and point mutations (Brent 1999). In experiments, adult mouse testes were subjected to irradiation with a single shot of 1 Gy or two shots of 1 Gy with 7 days interval (Shah et al. 2009). The researchers sampled the testes every third or fourth day postirradiation to follow the recovery pattern of spermatogenesis. Treatment with a single shot of 1 Gy radiation led to a gap in spermatogenesis noted by the loss of A1 to B-spermatogonia which lasted for approximately 10 days. As expected, treatment with two shots of 1 Gy had more severe effects on germ cell elimination compared to 1 Gy. Despite germ cell elimination, spermatogenesis recovered to normal values after 6–7 weeks of treatment in both groups (Shah et al. 2009). In another study, mice were irradiated with a dose of 2 Gy, and sperm recovery pattern was observed for 10 weeks posttreatment. In this study, spermatogenetic recovery was only 7 % at 7 weeks and reached to 84 % of the control values at 10 weeks after treatment (Searle and Beechey 1974). This shows that with a slightly higher dose of radiation, spermatogenetic recovery was much delayed. When mouse testes were irradiated with a slightly higher dose (2.4 Gy), testicular sperm count decreased significantly compared to controls at 30 days, while epididymis count decreased at 39 days after treatment (Meistrich and Samuels 1985). When using a 6 Gy dose of radiation, spermatogonial number did not recover completely but reached 90 % of the control values at 16 weeks after irradiation treatment (Erickson and Hall 1983).

Rat testis appears relatively more sensitive to irradiation damage compared to mouse testis and hence exhibits delayed spermatogenetic recovery. However, in the most widely studied and resistant strain of rats, i.e., Sprague-Dawley, the number of spermatogonia recovered to control levels within 5 weeks after 3 Gy radiation, and epididymal sperm count reached to 40 % of control after 19 weeks (Dym and Clermont 1970; Jegou et al. 1991). With treatment of 6 Gy radiations, the spermatogenetic recovery in rat was severely delayed, and 44 % of the tubules exhibited incomplete spermatogenesis even after 16 weeks of treatment (Erickson and Hall 1983). In cases of higher doses (>6 Gy), even at 26 weeks after treatment, spermatogenetic recovery was only 10 % compared to controls (Delic et al. 1986; Pinon-Lataillade et al. 1991).

12.4.1.2 Nonhuman Primates

Compared to humans, the recovery of spermatogenesis after testicular exposure to radiations is faster in rodents (Abuelhija et al. 2013). In order to have a better understanding of the process of postirradiation spermatogenic recovery, an animal model that simulates the response of human testis to radiation is needed. Nonhuman primates show much similarity to the human testis including similarities in histological stages of spermatogonia (Ehmcke and Schlatt 2006), with dramatic decrease in spermatogonial number after 2 or 4 Gy. Such decline in spermatogonial number was persistent until 6 months postirradiation, and incomplete recovery began only at 18 months of treatment (Foppiani et al. 1999; Kamischke et al. 2003). After irradiation with 0.4–0.5 Gy of X-rays, the number of A_{pale} spermatogonia (A_p) decreased to 13 % compared to control values after 11 days of treatment; however, the number of A_{dark} spermatogonia (A_d) showed no significant change at this time period but was decreased at day 14 postirradiation (van Alphen et al. 1988). Repopulation of seminiferous epithelium started from day 75 postirradiation when treated with 0.5, 1.0, and 2.0 Gy of X-rays. The number of spermatogonia (A_p and A_d) increased and reached 10 % of the control level at day 44 after treatment with 0.5 Gy dose and reached 90 % at day 200. Relatively higher doses (1.0 and 2.0 Gy) had more severe effects on spermatogonia recovery. After treatment with 1–2 Gy radiations, only 5 % of spermatogonia recovery was observed at day 44. Even at days 200 and 370 after treatment, the recovery was only 70 % (van Alphen et al. 1988). This suggests that in monkeys, the recovery of spermatogenesis is much delayed compared to rodents.

12.4.2 Human Studies

As mentioned earlier, human testes are relatively more sensitive to radiations compared to rodents. This means even subtle exposure to low-dose radiation can result in impairment of testicular function. For example, treatment with 1 Gy radiation showed significant reduction in the number of spermatocytes just after 14 day of treatment. The reduction in spermatocyte count was even more drastic at 25 days after treatment (Rowley et al. 1974). It was noted that reduction in spermatocytes count was not abrupt. Although radiation kills the cells immediately by necrosis and/or apoptosis or during their proliferation, the decline in spermatogonia number to their lowest level does not happen at once but instead occurs in a progressive manner. It may take several weeks to reach their lowest level depending upon the dose of irradiation (Rowley et al. 1974; Clifton and Bremner 1983). However, azoospermia is not achieved until 18 weeks of irradiation (Paulsen 1973). The actual reason of this gradual decline is not very clear, but one can speculate that a small population of non-cycling A-spermatogonia escapes the potential effects of radiation perhaps when they are in dormant phase of cell cycle (Meistrich 2013). Recovery of the A-spermatogonia starts after 21 weeks of irradiation which indicates that the self-renewal exceeds cell depletion at this time. As seen in animal studies, as well as in humans, the damage to spermatogenesis or testicular functions depends upon the radiation doses. High doses of radiation can result in permanent azoospermia leading to the killing of all spermatogonial stem cells. When a single dose of 10 Gy was given to the patients undergoing bone marrow transplantation, only 15 % of them regained their fertility (Meistrich 2013; Sanders et al. 1996).

The recovery of spermatogenesis after cancer treatment has been found to be linked to many factors such as the time of diagnosis, sperm parameters before the start of treatment, the nature of the treatment, both sperm parameters, and the nature of treatment, or sometimes no relation has been found with any of the above factors (Hansen et al. 1990; Petersen et al. 1999; Ishikawa et al. 2004; Bahadur et al. 2005; Pectasides et al. 2004; Eberhard et al. 2004; Lampe et al. 1997; Gandini et al. 2006). Therefore, regular cancer screening is imperative in patients with family history of cancer. This will allow the early detection and treatment of the disease with less severe effects on their future fertility.

12.5 Radiations and Sperm Parameters

12.5.1 Animal Studies

When mice were subjected to whole body irradiation of 2 Gy, a significant reduction in epididymal sperm count was observed in the irradiated group compared to the control, 28 days after treatment (Searle and Beechey 1974). This sperm concentration further reduced almost reaching zero at 42 and 49 days after treatment. Similar results in sperm count and morphology have been documented by others when testes of two different strains of mice (C_{57} BL and B_6C_3F1) were exposed to wider range (0, 0.3, 1.0, and 3 Gy) of X-rays. The highest dose (3 Gy) caused a drastic decrease in sperm number obtained from cauda epididymis of both the strains at 42 and 49 days postirradiation. Interestingly, the rise in percentage of sperm abnormalities was notable as early as 21 days and was seen in both groups (Bruce et al. 1974). In a recent study, treatment of mice with 2 Gy dose has shown significant reduction in cauda epididymal sperm count as well as percentage sperm viability in irradiated group compared with control group even after 24 h of treatment (Li et al. 2013).

When rats were irradiated (whole body irradiation), with a wider range of irradiation doses (0.675, 1.350, 2.700, and 4.050 Gy), abnormal sperm morphology was observed compared to control values in almost all doses. These abnormalities became more severe in 2.700 and 4.050 Gy groups, where most of the sperm tails were eroded out (Chatterjee et al. 1994).

In monkeys (*Macaca fascicularis*), when testes were irradiated with a single dose of 2 Gy X-rays, mean sperm concentration per ejaculate significantly decreased to $9.2 \pm 3.5 \times 10^6$ at day 35 postirradiation compared to pretreatment value ($60.3 \pm 15.5 \times 10^6$). The decrease in sperm count was more drastic at 60 days postirradiation, and some monkeys appeared with azoospermia beyond that period (Foppiani et al. 1999). The same study found reduction in percentage sperm morphology (71.4 ± 9.9) 42 days after irradiation compared to pretreatment values (89.8 ± 3.0).

12.5.2 Human Studies

A multicenter prospective study conducted at CECOS network of France has published interesting data on radiotherapy and sperm parameters. They recruited 129 testicular germ cell tumor (TGCT) patients. One semen sample was collected from each patient before starting the treatment to serve as his control, and then treatment was started. Subsequent semen samples were collected at 3, 6, 12, and 24 months postirradiation. The results showed significant reduction in sperm count and sperm motility at 3 months postirradiation, which remained significantly low until 12 months. The sperm count and motility reached control values only after 24 months postirradiation (Bujan et al. 2013; Di Bisceglie et al. 2013). In their study, sperm count decreased at 6 months after treatment and remained low compared to baseline values up to 12 months postirradiation. Eighteen months after treatment, almost all patients recovered normal sperm count, and their counts remained unchanged for the rest of study period (36 months).

Radiation effects are more severe if it involves total body irradiation (TBI) and/or combined with cyclophosphamide (CY). Out of 25 patients who underwent a combination of bone marrow transplantation and TBI/CY treatment, only one patient had recovered spermatogenesis levels to normal. The recovery time was much delayed (75 months) compared to those patients who had only radiation therapy (Jacob et al. 1998). The kinetics of recovery of spermatogenesis after radiation therapy is much more delayed compared to chemotherapy (Meistrich 2013; Bujan et al. 2013). In patients treated with hemi-pelvic or given pelvic radiotherapy, spermatogenic recovery did not start until 9 months postirradiation even with modest doses (0.5–0.8 Gy), and at higher dose (1.7 Gy), the delays were even more prolonged (Meistrich 2013).

12.6 Radiations and Sperm DNA

12.6.1 Animal Studies

Information on sperm DNA integrity after radiation treatment is scanty in animal models. Very few studies have been conducted on mouse. In one study, mice were subjected to acute testicular X-rays exposure with a maximum dose of 6 Gy. Spermatozoa were collected from epididymis 35 days postirradiation for DNA damage investigation. Analysis revealed that 30–40 % of spermatozoa had damaged DNA after the treatment. Some had chromosomal aneuploidy, and some others had DNA strand breaks (Pinkel et al. 1983). In an in vitro study, mouse spermatozoa recovered from epididymis were exposed to range of radiation doses (0–100 Gy). A linear dose-dependent DNA damage was observed in irradiated spermatozoa compared with controls (Haines et al. 1998). Further, in a more recent study on mice, Li et al. (2013) found a dose-dependent increase in sperm DNA fragmentation. They measured both sperm DNA fragmentation index (DFI) and high DNA stainability (HDS) through sperm chromatin structure assay (SCSA). The term DFI reflects the percentage of damaged DNA divided by the total sperm DNA which actually gives the loss of sperm DNA. HDS represents the immaturity and less condensed chromatin where sperm attain greater stainability. In these experiments, percentage of DFI was significantly higher in experimental group exposed to 2 Gy X-rays compared to control group (21.35 ± 0.78 vs 9.54 ± 0.31). Percentage HDS was also significantly higher in the experimental group compared to control group (12.03 ± 0.35 vs 3.90 ± 0.17). In another interesting study, sperm DNA damage was induced by exposing mice testicular region to different radiation doses (0.0, 2.5, 5.0, and 10.0 Gy). Comet assay was performed to quantify the sperm DNA damage. The percent tail DNA damage in spermatozoa exposed to 2.5 Gy was significantly higher compared to controls (7.98 ± 0.42 vs 5.44 ± 0.35). The difference became more significant at 5 Gy and 10 Gy (9.67 ± 0.44 and 12.14 ± 0.52) respectively (Kumar et al. 2013b).

12.6.2 Human Studies

Although sperm has highly compact DNA, it has to travel a long journey starting from testes all the way through male and female reproductive tracts before it reaches oocyte. This long passage makes it exposed to exogenous as well as endogenous threats including endogenous milieu of tracts and any foreign insult such as trauma, exposure to radiation, or toxic environment. Majority of the data available on sperm

DNA damage in cancer patients describe the effects of chemotherapy, and less is known about radiotherapy.

Some studies conducted on human sperm DNA integrity after radiotherapy report significant DNA damage compared to controls. An increase in high DNA stainability (HDS) was observed at 6 months after radiotherapy in 67 patients with pure seminoma. However, the values of sperm DNA fragmentation index (DFI) were not significantly higher than the control values (Bujan et al. 2013). Further, when patients with testicular carcinoma were treated with adjuvant radiotherapy, the DFI was significantly higher compared to the controls. The DFI was also higher compared to other treatments such as chemotherapy, which shows more drastic effects of radiation on sperm DNA. Interestingly, the increase in DFI was notable till 2 years posttreatment compared to non-treated patients (18 vs 13 %) (Stahl et al. 2004; Lord 1999).

12.7 Radiations and Sperm Fertilization Capacity

12.7.1 Animal Studies

Evidence exists that sperm can fertilize the oocyte with damaged DNA. When mice testes were irradiated with an acute dose of 2 Gy, no change in fertilization rates was observed in the irradiated group and control group at 4 weeks after treatment. However, from 4 weeks onward, the decline in fertilization rate was notable till week 7. The difference reached maximum significance at week 6 and then returned to control values after 8 weeks (Matsuda et al. 1985). In another mouse study, mice were subjected to whole body irradiation using a similar dose (2 Gy). The fertilization rates were not different in irradiated groups and the controls till 6 weeks after treatment. At weeks 7 and 8, the fertilization rates were significantly lower in irradiated groups compared to controls, and, after 9 weeks, these rates reached controls' levels (Searle and Beechey 1974). The delayed difference in fertilization rates in this study compared to the study of Matsuda and Colleagues (1985) could be because, in this earlier study, the whole body of mice was irradiated, while Matsuda et al. (1985) used acute testicular irradiation. Direct testicular irradiation may have a more severe impact on the quality of sperm compared to whole body irradiation. Interestingly, even fertilization rate was unaffected at 6 weeks in the irradiated groups (Searle and Beechey 1974); embryo implantation rate and number of live embryos were significantly lower at 6 weeks compared to controls. The difference reached the lowest value at 7 weeks and started increasing toward control values at 8 weeks (Searle and Beechey 1974). The reduction in embryo implantation rate and number of live embryos at 6 weeks in irradiated groups compared to controls reflects the damage to sperm DNA. This suggests that sperm with damaged DNA can fertilize the egg but may not support embryo development.

A recent study reported of similar results where male mice irradiated using higher doses (5–10 Gy) were mated with female mice, and the fertilization rate of the irradiated mice did not differ from the control (Kumar et al. 2013a). However, the average number of offspring per litter was significantly reduced in irradiated groups exposed to 5 and 10 Gy (6.0±0.3 and 3.3±0.2 respectively) doses as compared to control group (10.1±0.3). In the highest dose group (10 Gy), approximately 37 % offspring died within 10 weeks of age which shows teratogenicity of irradiation to testes (Kumar et al. 2013a).

12.7.2 Human Studies

No data is available on radiation therapy and fertilization rates in human. Scanty information is available on fertility outcome of the patients after radiation therapy used as cancer treatment. In comparison to radiation therapy, reasonable data is published on fertility outcome in patients after chemotherapy. Studies published on chemotherapy report a greater concern about fertility issues in patients after cancer treatment. A case-control American study showed that patients treated for testicular germ cell tumor were significantly more likely to experience fertility problems in terms of fathering a child compared to control population. Such cases had more consults for fertility distress as compared to the controls (Kim et al. 2010). The results of a more recent study showed that in patients with testicular tumor who attempted to conceive after radiotherapy alone or combined with chemotherapy (either naturally or through assisted reproductive techniques using fresh or frozen semen), live birth rates were as low as 32 % (9/28) and 28 % (2/7) respectively (Ping et al. 2014). The data also showed four miscarriages from the entire attempts made by 73 couples in all groups. However, there was no evidence of congenital abnormalities or any malignancies among the babies born after the treatment. The debate on the transgenerational effects of radiotherapy is going on and more data is required. Nevertheless, the deleterious effects of radiation therapy and its exposure should not be ignored, and effective protective measures must be adopted to safeguard male reproductive health.

12.8 Conclusions

Radiation therapy has negative impact on spermatogenesis and affects qualitative as well as quantitative sperm parameters in animals as well as humans. The extent to which the testes respond to radiation depends upon the dose and duration of exposure or treatment. Extreme care must be taken while treating cancer patients. Spermatozoa cryopreservation must be advised to all patients before treatment. It may be advisable to go for germ cell preservation in patients who have not achieved puberty and in whom spermatogenesis has not yet begun. In a multidisciplinary approach, patients must be counseled for the cryopreservation of gametes or tissues, and the options of assisted reproductive techniques should be well explained.

12.9 Future Directions

Although no abnormalities have been reported in children fathered by patients treated for cancer, larger prospective studies are required to represent the true data. Further, animal studies should be carried out to investigate the potential transgenerational effects of radiation therapy or male-mediated developmental toxicity. Couples should use contraceptive methods for 1–2 years after cancer treatment to avoid possible potential risk of DNA damage and aneuploidy caused by radiation therapy, which can affect embryo development.

References

Abuelhija M, Weng CC, Shetty G, Meistrich ML. Rat models of post-irradiation recovery of spermatogenesis: interstrain differences. Andrology. 2013;1:206–15.

Bahadur G, Ozturk O, Muneer A, Wafa R, Ashraf A, Jaman N, Patel S, Oyede AW, Ralph DJ. Semen quality before and after gonadotoxic treatment. Hum Reprod. 2005;20:774–81.

Brent RL. Utilization of developmental basic science principles in the evaluation of reproductive risks from pre- and postconception environmental radiation exposures. Teratology. 1999;59:182–204.

Bruce WR, Furrer R, Wyrobek AJ. Abnormalities in the shape of murine sperm after acute testicular x-irradiation. Mutat Res. 1974;23:381–6.

Bujan L, Walschaerts M, Moinard N, Hennebicq S, Saias J, Brugnon F, Auger J, Berthaut I, Szerman E, Daudin M, Rives N. Impact of chemotherapy and radiotherapy for testicular germ cell tumors on spermatogenesis and sperm DNA: a multicenter prospective study from the CECOS network. Fertil Steril. 2013;100:673–80.

Chatterjee J, De K, Basu SK, Das AK. Alteration of spermatozoal structure and trace metal profile of testis and epididymis of rat under chronic low-level X-ray irradiation. Biol Trace Elem Res. 1994;41:305–19.

Clifton DK, Bremner WJ. The effect of testicular x-irradiation on spermatogenesis in man. A comparison with the mouse. J Androl. 1983;4:387–92.

Delic JI, Hendry JH, Morris ID, Shalet SM. Dose and time relationships in the endocrine response of the irradiated adult rat testis. J Androl. 1986;7:32–41.

Di Bisceglie C, Bertagna A, Composto ER, Lanfranco F, Baldi M, Motta G, Barberis AM, Napolitano E, Castellano E, Manieri C. Effects of oncological treatments on semen quality in patients with testicular neoplasia or lymphoproliferative disorders. Asian J Androl. 2013;15:425–9.

du Plessis SS, Agarwal A, Sabanegh Jr ES. Male infertility: a complete guide to lifestyle and environmental factors. New York: Springer; 2014. ISBN 13: 978-1493910397.

Dym M, Clermont Y. Role of spermatogonia in the repair of the seminiferous epithelium following x-irradiation of the rat testis. Am J Anat. 1970;128:265–82.

Eberhard J, Stahl O, Giwercman Y, Cwikiel M, Cavallin-Stahl E, Lundin KB, Flodgren P, Giwercman A. Impact of therapy and androgen receptor polymorphism on sperm concentration in men treated for testicular germ cell cancer: a longitudinal study. Hum Reprod. 2004;19:1418–25.

Ehmcke J, Schlatt S. A revised model for spermatogonial expansion in man: lessons from non-human primates. Reproduction. 2006;132:673–80.

Erickson BH, Hall GG. Comparison of stem-spermatogonial renewal and mitotic activity in the gamma-irradiated mouse and rat. Mutat Res. 1983;108:317–35.

Foppiani L, Schlatt S, Simoni M, Weinbauer GF, Hacker-Klom U, Nieschlag E. Inhibin B is a more sensitive marker of spermatogenetic damage than FSH in the irradiated non-human primate model. J Endocrinol. 1999;162:393–400.

Gandini L, Sgro P, Lombardo F, Paoli D, Culasso F, Toselli L, Tsamatropoulos P, Lenzi A. Effect of chemo- or radiotherapy on sperm parameters of testicular cancer patients. Hum Reprod. 2006;21:2882–9.

Haines G, Marples B, Daniel P, Morris I. DNA damage in human and mouse spermatozoa after in vitro-irradiation assessed by the comet assay. Adv Exp Med Biol. 1998;444:79–91; discussion 92–3.

Hansen PV, Trykker H, Svennekjaer IL, Hvolby J. Long-term recovery of spermatogenesis after radiotherapy in patients with testicular cancer. Radiother Oncol. 1990;18:117–25.

Ishikawa T, Kamidono S, Fujisawa M. Fertility after high-dose chemotherapy for testicular cancer. Urology. 2004;63:137–40.

Jacob A, Barker H, Goodman A, Holmes J. Recovery of spermatogenesis following bone marrow transplantation. Bone Marrow Transplant. 1998;22:277–9.

Jegou B, Velez de la Calle JF, Bauche F. Protective effect of medroxyprogesterone acetate plus testosterone against radiation-induced damage to the reproductive function of male rats and their offspring. Proc Natl Acad Sci U S A. 1991;88:8710–4.

Kamischke A, Kuhlmann M, Weinbauer GF, Luetjens M, Yeung CH, Kronholz HL, Nieschlag E. Gonadal protection from radiation by GnRH antagonist or recombinant human FSH: a controlled trial in a male nonhuman primate (Macaca fascicularis). J Endocrinol. 2003;179: 183–94.

Kim C, Mcglynn KA, Mccorkle R, Zheng T, Erickson RL, Niebuhr DW, Ma S, Zhang Y, Bai Y, Dai L, Graubard BI, Kilfoy B, Barry KH, Zhang Y. Fertility among testicular cancer survivors: a case-control study in the U.S. J Cancer Surviv. 2010;4:266–73.

Kumar D, Upadhya D, Salian SR, Rao SB, Kalthur G, Kumar P, Adiga SK. The extent of paternal sperm DNA damage influences early post-natal survival of first generation mouse offspring. Eur J Obstet Gynecol Reprod Biol. 2013a;166:164–7.

Kumar D, Upadhya D, Uppangala S, Salian SR, Kalthur G, Adiga SK. Nuclear DNA fragmentation negatively affects zona binding competence of Y bearing mouse spermatozoa. J Assist Reprod Genet. 2013b;30:1611–5.

Lampe H, Horwich A, Norman A, Nicholls J, Dearnaley DP. Fertility after chemotherapy for testicular germ cell cancers. J Clin Oncol. 1997;15:239–45.

Lancranjan I, Maicanescu M, Rafaila E, Klepsch I, Popescu HI. Gonadic function in workmen with long-term exposure to microwaves. Health Phys. 1975;29:381–3.

Li HY, Zhang H, Miao GY, Xie Y, Sun C, Di CX, Liu Y, Liu YY, Zhang X, Ma XF, Xu S, Gan L, Zhou X. Simulated microgravity conditions and carbon ion irradiation induce spermatogenic cell apoptosis and sperm DNA damage. Biomed Environ Sci. 2013;26:726–34.

Lord BI. Transgenerational susceptibility to leukaemia induction resulting from preconception, paternal irradiation. Int J Radiat Biol. 1999;75:801–10.

Matsuda Y, Tobari I, Yamada T. *In vitro* fertilization rate of mouse eggs with sperm after X-irradiation at various spermatogenetic stages. Mutat Res. 1985;142:59–63.

Meistrich ML. Effects of chemotherapy and radiotherapy on spermatogenesis in humans. Fertil Steril. 2013;100:1180–6.

Meistrich ML, Samuels RC. Reduction in sperm levels after testicular irradiation of the mouse: a comparison with man. Radiat Res. 1985;102:138–47.

Paulsen CA. The study of hormonal aspects. Final progress report of AEC contract AT(45–1)-2225, task agreement 6. RLO-2225-2. U.S. Department of Energy; 1973.

Pectasides D, Pectasides M, Farmakis D, Nikolaou M, Koumpou M, Kostopoulou V, Mylonakis N. Testicular function in patients with testicular cancer treated with bleomycin-etoposide-carboplatin (BEC(90)) combination chemotherapy. Eur Urol. 2004;45:187–93.

Petersen PM, Skakkebaek NE, Rorth M, Giwercman A. Semen quality and reproductive hormones before and after orchiectomy in men with testicular cancer. J Urol. 1999;161:822–6.

Ping P, Gu BH, Li P, Huang YR, Li Z. Fertility outcome of patients with testicular tumor: before and after treatment. Asian J Androl. 2014;16:107–11.

Pinkel D, Gledhill BL, Van Dilla MA, Lake S, Wyrobek AJ. Radiation-induced DNA content variability in mouse sperm. Radiat Res. 1983;95:550–65.

Pinon-Lataillade G, Viguier-Martinez MC, Touzalin AM, Maas J, Jegou B. Effect of an acute exposure of rat testes to gamma rays on germ cells and on Sertoli and Leydig cell functions. Reprod Nutr Dev. 1991;31:617–29.

Rowley MJ, Leach DR, Warner GA, Heller CG. Effect of graded doses of ionizing radiation on the human testis. Radiat Res. 1974;59:665–78.

Sanders JE, Hawley J, Levy W, Gooley T, Buckner CD, Deeg HJ, Doney K, Storb R, Sullivan K, Witherspoon R, Appelbaum FR. Pregnancies following high-dose cyclophosphamide with or without high-dose busulfan or total-body irradiation and bone marrow transplantation. Blood. 1996;87:3045–52.

Searle AG, Beechey CV. Sperm-count, egg-fertilization and dominant lethality after X-irradiation of mice. Mutat Res. 1974;22:63–72.

Shah FJ, Tanaka M, Nielsen JE, Iwamoto T, Kobayashi S, Skakkebaek NE, Leffers H, Almstrup K. Gene expression profiles of mouse spermatogenesis during recovery from irradiation. Reprod Biol Endocrinol. 2009;7:130.

Stahl O, Eberhard J, Jepson K, Spano M, Cwikiel M, Cavallin-Stahl E, Giwercman A. The impact of testicular carcinoma and its treatment on sperm DNA integrity. Cancer. 2004;100:1137–44.

van Alphen MM, van de Kant HJ, de Rooij DG. Depletion of the spermatogonia from the seminiferous epithelium of the rhesus monkey after X irradiation. Radiat Res. 1988;113:473–86.

13 Aging and Male Reproduction

Shah Dupesh Khan

13.1 Introduction

We are currently looking at two fertility trends: number one is that women are having fewer children, and number two is that they are delaying the age of the first childbirth. There is an unprecedented growth in the number of older people especially those beyond 60 years of age (Daguet 2002). The concept of delaying the age of the first childbirth has its consequences; women may get disappointed with the delays and/or associated difficulties with conception they face as they get older due to the age-dependant decrease in their fecundity. A further consequence could be that this trend also contributes to an increase in the incidence of age-associated infertility (ESHRE Capri Workshop 2005).

Numerous demographic studies have shown that births seem to be more strictly planned. There has been a rise in the mean age of parity among numerous different cultural groups since the 1970s. Frequently, a woman at 35 is usually having her first child or a first child from a new union. Due to the well-established fact that fertility decline in the female begins from somewhere around the third decade, most couples trying at this age would frequently encounter delays and increasing time to pregnancy (Menken et al. 1986). A recent argument stated that with the availability of ART, postponing childbearing is not an issue; however, in an interesting simulation model constructed bearing in mind the monthly probability of conception and miscarriage and the probability of sterility, ART does not seem to compensate for the loss of fertility and/or fecundity with age (Leridon 2004).

S.D. Khan, MBBS, DCE, FASM, (PhD)
Department of Andrology and Sexual Medicine, Women's Center,
8A, Burkit Road, T. Nagar, Chennai 600017, India

Fortis Healthcare, Fortis Malar Hospital,
Adyar, Chennai 600020, India
e-mail: drsdk123@gmail.com

K. Gunasekaran, N. Pandiyan (eds.), *Male Infertility*,
DOI 10.1007/978-81-322-3604-7_13

13.2 Aging and Natural Selection

Aging remains an evolutionary paradox. Although many theories have tried to explain the reason behind aging, we are yet to come to a definitive conclusion. Why does an organism age? Unfortunately, we do not know the answer; most research suggests that reactive oxygen species or accumulation of deleterious mutations could be the possible reason for aging (Ashok and Ali 1999). While we have a lot of circumstantial evidence proving associations, a definitive cause-effect relationship remains to be proven. A high degree of variability in terms of aging is seen among different species in different environments. For instance, most mammals are outlived by birds of comparable sizes. Turtles seem to outlive other reptilian forms. In terms of fertility, in nature most males of lower species seem to follow a "live fast, die young strategy," i.e., males of lower species like the adult mayflies undergo rapid senescence postmating with the female. Males in these species have higher mortality and more rapid aging. Whether this scenario is applicable to human aging, fertility remains to be explored (Charlesworth 1980).

Thus, from an evolutionary perspective, "aging" or "senescence" is simply defined as a drop in the survival probability and/or fertility later in the life of the individual. Aging reduces the contribution an individual makes in terms of genetics to the future offspring by either reducing the individual's fitness or by reducing the number of successful coital attempts. Aging is programmed and nondirected. Although natural selection shapes life's history, genes for antiaging just do not exist. The aim of natural selection is to shape life history so as to achieve a delicate balance between somatic maintenance and reproductive fitness under strains imposed by the external environment of the organism in question. In the sense of a genetic program, aging can be characterized by the accumulation of molecular level damage to cell proteins, DNA, and lipids with mutation favored by natural selection (Finch 1990).

13.3 Is There an Andropause?

Male fertility seems to be well maintained very late into old age. In addition to numerous anecdotal reports, it has been scientifically documented till 94 years of age (Seymour et al. 1935). Several celebrities have become fathers at a relatively older age; Anthony Quinn and Pablo Picasso are commonly cited examples. Birth registry data from Germany and Japan and also other parts of the world clearly show that an increasing number of men father children beyond 50 years of age. Interestingly, older fathers seem to have younger partners. The German registry also shows that the mean age of men at their first marriage has risen from a median average of 26.6 years to 31.8 from 1985 to 2002 (Statistisches Bundesamt Deutschland 2004). This trend is definitely due to rising female awareness levels, female contraception, and postponed age of first marriage and/or childbearing. In females we know that aging is associated with a progressive loss of follicles, an increase in oocyte aneuploidy, and a miscarriage ultimately ending with menopause. This raises an important question; Does aging affect a man's fertility? Unlike female reproductive functions, male reproductive functions do not come to an abrupt halt, but on the other hand, spermatogenesis and androgen production continue lifelong. Thus, there is no "andropause" stating in the strictest sense. Notwithstanding though with increasing age, alterations in the male reproductive function are quite obvious (Lubna and Santoro 2003).

13.4 Aging and Male Fertility

Fertility and fecundity are terms used often interchangeably but are different. Fecundity refers to the ability to conceive within a specific time frame. Studies on the effect of male aging on fecundity are difficult to interpret due to numerous confounding variables, one of which is female age. Aging in a man is confounded also by the coital frequency which also depends on his period of cohabitation with his partner. The Avon Longitudinal Study of Pregnancy and Childhood (ALSPAC) assessed 12,106 couples (Ford et al. 2000). In this study, older men were less likely to be successful fathers in <6 or <12 months. Mean age of men who were 32.6 ± 5.91 years took >12 months to impregnate their partners, while men who had a mean age of 30.9 ± 5.27 years took less than 12 months to achieve the same. The results were statistically significant ($p<0.0001$). The European Fecundability Study of 7288 menstrual cycles from women participating across seven European centers also showed a trend for fertility decline from late 30s for men (Dunson et al. 2002) with no effect apparent up to 35 years of age. This study also showed that among women of 35 years of age, the proportion of couples who do not achieve conception within 12 menstrual cycles increases from 18 to 28 % if the male partner age is 35 years and 40 years, respectively. Interestingly, the observed effect on fertility is similar when the frequency of intercourse drops from twice per week to about once per week.

Descriptive birth data from the Irish population, data from the Mormon birth registry, and data from Kenya, Syria, and other developing countries all point to declining fertility with increasing male age (Goldman and Montgomery 1989). Another interesting study also found that in men >45 years of age, the time to pregnancy rates was 4.6 times likely to be prolonged beyond 12 months compared to men >25 years of age (Hassan and Killick 2003). In another European study, the risk of miscarriage and delay in pregnancy onset reached statistical significance especially when the fathers were > 40 years and the associated female partners were greater than 30 years of age (De la Prochebrochard and Thonneau 2003). The risk of pregnancy-related complications also was high in this age group compared with younger partners. Male age-based alterations are frequently masked by female age and its associated alterations.

Does male age affect ART outcomes? The answer is apparently no. The success rate of ICSI does not seem to be associated with male age (Spandorfer et al. 1998). To conclude, bearing in mind the studies discussed, it would seem male age affects fertility of the couples beginning from late 30s and that the effect of male age becomes more relevant with advancing age of the partner.

Table 13.1 The various histological changes seen in the aging testis along with the corresponding study

Histological changes	Reference
Physiological germ cell loss, Leydig cell loss	Holstein (1989)
Reduced dark A spermatogonia, giant spermatids, multinucleated spermatogonia	Johnson et al. (1990)
Lipid droplets in Sertoli cells, megalospermatocytes	Harbitz (1973)
Tubule involution	Panigua et al. (1987)
Defective vascularization of testicular parenchyma	Regadera et al. (1985)

13.5 The Aging Testis

In the aging male, testicular volume remains relatively constant with a very small decrease noted probably only in the eighth decade. Testicular histomorphological changes are also slow to develop. Histological studies on autopsied testes of older men sometimes reveal completely normal testicular structure. Changes are summarized below (Table 13.1).

The defective vascularization of testicular parenchyma is associated with systemic arteriosclerosis of the aging man.

13.6 Aging and Semen Parameters

Bearing in mind the various age-dependant changes taking place in the reproductive organs of men, expecting a high degree of variance in semen parameters is not surprising. Studies that have explored the effect of age on semen parameters are summarized in Table 13.2 below.

Most of the studies exploring the effect of age on semen parameters are limited in their ability to determine a suitable effect, as most of these studies are based on retrospective data further limited by a small sample size. To summarize the outcome of these studies, it would seem that the effect of aging on semen parameters is variable; no conclusion should be drawn in light of present evidence. Although a small effect is noted in different studies, the parameters measured were still within the normal reference ranges used in the studies. No threshold age is seen beyond which a rapid decline in semen parameters occurs. Much larger studies accounting for the inherent variability of semen parameters are required to come to any meaningful conclusions.

13.7 Effect of Paternal Aging on Genetics

Early observations have suggested that increasing male age is associated with certain syndromes. A possible reason is that, in males, there are a net higher number of germ cell divisions as compared to females, and male germ cells divide almost

Table 13.2 Studies mentioned in the table show the possible association of aging and it's impact on semen parameters

Study	No	Age	Effect on volume	Effect on concentration	Effect on motility	Effect on morphology
Studies on proven fertile males including sperm donors						
Dondero et al. (1985)	445	18–81	↓ NS after 40 years	↓ NS after 40 years	↓ NS after 40 years	No effect
Homonnai et al. (1982)	555	20–68	30 % decrease	No effect	↓ significant	No effect
Nieschlag et al. (1982)	43	24–88	↓ NS	Significant	↑ significant	No effect
Wang et al. 1985	1239	19–53	No effect	No effect	No effect	No effect
Bujan et al. (1996)	302	21–44	No effect	↑ 3.3 % per year but NS	No effect	No effect
Irvine et al. (1996)	577	18–53	No effect	↑ 2.1 % per year but HS	No effect	No effect
Eskenazi et al. (2003)	97	22–80	↑ 0.03 ml per year	↓ 2.5 % per year but significant	No effect	No effect
Fisch et al. (1996)	1283	34.3	$R=0.15$, weak effect	$R=0.03$, no effect	NS	No effect
Auger et al. (1995)	1351	19–59	No effect	↓ 3.3 % per year but NS	↓ 0.6 % per year	No effect
Schwartz et al. (1983)	809	26–50	No effect	No effect	↓ NS	↓ 0.9 % per year
Studies on men with infertility						
Mladenovic et al. (1994)	77	20–50	No effect	No effect	↓ significant	↓ significant
Berling and Wolner (1997)	718	21–54	No effect	No effect	No effect	No effect
Andolz et al. (1999)	20,411	15–74	↓ 0.5 % per year	↑ 0.7 % per year	↓ 0.3 % per year	↓ NS
Spandorfer et al. (1998)	821	39–50	NS	No effect	↓ NS	No effect
Rolf et al. (1996)	117	22–61	HS	↑ NS	↓ significant	No effect
Rolf et al. (2002)	3437	19–63	HS	No effect	No effect	No effect
Henkel et al. (1999)	90	22–57	No effect	No effect	No effect	No effect
Centola and Eberly (1999)	2065	19–67	↓ NS	No effect	No effect	↓ NS

↑ depicts an increase, ↓ depicts a decrease. *NS* non significant, *HS* highly significant continuously (Crow 2000). Bearing in mind this association, the age of semen donors in some countries has been capped at 40 years (ASRM 1998). No effect of age on aneuploidies of chromosomes 6, 8, 12, 13, 14, and 18 has been observed from previous studies. A paternal age effect on disomies XX, XY, or YY has been observed in a few studies (Asada et al. 2000; Lowe et al. 2001). No paternal age effect for Turner's syndrome as well as trisomy 13, 16, 18, and 21 (Hatch et al. 1990) is seen. However, larger studies clearly seem to show some effect as far as Down's syndrome is concerned, especially when combined with advanced maternal age >35 years (Fisch et al. 2003).

Structural chromosomal anomalies result due to chromosomal break followed by rearrangement within the same chromosome or between different chromosomes. Structural chromosomal anomalies are seen in the spermatozoa of aging men, although the numbers of studies are few (Sartorelli et al. 2001). Interestingly, no such increase in de novo structural chromosomal anomalies of newborns born to older fathers was observed (Hook et al. 1984). When we review autosomal dominant diseases, achondrodysplasia and Apert's syndrome have a high degree of relevance with respect to paternal age. Achondrodysplasia is a common form of dwarfism that afflicts 1 in 30,000 births (Vajo et al. 2000). It is caused by a mutation in FGF3 gene. Apert's syndrome, on the other hand, occurs to 1 in 70,000 births and is caused by a mutation in the FGF2 gene (Cohen et al. 1992). Both these conditions show an age-dependant increase in mutation of sperm, but peculiarly the number of sperm mutations does not correlate with the exponential increase in the number of reported cases. Other mutation with the FGF3 gene that shows an exponential rise with paternal age includes thanatophoric dysplasia and Crouzon's and Pfeiffer's syndrome (Glaser et al. 2003).

For diseases of complex etiology like Alzheimer's, cardiac defects like atrial septal defect (ASD) and ventricular septal defect (VSD), leukemia, and others, assessing the effect of paternal age is difficult due to the inherent genetic heterogeneity of the conditions. On the other hand, does the offspring of aging male have shorter life expectancy? In one interesting retrospective analysis of >8500 members of aristocratic families, it was found that daughters of fathers older than 50 years died 4.4 years earlier when compared to daughters of younger fathers between 20 and 30 years (Gavrilov et al. 1997). To conclude, genetics is complex. Only technical progress with in-depth understanding of sperm DNA damage, gene expression, epigenetics, and the mechanism that links them all will further our progress in unraveling any potential clinical benefits from a therapeutic viewpoint.

13.8 Effect of Aging on the HPT Axis

Aging male characteristics develop due to morphological changes in the organs linked with functional changes in the endocrine networks. The rate of aging greatly varies among individuals and is mainly influenced by the environment and lifestyle factors (Hermann et al. 2000). Late-onset hypogonadism (LOH) in the aging male is slow to develop and involves histological and functional changes in all three components of the hypothalamic-pituitary-testicular axis (Deslypere and Vermeulen 1984). Longitudinal results from the Massachusetts Male Aging Study (MMAS) clearly shows that with increasing age, total testosterone falls at 1.6 %/year, while LH and FSH rise at 0.9 %/year and 3.1 %/year. Sex hormone-binding globulin (SHBG) also increases at 1.2 %/year leading to further fall in free testosterone and bioavailable testosterone at approximately 2–3% per year (Feldman et al. 2002). The clinical relevance of serum steroid levels and their change with increasing age remains to be completely understood. Nevertheless, these findings have seemingly accelerated a significant worldwide increase in testosterone prescriptions (Handelsman 2012; Gan et al. 2012), despite the uncertainties and rises surrounding testosterone replacement therapies in aging men (Cunningham 2011).

A decline in total testosterone is accompanied by certain clinical symptoms that bear homology with hypogonadism; these are decreased bone and muscle mass, abdominal obesity, decreased beard growth, loss of sexual vigor along with a host of nonspecific symptoms like nervousness, depression, mood swings, and general fatigue (Schatzl et al. 2003). In the aging man, initially there is partial hypergonadotropic hypogonadism; with increasing age, a degree of central hypogonadotropic hypogonadism further eventually sets in due to secondary failure of the gonads and their feedback mechanism. There are a direct decrease of testicular steroidogenesis, LH cell inactivity, diminished testosterone secretory activity, decreased LH-stimulated testosterone rise, and a general decrease in GnRH-stimulated LH release and also disruption of testosterone feedback signaling (Keenan et al. 2006). One must also bear in mind that the abovementioned changes are applicable to the general population, but a word of caution is advised. It is important to understand that different components of the HPT axis would age differently. The degree of aging will further be influenced by lifestyle factors. Obese individuals would expect a greater drop in testosterone vs. nonobese physically active individuals. On these notes, results of the European Male Ageing Study that involved 2395 men from eight centers across Europe clearly showed that even 10 % drop in weight led to statistically significant rise in testosterone and free testosterone. A weight change of 15 % from baseline on the other hand was associated with a curvilinear change in free testosterone values (Camacho et al. 2013). Thus, bearing in mind the dynamic relationship between body weight and serum sex steroid levels, it would be prudent to encourage patients to maintain a healthy active lifestyle with suitable dietary modification (Mohr et al. 2006). One must exercise caution before hastily prescribing testosterone replacement therapies for the aging male.

Conclusion

Aging as a phenomenon is enigmatic. The aging male is susceptible to subtle but significant alterations in his reproductive functions. With increasing age there is definitely an increased risk of miscarriage and reduced fecundity while controlling for female factors. Aging is also associated with an increased risk of certain autosomal dominant diseases, although one must bear in mind that the absolute risk is low. A gradual change and/or fluctuation of semen parameters with age probably reflect and/or follow the histomorphological and functional changes in the HPT axis. The clinician is advised to exercise prudence while evaluating an aging male. Unnecessary and baseless testosterone replacement therapies should not be advocated as a first-line measure while treating late-onset hypogonadism. Weight reduction by diet and exercise and cessation of smoking and drinking may all play a significant role in preventing undue serum sex steroid level changes and also promoting a good quality of life.

References

American Society of Reproductive Medicine. Guidelines for therapeutic donor insemination: sperm. Fertil Steril. 1998;70 Suppl 3:1S–3.

Andolz P, Bielsa MA, Vila J. Evolution of semen quality in North-eastern Spain: a study in 22759 infertile men over a 36 year period. Hum Reprod. 1999;14:731–5.

Asada H, Sueoka K, et al. The effects of age and abnormal sperm count on the nondisjunction of spermatozoa. J Assist Reprod Genet. 2000;17:51–9.

Ashok BT, Ali R. The aging paradox: free radical theory of aging. Exp Gerontol. 1999;34(3):293–303.

Auger J, Kunstmann JM, et al. Decline in semen quality among fertile men in Paris during the last 20 years. N Eng J Med. 1995;332:281–5.

Berling S, Wolner P. No evidence of deteriorating semen quality among men in infertile relationships during the last decade: a study of males from Southern Sweden. Hum Reprod. 1997;12: 1002–5.

Bujan L, Mansat A, et al. Time series analysis of sperm concentration in fertile men in Toulouse, France between 1977 and 1992. Br Med J. 1996;312:471–2.

Camacho EM, Huhtaniemi IT, et al. Age associated changes in hypothalamic-pituitary-testicular function in middle aged and older men are modified by weight change and lifestyle factors: longitudinal results from the European Male Ageing Study. Eur Jr Endocrinol. 2013;168:445–55.

Centola GM, Eberly S. Seasonal variations and age related changes in human sperm count, motility and motion parameters, morphology and white blood concentration. Fertil Steril. 1999;72:803–8.

Charlesworth B. Evolution in age structured populations. Cambridge: Cambridge University Press; 1980.

Cohen MM, Kreiborg S, et al. Birth prevalence study of the Apert Syndrome. Am J Med Genet. 1992;42:655–9.

Crow JF. The origins, patterns and implications of human spontaneous mutation. Nat Rev Genet. 2000;1:40–7.

Cunningham GR, Toma SM. Why is androgen replacement in males controversial?. J Clin Endocrinol Metab. 2011;96(1):38–52.

Daguet F. Un siècle de fecondite francaise: 1901–1999. Paris: INSEE; 2002.

De la Prochebrochard E, Thonneau P. Paternal age>or=40 years: an important risk factor for infertility. Am J Obstet Gynecol. 2003;189:901–15.

Deslypere JP, Vermeulen A. Leydig cell function in normal men: effect of age, lifestyle, residence, diet, and activity. J Clin Endocrinol Metab. 1984;59:955–62.

Dondero F, Mazilli F, et al. Fertility in elderly men. J Endocrinol Invest. 1985;8 Suppl 2:87–91.

Dunson DB, Colombo B, Baird DD. Changes with age in the level and duration of fertility in the menstrual cycle. Hum Reprod. 2002;17:1399–403.

ESHRE Capri Workshop Group. Fertility and ageing. Hum Reprod Update. 2005;11(3):261–76.

Eskenazi B, Wyrobek AJ, et al. The association of age and semen quality in healthy men. Hum Reprod. 2003;18:447–54.

Feldman HA, Longcope C, et al. Age trends in the level of serum testosterone and other hormones in middle aged men: longitudinal results from the Massachusetts male ageing study. J Clin Endocrinol Metab. 2002;87:589–98.

Finch CE. Longevity, senescence and the genome. Chicago: University of Chicago Press; 1990.

Fisch H, Golubuff ET, et al. Semen analysis in 1283 men from the United States over a 25 year period: no decline in quality. Fertil Steril. 1996;65:1009–14.

Fisch H, Hyun G, et al. The influence of paternal age on down syndrome. J Urol. 2003;169:2275–8.

Ford WC, North K, et al. Increasing paternal age is associated with delayed conception in a large population of fertile couples: evidence for declining fecundity in older men. Hum Reprod. 2000;15:1703–8.

Gan E, Pattman S, et al. A U.K epidemic of testosterone prescribing 2000–2010 'never mind the testes'. Endocrine Abstr. 2012;28:39.

Gavrilov LA, Gavrilov NS, et al. Mutation load and human longevity. Mutat Res. 1997;377:61–2.

Glaser RL, Broman KW, et al. The paternal age effect in Apert syndrome is due, in part, to the increased frequency of mutations in sperm. Am J Hum Genet. 2003;73:939–47.

Goldman N, Montgomery M. Fecundability and husband's age. Soc Biol. 1989;36:146–66.

Handelsman DJ. Pharmacoepidemiology of testosterone prescribing in Australia. Med J Aust. 2012;192:642–5.

Harbitz TB. Morphometric studies of the Sertoli cells in elderly men with special reference to the histology of the prostate. Acta Pathol Microb Scand Sect A Patho. 1973;81:703–17.

Hassan MA, Killick SR. Effect of male age on fertility: evidence for the decline in male fertility with increasing age. Fertil Steril. 2003;79:1520–7.

Hatch M, Kline J, et al. Paternal age and trisomy among spontaneous abortions. Hum Genet. 1990;85:355–61.

Henkel R, Bitter J, et al. Relevance of zinc in human sperm flagella and its relation to motility. Fertil Steril. 1999;71:1138–43.

Hermann M, Untergasser G, et al. Ageing of the male reproductive system. Exp Gerontol. 2000;35:1267–79.

Holstein AF. Morphological evidence for the involution of spermatogenesis during senescence. Diesbach/Berlin/Germany: Reproductive Biology and Medicine; 1989. p. 66–77.

Homonnai ZT, Finman N, et al. Semen quality and sex hormone pattern of middle aged men. Andrologia. 1982;14:164–70.

Hook EB, Schreinemachers DM, et al. Inherited structural cytogenetic abnormalities detected incidentally in fetuses diagnosed prenatally: frequency, parental age associations, sex ratio trends, and comparison with rates of mutants. Am J Hum Genet. 1984;36:422–43.

Irvine S, Cawood E, et al. Evidence of deteriorating semen quality in the United Kingdom: birth cohort study of 577 men in Scotland over 11 years. Br Med J. 1996;312:467–77.

Johnson L, Grumbles JS, et al. Increased germ cell degeneration during postprophase of meiosis is related to increased serum follicle –stimulating hormone concentrations and reduced daily sperm production in aged men. Biol Reprod. 1990;42:281–7.

Keenan DM, Takahashi PY, et al. An ensemble model of the male gonadal axis: illustrative application in ageing men. Endocrinology. 2006;147:2817–28.

Leridon H. Can assisted reproduction technology compensate for natural decline in fertility with age? A model assessment. Hum Reprod. 2004;19:1548–53.

Lowe X, Eskenazi B, et al. Frequency of XY sperm increases with age in fathers of boys with Klinefelter's syndrome. Am J Hum Genet. 2001;69:1046–54.

Lubna P, Santoro N. Age related decline in fertility. Endo Metab Clin N Am. 2003;32:669–88.

Menken J, Trussel J, Larsen U. Age and infertility. Science. 1986;233:1389–94.

Mladenovic I, Micic S, et al. Sperm morphology and motility in different age populations. Arch Androl. 1994;32:197–205.

Mohr BA, Bhasin S, et al. The effect of changes in adiposity on testosterone levels in older men: longitudinal results from the Massachusetts Male Ageing Study. Clin Endocrinol (Oxf). 2006;155:443–52.

Nieschlag E, Lammers U, et al. Reproductive functions in young fathers and grandfathers. J Clin Endocrinol Metab. 1982;55:676–81.
Panigua R, Nistal M, et al. Seminiferous tubule involution in elderly men. Biol Reprod. 1987;36:939–47.
Regadera J, Nistal M, Panigua R. Testis, epididymis, and spermatic cord in elderly men. Correlation of angiographic and histologic studies with systemic arteriosclerosis. Arch Pathol lab Med. 1985;109:663–7.
Rolf C, Behre HM, Nieschlag E. Reproductive parameters of older couples compared to younger men of infertile couples. Int J Androl. 1996;19:135–42.
Rolf MP, Feingold J, et al. Age related disease pattern in infertile men: increasing incidence of infections in older men. Andrologia. 2002;34:209–17.
Sartorelli EM, Mazzucatto LF, et al. Effect of paternal age on human chromosomes. Fertil Steril. 2001;76:1119–23.
Schatzl G, Madersbacher S, et al. Serum androgen levels in men: impact of health status and age. Urology. 2003;61:629–33.
Schwartz D, Maytaux MJ, et al. Semen characteristics as a function of age in 833 fertile men. Fertil Steril. 1983;39:530–5.
Seymour FI, Duffy C, Koerner A. A case of authenticated fertility in a man, aged 94. J Am Med Assoc. 1935;105:1423–4.
Spandorfer SD, Avrech OM, et al. Effect of parental age of fertilization and pregnancy characteristics in couples treated by intracytoplasmic sperm injection. Hum Reprod. 1998;13:334–8.
Statistisches Bundesamt Deutschland. 2004. http://www.destatis.de/basis/dbevoc/bevoctabl.htm
Vajo Z, Francomano CA, Wilkin DJ. The molecular and genetic basis of fibroblast growth factor receptor three disorders: the achondroplasia family of skeletal dysplasias, Muenke craniosynostosis and Crouzon syndrome with acanthosis nigricans. Endocr Rev. 2000;21:23–39.
Wang C, Chan SY, et al. Cross sectional study of semen parameters in a large group of normal Chinese men. Int J Androl. 1985;8:257–74.

Cryopreservation of Human Semen 14

Sasikala Natarajamani

14.1 Introduction

Spallanzani, the famous Italian biologist in 1776, reported the maintenance of motility of human spermatozoa after exposure to low temperatures. Researchers and embryologists were keen to observe the effect of freezing on sperm viability. Later, (Mantegazza 1866) proposed sperm banks for frozen human sperm. But it was Polge's accidental discovery of glycerol (1949) as a cryoprotectant that laid the foundation for modern sperm cryobiology which accelerated the application of cryopreservation techniques. This was shortly followed by the work of (Sherman and Bunge 1953) who observed that human spermatozoa after freeze-drying were able to support normal embryonic development. The first live birth using frozen ejaculated sperm was reported in the year 1953 by Sherman who is also known to have first described liquid nitrogen vapor freezing in the early 1960s (Sherman 1973).

Though the first commercial human semen banks were started in the USA during the early 1970s, the first organized cryobank was set up in France, at the Center d'Etude et de Conservation du Sperme, in 1973. Later, in 1976, the American Association of Tissue Banks was started that included cryopreservation of gametes (Ozkavukcu and Erdemli 2002):

S. Natarajamani, MBBS, MMEDSCI (ART), EMB (ACE)
American College of Embryologists Certified Lab,
Crea Conceptions (ACE Certified) (P) Limited, Chennai, India
e-mail: sasikala@creaconceptions.com; http://www.creaconceptions.com

K. Gunasekaran, N. Pandiyan (eds.), *Male Infertility*,
DOI 10.1007/978-81-322-3604-7_14

Development of human semen cryobanking (1776–1964) (Sherman 1980)		
Date	Contributor	Contribution
1776	Spallanzani	First low-temperature observations
1866	Mantegazza	First suggestion of frozen semen bank
1938	Jahnel	−269 °C survival, storage at −79 °C
1940	Shettles	Individual variation, aging, and thawing
1945	Parkes	Survival better in greater volumes
1949	Polge et al.	Glycerol as cryoprotectant agent
1953–1955	Sherman	Freezing rates, glycerol, preservation
1953–1955	Bunge et al.	First progeny from stored spermatozoa, dry ice method
1954–1959	Keetel et al.	Sixteen births from stored spermatozoa
1958–1959	Sawada et al.	Six births with stored spermatozoa
1962–1963	Sherman	Survival factors, banking applications, nitrogen vapor technique
1964	Perloff et al.	Four births with nitrogen vapor technique

14.2 Cryopreservation

Cryopreservation is defined as the frozen storage of sperms, eggs, embryos, or ovarian and testicular tissues (ART glossary – ESHRE).

Cryopreservation, in general, is a process where cells, whole tissues, or any other substances susceptible to damage caused by chemical reactivity or time are preserved by cooling to subzero temperatures.

14.3 Cryoprotectants

Following ice formation in an aqueous solution like growth media, the ionic composition increases dramatically which is lethal to cells. Cryoprotectants are low-molecular-weight and highly permeable chemicals used to protect spermatozoa from freeze damage during ice crystallization by increasing the unfrozen fraction at a given temperature and hence reduce the ionic composition. Cryoprotectants act by decreasing the freezing point of a substance, reducing the amount of salts and solutes present in the liquid phase of the sample, and also by decreasing ice formation within the spermatozoa (Royere et al. 1996).

They can be classified as follows based on their ability to diffuse across cell membranes:

- *Permeating* – That which cross the plasma membrane into the cytoplasm
- (e.g., glycerol, 1,2-propanediol, DMSO)
- *Non-permeating* – That which does not cross the plasma membrane
- (e.g., proteins, sucrose)

Lovelock suggested that the mechanism of action of cryoprotectants was due to their colligative properties (the collective properties that a solution has when these compounds are present). In particular, it was the reduction in salt concentration at a given temperature that allowed cells to suffer less injury at that temperature. An effective penetrating cryoprotectant should provide colligative properties in which the salt is buffered down to low temperatures. It should also be freely permeable across the cell membrane so that it can buffer the intracellular salt as well, thereby reducing the damage caused to the plasma membrane (Holt 2000; McGann 1979, 1988).

Non-penetrating cryoprotectants act by dehydrating the cell at high subfreezing temperatures, thereby allowing them to be rapidly cooled before the solution effects injury of slow cooling can lead to extensive damage. These compounds are generally polymers and form extensive hydrogen bonds with water, reducing the water activity to a greater extent.

It is necessary that the medium interacts with the cells. The effectiveness of cryoprotecting substances is a function of the time of interaction between the cryoprotectants and the cells. Glycerol is a permeating cryoprotectant most widely used for human sperm cryopreservation. It acts by depressing the freezing point and the consequent lowering of electrolyte concentrations in the unfrozen fraction at any given temperature that would help to counter the harmful "solution effects" imposed during the freezing process.

14.4 Methods of Semen Freezing

Freezing semen can be done by slow freezing, rapid freezing, or vitrification.

14.4.1 Slow Freezing

This conventional technique was given by Behrman and Sawada (1966). Done either manually or automatically by programmed freezers, this method consists of cooling semen over a period of 2–4 h in stepwise manner by adding cryoprotectants (Said et al. 2010). Samples are cooled at a rate of 0.5–1 ° C/min for initial cooling from room temperature to 5 °C. This is followed by freezing from 5 to −80 °C at a rate of 1–10 °C/min. The sample is then plunged in liquid nitrogen at −196 °C (Thachil and Jewett 1981).

Because of the reproducibility issues with this technique, programmable freezers are sometimes used (Holt 2000). Samples are kept on a plate which is placed above a storage tank of liquid nitrogen. The machine once programmed uses software data to cool the sample at the set rate of fall in temperature. Once the decided temperature is achieved, the samples are removed and stored in liquid nitrogen tanks. Some authors believe that conventional freezing techniques result in extensive damage due to formation of ice crystals (Mazur et al. 1981).

14.4.2 Rapid Freezing

Sherman was the first to propose the rapid freezing technique (Sherman 1990) where equal volumes of cryoprotectant and the sample are mixed in a dropwise manner. The sample is then loaded in straws and left to incubate at 4 ° C for 10 min. This is followed by placing the straws at a distance of 15–20 cm above liquid nitrogen with a temperature of −80 °C for 15 min and then plunging them into liquid nitrogen at −196 °C. In this method, there is direct contact between the samples and liquid nitrogen vapor. It might be beneficial to place the straws in a horizontal manner so that the heat difference between the ends is minimal.

The disadvantages of this technique include (Fabbri et al. 2004):

1. Low reproducibility
2. Difficulties in temperature drop control
3. Varying freezing temperature

14.5 Effects of Cryopreservation on Semen Parameters

Cryopreservation has proven to be a very useful technique in the management of infertility, and the success of the technique has an impact on the reproductive outcome of the couple, though the process of cryopreservation itself has a deleterious effect on the structure and function of sperm. Cryopreservation is said to reduce sperm motility and fertility rates by the deleterious effects on sperm membranes, acrosomal structure, and acrosin activity. Many studies have proven the deleterious effect of freezing on motility.

It is said that spermatozoa are less sensitive to cryodamage when compared to other cell types. This can be attributed to the high fluidity of the membrane and low water content. Despite this, there tend to be significant deleterious changes that have been observed in sperm characteristics. It has been reported that several damaging processes can occur during the freezing and thawing of human spermatozoa due to thermal shock with the formation of intracellular and extracellular ice crystals, cellular dehydration, and osmotic shock. The intracellular ice crystals thus formed may breach the membranes and affect the functioning of the organelles. This can lead to impaired cell survival. Cryoinjury is not only limited to the freezing process but it may also occur during the thawing process. Moreover, the survival of sperm after cryopreservation exhibits large male-to-male variability.

14.6 Effect on Sperm Motility

Sperm motility is one of the important parameters that determine the success rate of cryopreservation. The motility of sperms is found to decrease after cryopreservation. The decrease in motility of the spermatozoa has been attributed to the damage caused to the mitochondrial membrane. The greatest amount of energy necessary for sperm motility is provided by ATP molecules. The ATP generated by oxidative phosphorylation in the inner mitochondrial membrane is transferred to the microtubules, to drive motility. Therefore an impairment of mitochondrial activity may explain the reduction in motility. However, with progression of time, significant recovery of sperm motility was reported during the post-thaw period. Though there is no direct link between motility and fertilizing capacity of the sperm, it is one of the important factors that affects sperm quality. The quality of motility had greater impact on the fertility outcome rather than the percentage of motility (Oberoi et al. 2014).

14.7 Effects on Sperm Morphology

The morphological effects of cryopreservation that have been noticed are flattening, cupping, and wrinkling of the head and tail regions. The reasons attributed to the shrinkage are an interaction between the cooling and warming rates. When exposed to hyperosmotic solutions such as glycerol, sperms first shrink because of dehydration and then increase in volume as the glycerol permeates and water concomitantly reenters the cell. The sperm cells maintain membrane integrity in the shrunken state, and serious cell membrane damage can be detected only after returning to isotonic solutions. Also, the post-hypertonic injury of sperm was shown to be a function of time, that is, the shorter the time of exposure to hypertonic solution, the higher the percentage of cell survival (Gao et al. 1993).

14.8 Effects on DNA Integrity

There have been studies suggesting that there is significant damage to DNA leading to fragmentation following cryopreservation. (Donnelly et al. 2001) reported that only spermatozoa from subfertile males and not from fertile males demonstrated a significant increase in DNA fragmentation following cryopreservation (Baumber et al. 2003). Also, studies have suggested that morphologically abnormal sperm are more prone to cryodamage than normal sperm (Kalthur et al. 2008).

The main reasons that lead to DNA fragmentation include increase in the oxidative stress (Said et al. 2010) during cryopreservation. The alteration in the mitochondrial membrane fluidity leads to rise in the mitochondrial membrane potential and subsequent release of reactive oxygen species. This release of reactive oxygen species causes DNA damage that presents with high frequencies of single- and double-strand DNA breaks. The source of ROS include human spermatozoa and seminal leukocytes. Thus cryopreserved samples containing leukocytes are more prone to DNA damage. Besides, cryopreservation process by itself diminishes the antioxidant activity of the spermatozoa making them more susceptible for DNA damage.

14.9 Mazur's Two-Factor Hypothesis (Mazur et al. 1972)

At slow cooling rates, cryoinjury occurs due to solution effects (i.e., the solute/electrolyte concentration, the severe cell dehydration, and the reduction of unfrozen fraction in the extracellular space); and at high cooling rates, cryoinjury occurs due to the lethal intracellular ice formation. The optimal cooling rate for cell survival should be low enough to avoid intracellular ice formation but high enough to minimize the solution effects. Hence an optimal freezing rate has to be established in order to prevent cell damage (Mazur et al. 1972).

14.10 Freezing Surgically Retrieved Sperm

In the initial days of ART, treating azoospermic men involved reconstructive surgery, in the case of an obstruction or donor insemination. But with the advancement of treatment options such as intracytoplasmic sperm injection (ICSI) technique, men with azoospermia can become biological fathers using sperm obtained from their epididymis or testis (Shah 2011).

Azoospermia is the complete absence of spermatozoa in the ejaculate. The two forms of azoospermia are obstructive and nonobstructive azoospermia (Schill). Obstructive azoospermia has been attributed to a mechanical blockage that can occur anywhere along the reproductive tract, including the vas deferens, epididymis, and ejaculatory duct. On the other hand, the conditions that may cause NOA include genetic and congenital abnormalities, postinfectious issues, exposure to gonadotoxins, medications, varicocele, trauma, endocrine disorders, and idiopathic causes (Esteves and Agarwai 2013).

Retrieval of epididymal or testicular sperm for ICSI is indicated in the following conditions:

- Obstructive azoospermia
- Nonobstructive azoospermia
- Failure to ejaculate during an ICSI procedure
- Total astheno-/necrozoospermia

The various surgical techniques employed in sperm retrieval are as follows (Practice Committee of the American Society for Reproductive Medicine 2006):

- Microsurgical epididymal sperm aspiration (MESA)
- Testicular epididymal sperm aspiration (TESA)
- Percutaneous epididymal sperm aspiration (PESA)
- Testicular epididymal sperm extraction (TESE)
- Percutaneous testicular biopsy (PercBiopsy)
- Testicular fine-needle aspiration (TEFNA)

14.11 Importance of Freezing Surgically Retrieved Sperm

Efficient cryopreservation of surgically retrieved spermatozoa reduces the number of surgical interventions and avoids the logistic problems associated with coordinating the women's oocyte retrieval and also the risk of no sperm being found on the day of oocyte retrieval. The conventional methods of sperm cryopreservation are not ideal to cryopreserve small number of cells, such as epididymal and testicular spermatozoa; hence novel approaches have been designed to cryopreserve limited number of motile sperms in a very small volume.

14.12 Freezing Small Number of Spermatozoa

Various attempts have been made to check if freezing sperms in small numbers aids in better recovery rates. Also during surgical sperm recovery, there might be situations where there are very few sperms recovered which might have to be frozen for usage at a later date. Many methods have been adopted including using empty zonae, ICSI needles, etc.

14.13 Fertility Preservation in Prepubertal Cancer Patients

Of all the tissues in the human body, the testis has been shown to be highly susceptible to the toxic effects of cancer therapy at all stages of life. Advances in the management of malignancies in childhood and in the early reproductive phase have made the long-term survival of cancer patients a reality. However, with increasing survival rates, treatment-related morbidity has become an issue among the survivors. Fertility preservation techniques such as spermatogonial stem cell transplantation (Struijk et al. 2013) and freezing testicular tissue are option to biologically father a child in the later years. As the production of spermatozoa begins at puberty, it is not possible to obtain sperm before the age of 12–13 years, and hence cryopreservation of immature testicular tissue has been advocated. However, freezing testicular tissue in prepubertal boys is only an experimental technique, and further evidence and research are required (Orwig and Schlatt 2005).

14.14 Freezing Limited Number of Spermatozoa (Di Santo et al. 2012)

Cryopreservation techniques	Principle	Advantages	Limitations
Empty zona pellucida	Storage of individual spermatozoa in animal or human empty zona pellucida	Avoid waste of time in screening to locate motile sperm; cryoprotectants can be added and removed without loss of spermatozoa sequestered in the zona	Risk of biological contamination

Cryopreservation techniques	Principle	Advantages	Limitations
Microdroplets	Storage of droplets of sperm/cryoprotectant mixture on the surface of dry ice and directly plunged into liquid nitrogen	Avoid sperm loss through adherence to the vessel	Risk of cross contamination; shape and size of dishes make it difficult to handle and store in conventional freezers and liquid nitrogen tanks
ICSI pipette	Storage of spermatozoa in ICSI pipettes	Sterile, simple, and convenient system	Not practical for long-term storage, fragility of ICSI pipettes, risk of cross contamination
Volvox globator spheres	Storage of sperm into spheres of *Volvox globator*	Significant post-thaw recovery of motile sperm	Exposure to genetic material from the algae, constant source of algae
Alginate beads	Microencapsulation in alginate beads	Inert nature of alginate beads	Decrease sperm motility with encapsulation
Cryoloop	Individual spermatozoa deposited directly on cryoprotectant film covering the nylon loop and immersed in liquid nitrogen	Excellent vessel for vitrification, no additional preparation	Open system: risk of cross contamination
Agarose microspheres	Storage of sperm loaded in agarose microspheres	Nonbiological carrier	Clinical value of this approach not evaluated
Straws	Sperms/cryoprotectants loaded into the ministraw	Sterile, simple, and convenient system	Not ideal for severely impaired specimens, sperm loss due to adherence to the vessel

14.15 Post-thaw Survival of Sperms

Factors affecting post-thaw survival rate of spermatozoa are as follows:

1. Cooling/freezing rate
2. Thaw rate
3. Quality of sperm

14.15.1 Cooling/Freezing Rate

The optimal cooling rate from room temperature to 5 °C is 0.5–1 °C/min. The optimal freezing rate observed to be is 10 °C from 5 to −80 °C. Cooling and freezing rates any lesser or higher have been known to adversely affect the post-thaw survival of sperms (Gardner et al. 2002).

14.15.2 Thaw rate

Thaw rate is an important factor that affects the survival of sperms. Since most of the deleterious changes are found to occur in the post-thaw period, an optimal thaw rate is highly essential. Slow thawing in 20 or 30 °C at a rate of 1 °C/min [2] resulted in better survival than other slower or faster thawing methods used (Mahadevan and Trounson 1984).

14.15.3 Quality of Spermatozoa

The quality of sperm, pre-freeze, is also known to affect the post-thaw results. Sperms that have better pre-freeze parameters are known to have better post-thaw survival (Keel and Karow 1980).

Also, it is known that there is significant inter-sample variability, in post-thaw sperm characteristics that have been reported in semen samples collected from healthy men, subfertile men, and men with cancer (Nallella et al. 2004).

14.16 Use of Frozen Sperm in ART and Pregnancy Outcome

Studies have shown that the pregnancy outcomes in ART treatment using fresh and frozen sperm are similar. In men with obstructive azoospermia, no statistical difference was observed between the use of fresh and cryopreserved-thawed testicular sperm when assessing clinical pregnancy or fertilization rates in couples undergoing ICSI (Ohlander et al. 2014).

Researchers say the findings suggest that attempts to coordinate the timing of sperm acquisition for intracytoplasmic sperm injection (ICSI) and in vitro fertilization (IVF) cycle may be unnecessary. The use of cryopreserved sperm also allows clinicians to know whether sperm is available for assisted reproduction.

14.17 Screening of Patients and Donors

Screening of patients and donors is absolutely important before semen freezing, in order to minimize the risk of potentially infecting other samples in the case of leakage of contents into liquid nitrogen. The mandatory screening tests are as follows: HIV-1 and HIV-2 antibodies, hepatitis B surface antigen (HBsAg), hepatitis C virus (HCV) antibodies, and syphilis (Gardner et al. 2002).

14.18 Requirements for a Sperm Donor: ASRM Guidelines

14.18.1 American Society for Reproductive Medicine (The Practice Committee of the American society for Reproductive Medicine and the Practice Committee of the Society for Assisted Reproductive Technology 2013)

14.18.1.1 Selection of Donor

1. Good health status and the absence of known genetic abnormalities.
2. The donor should be of legal age and, ideally, less than 40 years of age.
3. Established fertility status desirable but not required.
4. Psychological evaluation and counseling by a qualified mental health professional. The assessment includes a clinical interview and, where appropriate, psychological testing. Psychological consultation should be required for individuals in whom there appear to be factors that warrant further evaluation. In cases of directed donation, psychological evaluation and counseling are strongly recommended for the donor and his partner (if applicable) as well as for the recipient female and her partner (if applicable). The potential impact of the relationship between the donor and recipient should be explored.

   The psychological assessment also should address the potential psychological risks and evaluate for evidence of coercion financially or emotionally. It is important to ascertain whether the donor is well informed about the extent to which information about him might be disclosed and about any plans that may exist relating to future contact.
5. No owner, operator, laboratory director, or employee of a facility performing TDI may serve as a donor in that practice.
6. Neither the patient's physician nor the individual performing the actual insemination can be the sperm donor.

14.19 WHO Criteria for Normal Semen Quality (WHO Laboratory Manual for the examination of human semen and sperm cervical mucus interaction)

	WHO 2010
Semen volume	1.5
Sperm concentration (10^6/ml)	15
Total number (10^6/ejaculate)	39
Total motility (% a + b + c)	40
Progressive motility (% a + b)	32
Morphology (% normal)	4
Vitality (% live)	58
White blood cells (10^6/ml)	<1.5

Risk assessment of cryopreservation and storage of human semen (WHO Laboratory manual for examination and processing of human semen) *WHO guidelines*
In assessing the risks associated with cryopreservation and storage of semen, the following issues should be considered
Resources
Physical security of the vessels, specimens, and storage room, to reduce risk of loss by theft or fire or failure of cryopreservation straws, ampoules, and vessels or liquid nitrogen supply
Suitability of equipment for proposed use
System of containment and removal of nitrogen
Staff safety and protection
Personal protective equipment
Alarm systems for detection of low liquid nitrogen and low atmospheric oxygen levels
Risk of cross contamination
To reduce the risk of cross contamination with infectious agents between samples in the storage (e.g., transmission of HIV or hepatitis B or C via a cryopreservation vessel), consider
Type of storage container: vials or straws and method of sealing straws (heat or polymer)
Nature of storage: liquid nitrogen or vapor phase
Protocol and method of storage of high-risk samples (samples known or suspected to contain viruses)
Security of frozen samples
Split samples and store at different sites to reduce risk of total loss
Double-check identity of samples at each step
Use robust labeling and identifying codes
Have procedures for regular audit of the use of material and samples remaining in storage

14.20 Current Status of Semen Freezing

Cryopreserving male gamete and its effective usage has revolutionized the field of reproductive medicine. With the increase in malignancies through the recent years, fertility preservation in cancer survivors becomes an important issue to be addressed (Tournaye et al. 2004). Also, freezing sperm avoids the need for additional surgery (azoospermic males) in couples undergoing repeated in vitro fertilization/intracytoplasmic sperm injection cycles and the difficulty of unavailability of male partner during the treatment cycle.

References

Baumber J, Ball BA, Linfor JJ, Meyers SA. Reactive Oxygen Species and Cryopreservation Promote DNA Fragmentation in Equine Spermatozoa. J Androl. 2003;24(4):621–8. Copyright American Society of Andrology.

Behrman SJ, Sawada Y. Heterologous and Homologous inseminations with human semen frozen and stored in liquid nitrogen refrigerator. Fertil Steril. 1966;17(4):457–66.

Bunge RG, Sherman JK. Fertilizing capacity of frozen human spermatozoa. 1953.

Di Santo M, et al. Human Sperm Cryopreservation: Update on Techniques, Effect on DNA Integrity, and Implications for ART. Adv Urol. 2012;2012:854837. doi:10.1155/2012/854837.

Donnelly ET, McClure N, Lewis SE. Cryopreservation of human semen and prepared sperm: effects on motility parameters and DNA integrity. Fertil Steril. 2001;76(5):892–900.

Esteves SC, Agarwai A. The azoospermic male: current knowledge and future perspectives. Clinics (Sao Paulo). 2013;68 Suppl 1:1–4. doi:10.6061/clinics/2013(Sup01)01, PMCID: PMC3583158.

Fabbri R, Ciotti P, Di Tommaso B, et al. Technie di crioconservazione riproduttiva. RivistaItaliana di Ostetricia e Ginecologia. 2004;3:33–41.

Gao DY, Ashworth E, Watson PF, Kleinhans FW, Mazur P, Critser JK. Hyperosmotic Tolerance of Human Spermatozoa: Separate Effects of Glycerol, Sodium Chloride, and Sucrose on Spermolysis. Biol Reprod. 1993;49(1):112–23.

Gardner DK, Lane M, Schoolcraft WB. Physiology and culture of the human blastocyst. J Reprod Immunol. 2002;55(1):85–100.

Holt WV. Basic Aspects of frozen storage of semen. Anim Reprod Sci. 2000;62:3–22.

Kalthur G, Adiga SK, Upadhya D, Rao S, Kumar P. Effect of cryopreservation on sperm DNA integrity in patients with Teratospermia. Fertil Steril. 2008;89(6):1723–7.

Keel BA, Karow Jr AM. Motility characteristics of human sperm, nonfrozen and cryopreserved. Arch Androl. 1980;4(3):205–12.

Mahadevan M, Trounson AO. Effect of cooling, freezing and thawing rates and storage conditions on preservation of human spermatozoa. Andrologia. 1984;16(1):52–60.

Mazur P, Leibo SP, Chu EHY. A two-factor hypothesis of freezing injury. Exp Cell Res. 1972;71:345–55.

Mazur P, RAll WF, Rigopolous N. Relative contributions of unfrozen water and salt concentration to the survival of slowly frozen human erythrocytes. Biophys J. 1981;36(3):653–75.

McGann LE. Optimal Temperature Ranges for Control of Cooling Rate. Cryobiology. 1979;16:211–6.

McGann LE, Yang H, Walterson M. Manifestations of cell damage after freezing and thawing. Cryobiology. 1988;25:178–85.

Mantegazza P. Fisiologia sullo sperma umano. Rendic Reale Instit Lomb. 1866;3:183–6.

Nallella KP, Sharma RK, Said TM, Agarwal A. Inter-sample variability in post-thaw human spermatozoa. Cryobiology. 2004;49:195–9.

Oberoi B, Kumar S, Talwar P. Study of human sperm motility post cryopreservation. Med J Armed Forces India. 2014;70(4):349–53.

Ohlander S, Hotaling J, Kirshenbaum E, Niederberger C, Eisenberg ML. Impact of fresh versus cryopreserved testicular sperm upon intracytoplasmic sperm injection pregnancy outcomes in men with azoospermia due to spermatogenic dysfunction: a meta-analysis. Fertil Steril. 2014;101(2):344–9. doi:10.1016/j.fertnstert.2013.10.012. Epub 2013 Dec 9.

Orwig KE, Schlatt S. Cryopreservation and transplantation of spermatogonia and testicular tissue for preservation of male fertility. J Natl Cancer Inst Monogr. 2005;34:51–6.

Ozkavukcu S, Erdemli E. Cryopreservation: basic knowledge and biophysical effects. J Ankara Med School. 2002;24:187–96.

Practice Committee of the American Society for Reproductive Medicine. Sperm retrieval for obstructive azoospermia. Fertil Steril. 2006;86(5 Suppl 1):S115–20.

Royere D, Barthelemy C, Hamamah S, Lansac J. Cryopreservation of spermatozoa: a 1996 review. Hum Reprod Update. 1996;2(6):553–9. View.

Said TM, Gaglani A, Agarwal A. Implication of apoptosis in sperm cryoinjury. Reprod Biomed Online. 2010;21(4):456–62.

Schill WB, Comhaire FH, Hargreave TB, editors. Andrology for the Clinician. Springer Science & Business Media; 2006.

Shah R. Surgical sperm retrieval: Techniques and their indications. Indian J Urol. 2011;27(1):102–9. doi:10.4103/0970-1591.78439, PMCID: PMC3114571.

Sherman J. Synopsis of the use of frozen human semen since 1964: state of the art of human banking. Fertil Steril. 1973;24(5):397–412.

Sherman J. Cryopreservation of human semen. In: Keel B, Webster BW, editors. Handbook of the laboratory diagnosis and treatment of Infertility. Boca Raton: CRC Press; 1990.

Sherman JK. Historical synopsis of human semen cryobanking. In Human artificial insemination and semen preservation. Springer US; 1980. pp. 95–105.

Struijk RB, Mulder CL, van der Veen F, van Pelt AM, Repping S. Restoring Fertility in Sterile Childhood Cancer Survivors by Autotransplanting Spermatogonial Stem Cells: Are We There Yet? Biomed Res Int. 2013;2013:903142. doi:10.1155/2013/903142.

Thachil JV, Jewett MAS. Preservation techniques for human semen. Fertil Steril. 1981;35(5):546–8.

The Practice Committee of the American society for Reproductive Medicine and the Practice Committee of the Society for Assisted Reproductive Technology. Recommendations for gamete and embryo donation: a Committee opinion. Fertil Steril. 2013;99:47–62 by ASRM.

Tournaye H, Goossens E, Verheyen G, Frederickx V, De Block G, Devroey P, Van Steirteghem A. Preserving the reproductive potential of men and boys with cancer: current concepts and future prospects. Hum Reprod Update. 2004;10(6):525–32. Epub 2004 Aug 19.

WHO Laboratory manual for examination and processing of Human semen. p. 169–76.

Who Laboratory Manual for the examination of human semen and sperm-cervical mucus interaction. 4th edn.

Fertility Preservation in Men and Prepubertal Boys

15

Shubhashree Uppangala, Guruprasad Kalthur, and Satish Kumar Adiga

15.1 Introduction

Managing the fertility potential has emerged as a major concern for young men who receive gonadotoxic therapy for various malignant and nonmalignant conditions. One of the major causes of non-accidental mortality worldwide is cancer. Over the past few decades, due to the development of reasonably effective cancer treatment regimens, survival rate among childhood cancer patients has increased (Smith et al. 2014). A recent estimate suggests that ~1 in 530 young adults between the ages of 20 and 39 years is a childhood cancer survivor (Ward et al. 2014). Unfortunately, the different cancer regimens like radiotherapy and/or chemotherapy employed to cure cancer also damage other healthy rapidly dividing cells such as the spermatogonial stem cells. Thus, cancer treatments become gonadotoxic and render patients to suffer subfertility or infertility. Infertility or subfertility due to cancer treatment may be reversible in some cases, whereas persistent infertility may occur in 50–95 % of malignancies. Hence, maintaining reproductive health or the ability to father a normal biological child post-cancer treatment becomes of paramount concern in cancer survivors. To tackle these issues the area of fertility preservation has emerged as an option to maintain reproductive potential to all those who receive gonadotoxic treatments.

In order to protect the fertility of the patients, several strategies have been developed. Cryopreservation of sperm has been established in case of adult men (Sharma 2011). Testicular tissue freezing and cryopreservation of stem cells have been proposed as an experimental procedure in case of prepubertal boys who cannot produce sperm (Jahnukainen et al. 2011). Fertility preservation is a combined effort of both clinicians and the fertility specialists on improving reproductive function in cancer

S. Uppangala • G. Kalthur • S.K. Adiga (✉)
Division of Clinical Embryology, Kasturba Medical College, Manipal University, Manipal 576 104, India
e-mail: satish.adiga@manipal.edu

K. Gunasekaran, N. Pandiyan (eds.), *Male Infertility*,
DOI 10.1007/978-81-322-3604-7_15

patients and also maintaining the existing efficacy of available cancer therapies. With respect to the role of fertility preservation in cancer treatment, recommendations have been established by the American Society of Clinical Oncology (ASCO) and American Society for Reproductive Medicine (ASRM) for oncologists managing malignancy (Ethics Committee of the American Society for Reproductive Medicine 2005; Lee et al. 2006) including childhood cancers. These committees have recommended clinicians to address the topic of fertility preservation at the earliest opportunity, with in-depth discussions of the available options, and to consider referring patients to a qualified fertility specialist. Although fertility preservation has been recognized as an important issue, numerous aspects continue to impede its incorporation in routine clinical practice. These factors include time restrictions, lack of knowledge, financial burden, lack of available fertility preservation services, and discomfort in discussing the topic.

Although the consequences of gonadotoxic treatments on male fertility has been an important aspect of patient care since several years (Woodruff 2007), the field of fertility preservation gained importance only recently. As an emerging field, fertility preservation has resulted in an increasingly available network of resources to both clinicians and patients with the aim of preserving both the quantity and quality of life of patients undergoing gonadotoxic treatments.

Given the broad scope of fertility preservation in male individuals, this chapter will focus predominantly on fertility preservation in males with an emphasis on different indications for fertility preservation and available treatment strategies. In addition, the ethical issues to be considered during fertility preservation as well as brief overview of future directions in male fertility preservation techniques will also be considered.

15.2 Indications for Male Fertility Preservation

15.2.1 Cancer Patients

The major beneficiaries from fertility preservation are cancer patients. Cancer and its treatment have a detrimental impact on systemic health since many biological processes, cells, and tissues become affected. In the testis, rapidly dividing germ cells are highly sensitive to cytotoxic agents such as chemotherapeutic drugs and radiation (Meistrich 2013). Thus, cancer treatments not only damage cancer cells but also target the germ cells. Low-dose treatments may destroy the differentiating spermatogonia, whereas less sensitive spermatogonial stem cells survive, and other population such as spermatocytes and spermatids complete the maturation process to produce sperm (van Alphen et al. 1988).

Testicular recovery after such treatments has been found to be a slow process which may extend for several weeks, until either temporary or permanent azoospermic condition sets in at least among adult men. Even in prepubertal boys, spermatogonial cells divide (Wyns et al. 2008) and increase in number over time (Paniagua and Nistal 1984). Thus, chemotherapy and radiotherapy can cause either temporary,

Table 15.1 Nonmalignant diseases requiring fertility preservation

Nonmalignant diseases
1. Adrenoleukodystrophy
2. Alpha-mannosidosis
3. Aplastic anemia
4. Aspartylglucosaminuria
5. Ataxia telangiectasia
6. DiGeorge syndrome
7. Galactosemia
8. Hurler syndrome
9. Inflammatory bowel disease (IBD)
10. Klinefelter syndrome
11. Sickle cell anemia
12. Systemic lupus erythematosus (SLE)

long-term, or permanent gonadal toxicity depending on the dose and type of treatment in both adult men and prepubertal boys (Meistrich 2009, 2013). Therefore, in clinical practice, depending on the type of cancer and treatment protocols, it is important to estimate infertility risk for each patient and consult with him and his parents (for prepubertal and adolescent patients) on his infertility risk (Wyns et al. 2011).

15.2.2 Nonmalignant Diseases

In addition to malignant diseases, certain other disease conditions require high-dose chemotherapy and/or irradiation. Certain benign hematological conditions, such as aplastic anemia, sickle cell disease, Fanconi anemia and thalassemia major, and severe autoimmune diseases unresponsive to immunosuppressive therapy, such as juvenile idiopathic arthritis, juvenile systemic lupus erythematosus (SLE), systemic sclerosis, and immune cytopenias, necessitate administration of high-dose chemotherapy (Anserini et al. 2002; Berthaut et al. 2008; Oktay and Oktem 2009). Total body irradiation is required before hematological stem cell transplantation which is associated with significant germ cell failure (Sarafoglou et al. 1997). This often leads to severe, dose-dependent, and sometimes irreversible spermatogenic damage (David et al. 1993). Therefore, these patients may also need to be counseled for fertility preservation. A list of nonmalignant conditions where fertility preservation is opted is given in Table 15.1.

15.3 Strategies for Male Fertility Preservation

Different strategies are being used to preserve fertility in males. The protocols such as semen collection and sperm cryopreservation have been clinically validated. Recently, cryopreservation of immature testicular tissue has been adopted as an experimental approach to preserve the fertility potential of prepubertal boys (Wyns et al. 2010). Other strategies such as hormonal therapy and use of anti-apoptotic agents such as sphingosine-1-phosphate have been shown to be of limited value (Suomalainen et al. 2003; Shetty and Meistrich 2005).

15.3.1 Semen Cryopreservation

The most routinely used strategy for fertility preservation in pubertal and adult patients is semen cryopreservation (Sharma 2011). For adult men, semen cryopreservation before their gonadotoxic treatment has been clinically validated as an efficient method to preserve fertility using ART procedures. Live births have been reported after insemination of stored sperm even after freezing for a period of 28 years (Feldschuh et al. 2005). For semen collection, masturbation is recommended. However, some patients may not be able to collect ejaculate by masturbation due to stress or because of certain medical conditions or treatment. These patients include those who have ejaculatory dysfunction, psychogenic anejaculation, and peripubertal adolescents unfamiliar with masturbation. For individuals with ejaculatory dysfunction and anejaculation, penile vibratory stimulation (PVS) or electroejaculation (EEJ) methods can be employed. The optimized environment should be provided by eliminating time constraints for sample production, and the appropriate stimulating materials should be arranged. In case of adolescent patients, before their treatment clinicians are recommended to give information regarding the need for fertility preservation and they should explain all available options as early as possible (Lee et al. 2006). If the patients can produce an ejaculate, semen samples are cryopreserved in case of adolescent boys also (Daudin et al. 2015), and it is recommended that parents should not be allowed to attend the appointment for sample collection.

15.3.2 Testicular Sperm Cryopreservation

In addition to semen samples, testicular sperm extraction (TESE) and storage is the only method available for cancer patients (adolescent or adult) with azoospermia. The TESE procedure is a surgical intervention. This procedure is done either with local or general anesthesia. However, higher recovery rates were obtained following microsurgical techniques (Donoso et al. 2007; Colpi et al. 2009). Testicular sperm extraction has been used successfully to obtain sperm in approximately 50 % of cases of persistent azoospermia post-cancer therapy with previous failure of cryopreservation or when cryopreservation strategy has not been considered (Hsiao et al. 2011).

15.3.3 Testicular Tissue Cryopreservation

In prepubertal boys, when there is no evidence of presence of spermatozoa, immature testicular tissue cryopreservation method is considered as a strategy of fertility preservation. There is increasing trend in the use of testicular tissue cryopreservation before the cancer treatment as a means to preserve the fertility of prepubertal and peri-pubertal boys to 16 years of age (Wyns et al. 2011). This is an experimental approach. Since testicular tissue recovery is a surgical procedure, in order to minimize the trauma to the patient and also to minimize the risk of anesthesia in children, the surgical recovery of testicular tissue should be combined with other interventions requiring anesthesia, such as bone marrow sampling or implantation of venous ports. In order to minimize the manipulation and trauma, retrieving tissue from only one testis is suggested to minimize manipulation (Wyns et al. 2011), and the size of tissue may vary between 80 and 250 mm^3 based on testicular size in the different age groups (Goede et al. 2011).

Till date, there is no optimized freezing protocol for human immature testicular tissue. Different freezing protocols have been used such as slow freezing and vitrification. Studies have shown that vitrification may be as effective as slow freezing in preserving testicular tissue (Curaba et al. 2011; Poels et al. 2013). Different cryoprotectants have been used such as ethylene glycol and sucrose (Kvist et al. 2006), DMSO (Keros et al. 2005, 2007), and also DMSO in combination with sucrose (Wyns et al. 2007, 2008; Poels et al. 2014). In order to maximize the quality and viability of human testicular tissue post-thaw, all aspects of the tissue collection and processing, the type and concentration of cryoprotectant used, as well as the cooling and warming protocols must be fully optimized. Since the reproductive potential of cryopreserved immature testicular tissue has still to be proven in humans, the technique remains experimental, and no one preservation protocol has been shown to be superior over any other published methods (Kvist et al. 2006; Keros et al. 2007; Wyns et al. 2008; Baert et al. 2013; Goossens et al. 2013; Poels et al. 2013).

15.4 Strategies to Restore Fertility from Cryopreserved Testicular Tissue

Several methods have been considered for the restoration of fertility from cryopreserved testicular tissue. These procedures are in experimental stage, and they are far less advanced than the methods used to preserve testicular tissue and spermatogonial stem cells. Some of the methods which can be used to restore fertility are autotransplantation/autografting of SSC suspension or testicular graft and in vitro spermatogenesis. Till now none of the techniques have been proven to be clinically safe, and extensive research has to be done in this regard.

15.4.1 Male Germ Cell Transplantation

Male germ cell transplantation technique was originally described in the mouse model (Brinster and Zimmermann 1994). In this method, SSC cell suspensions were infused through the efferent duct into the rete testis of sterile recipients with the successful reinstatement of spermatogenesis and finally the restoration of fertility. However, studies have shown that injection of SSC via the rete testis has proved to be a better treatment site for species such as the bovine, primate, and human because of differences in anatomy and consistency and the larger testis size (Schlatt et al. 1999; Ning et al. 2012). At present, SSC injection is considered the most promising method for fertility restoration in prepubertal cancer patients. For this purpose, SSC propagation has to be done *in vitro.* Studies have shown the ability of SSC propagation in several species (Schlatt et al. 1999; Honaramooz et al. 2002; Kanatsu-Shinohara et al. 2003; Aponte et al. 2008; Nobrega et al. 2010). However, recent study has demonstrated spermatogenesis *in vivo* after germ cell transplantation and confirmed fertilizing ability of those spermatozoa by ICSI in primates (Hermann et al. 2012). Though this study is a milestone toward restoring fertility in humans, whether epigenetic programming and stability of SSC are not compromised following cryopreservation, culture, and transplantation in humans is yet to be elucidated (Struijk et al. 2013).

15.4.2 Autotransplantation of Testicular Tissue

Transplantation of testicular tissue fragments is an alternative strategy to the use of SSC suspensions. This approach maintains the SSCs within their natural niche, thus preserving the interactions between the germ cells and their supporting somatic cells. Nutrients and hormones from the body will reach the graft and induce spermatogenesis, and the resultant sperm can be extracted and used in ICSI procedures. Autologous transplantation of the testicular biopsy back into the testis (Van Saen et al. 2009), scrotum (Wyns et al. 2007), or ectopically under the skin (Jahnukainen et al. 2007) can however only be used to restore spermatogenesis if the presence of malignant cells can be excluded.

15.4.3 In Vitro Spermatogenesis

Spermatogenesis in a culture system provides the one of the best perspectives of fertility preservation. In other methods described in the above sections, there is a chance of reintroducing malignant cells, which can be avoided by the technique of producing sperm in vitro. Several methods have been employed to produce sperm in vitro. However, very little progress has been made in this regard. Conventional testicular cell culture was not successful in differentiating spermatogonia into mature spermatozoa. Recently three-dimensional culture systems have been developed which could successfully generate morphologically mature spermatozoa (Stukenborg et al. 2008, 2009). Major breakthrough in this regard is the production of live offspring in mouse through organ culture systems (Sato et al. 2011a, b). Nevertheless, effective spermatogenesis in vitro still remains to be established.

15.5 Ethical Considerations During Fertility Preservation

The setting and implementing fertility preservation for malignancy-related cases raises complex ethical and legal issues. Care must be taken to distinguish between established fertility preservation protocols and experimental interventions. Young patients present further ethical issues related to age of assent and consent to procedures and rights of ownership of preserved specimens. Additional challenges include concerns over potential delay of cancer treatment for cryopreservation, postmortem disposition of sperm, and rights attributed to banked testicular material (Picton et al. 2015). Each of these issues should be considered and addressed when appropriate, preferably at the time of initial fertility preservation consultation. In all cases informed consent from parents or legal guardians should be taken before tissue is harvested. Even when minors are legally incompetent, an effort should be made to inform them about the implications of the procedure (at a level appropriate for their age and maturity) and to obtain assent (Bahadur et al. 2001). The risks of fertility loss must be balanced against the potential for fertility restoration from stored samples and explained to each individual child and his parents to make sure that they understand that there is no guarantee of success.

15.6 Future Challenges

The development of strategies for fertility preservation in prepubertal boys and adolescents is still in its infancy and represents a balance between biological, clinical, and technical knowns, technological unknowns, and ethical and legal questions. There are many unanswered questions in regard with the immature testicular tissue cryopreservation. Optimization of protocols for tissue retrieval, processing, freezing, and thawing has to be carried out. Fertility restoration methods have to be established. Safety of cryopreserved samples in terms of genetic and epigenetic stability has to be elucidated. Progress in this field is encouraging; however, there is requirement of safe validated methods to incorporate in routine clinical practice to restore fertility of patients undergoing gonadotoxic treatments.

References

Anserini P, Chiodi S, Spinelli S, Costa M, Conte N, Copello F, Bacigalupo A. Semen analysis following allogeneic bone marrow transplantation. Additional data for evidence-based counselling. Bone Marrow Transplant. 2002;30:447–51.

Aponte PM, Soda T, Teerds KJ, Mizrak SC, van de Kant HJ, de Rooij DG. Propagation of bovine spermatogonial stem cells in vitro. Reproduction. 2008;136:543–57.

Baert Y, Van Saen D, Ning L, Haentjens P, Tournaye H, Goosens E. What is the best cryopreservation protocol for human testicular tissue banking? Hum Reprod. 2013;28:1816–26.

Bahadur G, Whelan J, Ralph D, Hindmarsh P. Gaining consent to freeze spermatozoa from adolescents with cancer: legal, ethical and practical aspects. Hum Reprod. 2001;16:188–93.

Berthaut I, Guignedoux G, Kirsch-Noir F, de Larouziere V, Ravel C, Bachir D, Galactéros F, Ancel PY, Kunstmann JM, Levy L, Jouannet P, Girot R, Mandelbaum J. Influence of sickle cell disease and treatment with hydroxyurea on sperm parameters and fertility of human males. Haematologica. 2008;93:988–93.

Brinster RL, Zimmermann JW. Spermatogenesis following male germ-cell transplantation. Proc Natl Acad Sci USA. 1994;91:11298–302.

Colpi GM, Colpi EM, Piediferro G, Giacchetta D, Gazzano G, Castiglioni FM, Magli MC, Gianaroli L. Microsurgical TESE versus conventional TESE for ICSI in non-obstructive azoospermia: a randomized controlled study. Reprod Biomed Online. 2009;18:315–9.

Curaba M, Poels J, Van Langendonckt A, Donnez J, Wyns C. Can prepubertal human testicular tissue be cryopreserved by vitrification? Fertil Steril. 2011;95:2123.e9–e12.

Daudin M, Rives N, Walschaerts M, Drouineaud V, Szerman E, Koscinski I, Eustache F, Saïas-Magnan J, Papaxanthos-Roche A, Cabry-Goubet R, et al. Sperm cryopreservation in adolescents and young adults with cancer: results of the French national sperm banking network (CECOS). Fertil Steril. 2015;103:478–86.

David J, Vouyiouka O, Ansell BM, Hall A, Woo P. Amyloidosis in juvenile chronic arthritis: a morbidity and mortality study. Clin Exp Rheumatol. 1993;11:85–90.

Donoso P, Tournaye H, Devroey P. Which is the best sperm retrieval technique for non-obstructive azoospermia? A systematic review. Hum Reprod Update. 2007;13:539–49.

Ethics Committee of the American Society for Reproductive Medicine. Fertility preservation and reproduction in cancer patients. Fertil Steril. 2005;83:1622–8.

Feldschuh J, Brassel J, Durso N, Levine A. Successful sperm storage for 28 years. Fertil Steril. 2005;84:1017.

Goede J, Hack WW, Sijstermans K, van der Voort-Doedens LM, Van der Ploeg T, Meij-de Vries A, Delemarre-van de Waal HA. Normative values for testicular volume measured by ultrasonography in a normal population from infancy to adolescence. Horm Res Paediatr. 2011;76:56–64.

Goossens E, Van Saen D, Tournaye H. Spermatogonial stem cell preservation and transplantation: from research to clinic. Hum Reprod. 2013;28:897–907.

Hermann BP, Sukhwani M, Winkler F, Pascarella JN, Peters KA, Sheng Y, Valli H, Rodriguez M, Ezzelarab M, Dargo G, et al. Spermatogonial stem cell transplantation into rhesus testes regenerates spermatogenesis producing functional sperm. Cell Stem Cell. 2012;11:715–26.

Honaramooz A, Megee SO, Dobrinski I. Germ cell transplantation in pigs. Biol Reprod. 2002;66:21–8.

Hsiao W, Stahl PJ, Osterberg EC, Nejat E, Palermo GD, Rosenwaks Z, Schlegel PN. Successful treatment of postchemotherapy azoospermia with microsurgical testicular sperm extraction: the Weill Cornell experience. J Clin Oncol. 2011;29:1607–11.

Jahnukainen K, Ehmcke J, Hergenrother SD, Schlatt S. Effect of cold storage and cryopreservation of immature non-human primate testicular tissue on spermatogonial stem cell potential in xenografts. Hum Reprod. 2007;22:1060–7.

Jahnukainen K, Ehmcke J, Hou M, Schlatt S. Testicular function and fertility preservation in male cancer patients. Best Pract Res Clin Endocrinol Metab. 2011;25:287–302.

Kanatsu-Shinohara M, Ogonuki N, Inoue K, Miki H, Ogura A, Toyokuni S, Shinohara T. Long-term proliferation in culture and germline transmission of mouse male germline stem cells. Biol Reprod. 2003;69:612–6.

Keros V, Rosenlund B, Hultenby K, Aghajanova L, Levkov L, Hovatta O. Optimizing cryopreservation of human testicular tissue: comparison of protocols with glycerol, propanediol and dimethylsulphoxide as cryoprotectants. Hum Reprod. 2005;20:1676–87.

Keros V, Hultenby K, Borgström B, Fridström M, Jahnukainen K, Hovatta O. Methods of cryopreservation of testicular tissue with viable spermatogonia in pre-pubertal boys undergoing gonadotoxic cancer treatment. Hum Reprod. 2007;22:1384–95.

Kvist K, Thorup J, Byslov AG, Hoyer PE, Mollgard K, Yding AC. Cryopreservation of intact testicular tissue from boys with cryptorchidism. Hum Reprod. 2006;21:484–91.

Lee SJ, Schover LR, Partridge AH, Patrizio P, Wallace WH, Hagerty K, Beck LN, Brennan LV, Oktay K. American Society of Clinical Oncology recommendations on fertility preservation in cancer patients. J Clin Oncol. 2006;24:2917–31.
Meistrich ML. Male gonadal toxicity. Pediatr Blood Cancer. 2009;53:261–6.
Meistrich ML. Effects of chemotherapy and radiotherapy on spermatogenesis in humans. Fertil Steril. 2013;100:1180–6.
Ning L, Meng J, Goossens E, Lahoutte T, Marichal M, Tournaye H. In search of an efficient injection technique for future clinical application of spermatogonial stem cell transplantation: infusion of contrast dyes in isolated cadaveric human testes. Fertil Steril. 2012;98:1443–8.
Nobrega RH, Greebe CD, van de Kant H, Bogerd J, de Franca LR, Schulz RW. Spermatogonial stem cell niche and spermatogonial stem cell transplantation in zebrafish. PLoS One. 2010;5:2010.
Oktay K, Oktem O. Fertility preservation medicine: a new field in the care of young cancer survivors. Pediatr Blood Cancer. 2009;53:267–73.
Paniagua R, Nistal M. Morphological and histometric study of human spermatogonia from birth to the onset of puberty. J Anat. 1984;139:535–52.
Picton HM, Wyns C, Anderson RA, Goossens E, Jahnukainen K, Kliesch S, Mitchell RT, Pennings G, Rives N, Tournaye H, van Pelt AM, Eichenlaub-Ritter U, Schlatt S, ESHRE Task Force On Fertility Preservation In Severe Diseases. A European perspective on testicular tissue cryopreservation for fertility preservation in prepubertal and adolescent boys. Hum Reprod. 2015;30:2463–75.
Poels J, Van Langendonckt A, Many MC, Wese FX, Wyns C. Vitrification preserves proliferation capacity in human spermatogonia. Hum Reprod. 2013;28:578–89.
Poels J, Abou-Ghannam G, Herman S, Van Langendonckt A, Wese F-X, Wyns C. In search of better spermatogonial preservation by supplementation of cryopreserved human immature testicular tissue xenografts with N-acetylcysteine and testosterone. Front Surg. 2014;1:47.
Sarafoglou K, Boulad F, Gillio A, Sklar C. Gonadal function after bone marrow transplantation for acute leukemia during childhood. J Pediatr. 1997;130:210–6.
Sato T, Katagiri K, Gohbara A, Inoue K, Ogonuki N, Ogura A, Kubota Y, Ogawa T. In vitro production of functional sperm in cultured neonatal mouse testes. Nature. 2011a;471:504–7.
Sato T, Katagiri K, Yokonishi T, Kubota Y, Inoue K, Ogonuki N, Matoba S, Ogura A, Ogawa T. In vitro production of fertile sperm from murine spermatogonial stem cell lines. Nat Commun. 2011b;2:472.
Schlatt S, Rosiepen G, Weinbauer GF, Rolf C, Brook PF, Nieschlag E. Germ cell transfer into rat, bovine, monkey and human testes. Hum Reprod. 1999;14:144–50.
Sharma V. Sperm storage for cancer patients in the UK: a review of current practice. Hum Reprod. 2011;26:2935–43.
Shetty G, Meistrich ML. Hormonal approaches to preservation and restoration of male fertility after cancer treatment. J Natl Cancer Inst Monogr. 2005;34:36–9.
Smith MA, Altekruse SF, Adamson PC, Reaman GH, Seibel NL. Declining childhood and adolescent cancer mortality. Cancer. 2014;120:2497–506.
Struijk RB, Mulder CL, van der Veen F, van Pelt AM, Repping S. Restoring fertility in sterile childhood cancer survivors by autotransplanting spermatogonial stem cells: are we there yet? Biomed Res Int. 2013;2013:903142.
Stukenborg JB, Wistuba J, Luetjens CM, Elhija MA, Huleihel M, Lunenfeld E, et al. Coculture of spermatogonia with somatic cells in a novel three-dimensional soft-agar-culture-system. J Androl. 2008;29:312–29.
Stukenborg JB, Schlatt S, Simoni M, Yeung CH, Elhija MA, Luetjens CM, et al. New horizons for in vitro spermatogenesis? An update on novel three-dimensional culture systems as tools for meiotic and post-meiotic differentiation of testicular germ cells. Mol Hum Reprod. 2009;15:521–9.
Suomalainen L, Hakala JK, Pentikäinen V, Otala M, Erkkilä K, Pentikäinen MO, Dunkel L. Sphingosine-1-phosphate in inhibition of male germ cell apoptosis in the human testis. J Clini Endocrinol Metab. 2003;88:5572–9.

van Alphen MM, van de Kant HJ, de Rooij DG. Depletion of the spermatogonia from the seminiferous epithelium of the rhesus monkey after X irradiation. Radiat Res. 1988;113:473–86.

Van Saen D, Goossens E, De Block G, Tournaye H. Regeneration of spermatogenesis by grafting testicular tissue or injecting testicular cells into the testes of sterile mice: a comparative study. Fertil Steril. 2009;91:2264–72.

Ward E, De Santis C, Robbins A, Kohler B, Jemal A. Childhood and adolescent cancer statistics, 2014. CA Cancer J Clin. 2014;64:83–103.

Woodruff TK. The emergence of a new interdiscipline: oncofertility. Cancer Treat Res. 2007;138:3–11.

Wyns C, Curaba M, Martinez-Madrid B, Van Langendonckt A, Wese F-X, Donnez J. Spermatogonial survival after cryopreservation and short-term orthotopic immature human cryptorchid testicular tissue grafting to immunodeficient mice. Hum Reprod. 2007;22:1603–11.

Wyns C, Van Langendonckt A, Wese FX, Donnez J, Curaba M. Long-term spermatogonial survival in cryopreserved and xenografted immature human testicular tissue. Hum Reprod. 2008;23:2402–14.

Wyns C, Curaba M, Vanabelle B, Van Langendonckt A, Donnez J. Options for fertility preservation in prepubertal boys. Hum Reprod Update. 2010;16:312–28.

Wyns C, Curaba M, Petit S, Vanabelle B, Laurent P, Wese JF, Donnez J. Management of fertility preservation in prepubertal patients: 5 years' experience at the Catholic University of Louvain. Hum Reprod. 2011;26:737–47.

Sexual Dysfunction and Infertility

16

Narayana Reddy, Varsha Swamy, N. Pandiyan, and Shah Dupesh

16.1 Introduction

Human sexual behaviour seems to be different from other species. Humans do not engage in *sex just for reproduction*, but on the other hand, there seems to be a variety of complex factors driving people towards it. Why do humans engage in sex? The answer would seem quite obvious for some, such as, to reproduce, to experience pleasure, to relieve tension and to make a short-term relationship long term; for some sex could be a tool utilized for 'mate guarding' and among other reasons which would seem too simple to comprehend. Sex is a fungible resource; in some settings, sex is exchanged for money, and in some hunter groups like the Ache of Paraguay, sex is exchanged for meat (Meston and Buss 2007). Thus from a much broader social and cultural view point, humans engage in sex for a myriad of

N. Reddy, MBBS, PhD (✉)
(University of Madras), AASECT (American Association of Sexuality Educators Counsellors and Therapists), Dega Institute of Sexual Medicine,
A2 Ravi Towers, 53/22 Hindi Prachar Sabha Street, T-Nagar 600017, India
e-mail: deganr@gmail.com

V. Swamy, MSc
Bloom Fertility Center, No.32, Taramani Link Road, Velachery 600 042, India

N. Pandiyan
Department of Reproductive Medicine, Chettinad Hospital and Research Institute,
International Academic Affiliations, Chettinad University,
Rajiv Gandhi Salai, Kelambakkam, Tamil Nadu 603103, India

S. Dupesh
Centre of Excellence for Men's health, The Women's Infertility Clinic, Women's centre,
8A, Burkit Rd, CIT Nagar East, T Nagar, Tamil Nadu 600017, India

Fortis Healthcare, Fortis Malar Hospitals, Adyar, India

K. Gunasekaran, N. Pandiyan (eds.), *Male Infertility*,
DOI 10.1007/978-81-322-3604-7_16

reasons. Human sexuality plays an important role in determining a person's sexual behaviour and is greatly influenced by a person's societal, religious, cultural and personal beliefs. Human sexuality is often for recreation, and procreation is a by-product (Abramson et al. 2002). Much of our current-day understanding on human sexual function comes from the pioneering work of Masters and Johnson's previous work where they observed and documented 10,000 cycles of sexual response (Masters and Johnson 1986) which included homosexuals. Perusal of data from large-scale population studies indicates that sexual dysfunction is increasingly common. At a primary care level, sexual dysfunction affects 30–40 % of either partner in a couple (Read et al. 1997). Interestingly in a large multinational survey involving 12,815 participants between the age groups of 50–80, 71 % of men reported at least one episode of sexual dysfunction, in the preceding 4 weeks. More importantly, the severity of the dysfunction correlated with increasing age and lower urinary tract symptoms and was also independent of associated comorbidities like hypertension, dyslipidemia, diabetes and cardiac disease (Rosen et al. 2003). This clearly indicates that sexual dysfunction represents a complex problem with a multifactorial aetiology. From a clinical standpoint, the treating physician should be sagacious enough to differentiate *a* 'sexual dysfunction' *from* 'sexual difficulties' since sexual difficulties like a lack of interest or an inability to relax are more consistently related to the degree of sexual dissatisfaction as when compared to sexual dysfunction (Frank et al. 1978). A key point to be borne in mind is that, only 23 % of men and about 56 % of women initiate discussions about their sexual problems. Eliciting a sexual history from the patient must be physician initiated (Halvorsen and Metz 1992). For many adults talking about sex in itself is a new experience, as most adults discuss sex only from a third-person perspective. While eliciting a sexual history, one must start from a broad sexual topic and then progress towards the patient's specific sexual problem. Every patient should be asked some basic questions, like 'What problems do you have with sex?' or 'Has your illness affected your sex life?' A sexual history outline is given in Table 16.1.

Whenever a sexual dysfunction is identified, clinical acumen would involve eliciting a detailed history and physical exam of the partner, since all sexual dysfunctions are potentially relationship issues. Immediate involvement of the partner gives a different perspective and helps redesigning therapeutic strategies. The couple should be reassured that sexual problems are treatable. This very statement can unburden the couple and allow them to focus towards therapeutic goals

16.2 Definition and Classification of Sexual Dysfunctions

The definition of sexual dysfunction from a psychological perspective is derived from the four-phase model of the human sexual response cycle proposed by Masters and Johnson and Kaplan (1980). The first phase, termed the arousal phase, encompasses the appetitive or motivational aspect of sexual response and includes a person's sexual fantasies and urges. The second phase called the excitement phase, is the subjective sense of pleasure felt and is accompanied by erection and increased

Table 16.1 An outline of the various components involved in eliciting a sexual history

Sexual history outline	Subcomponents
History of the presenting complaint	Date/mode of onset, situational or global, effect of ongoing/past treatment on sexual function, exacerbations/remissions, any other symptoms in other body systems
Marital history	Stability in the marriage, interpersonal communications, conflicts and misunderstanding in the current relationship, feelings towards the current partner, problems with fidelity
Sexual history	Intercourse frequency, time of intercourse, frequency and preference of each partner, sexual fantasies of each partner, foreplay duration, types of sex play preferred by each partner, history of pain during sex, privacy during sex, time of intercourse and associated fatigue, any associated difficulties in both non-verbal and verbal communications during intercourse, masturbatory practices
Potential stressors	Infertility and its treatment, death of a loved one, financial stressors, etc.
Familial and cultural beliefs	Religious beliefs on sex, joint/nuclear family, privacy if living as a joint family, presence of siblings in the household
Medical history	Complete review of all body systems, medical illness and surgery, history of alcohol, drugs, smoking and medications

vaginal congestion and lubrication. The third phase is called orgasm or climax phase and encompasses peak sexual pleasure felt, associated with rhythmic contracture of the musculature around the genital area and ejaculatory inevitability culminating in ejaculation in men. The final phase is the phase of resolution, where there is a relief of sexual tension and general sense of well-being felt by both partners. Post the orgasm phase, women still remain receptive to stimulation. In men, after the phase of resolution, a period of refractoriness for both erection and ejaculation follows; nevertheless, the literature reports a few men report having multiple orgasms without refractory latency both with and without ejaculation (Dunn and Trost 1989).

A sexual dysfunction is defined as a problem affecting any one of the four phases of the sexual response cycle. Strictly stating, only the first three phases are of clinical significance. A sexual dysfunction may be situational (defined as occurring with a specific partner or situation or circumstance) or global. Sexual dysfunction can also be classified as either primary (present lifelong) or secondary (developing secondary to a particular pathology/medical condition). A sexual dysfunction can significantly affect a person's mood, self-esteem, interpersonal relationship and quality of life. Recently, the DSM-IV criteria (Diagnostic and statistical manual of mental disorders) was revised. The DSM-V criteria were published in May 2013 and incorporate several changes. For a person to be diagnosed with sexual dysfunction, the dysfunction should have been present at least for a period of 6 months with a frequency between 75 and 100 % (DSM V 2013). Exceptions to the rule include disorders caused by medications and substance abuse. Importantly the dysfunction should have caused considerable *distress* to both partners. As per the revised

Table 16.2 Revised classification of male and female sexual dysfunction as per DSM-V diagnostic criteria

Male sexual dysfunction	Female sexual dysfunction
Erectile disorder	Female sexual interest/arousal disorder
Male hypoactive sexual desire disorder	Genitopelvic pain/penetration disorder (includes both dyspareunia and vaginismus)
Premature ejaculation	Female orgasmic disorder
Delayed ejaculation	
Substance-/medication-induced sexual dysfunction	
Unspecified sexual dysfunction	

guidelines, there are now three female sexual dysfunctions and four male sexual dysfunctions. Table 16.2 outlines both the male and female sexual dysfunctions as per the revised DSM-V criteria.

An important change of notable mention in the DSM-V guideline is the inclusion of both dyspareunia and vaginismus as a single entity titled genitopelvic pain/penetration disorder. This is because both the conditions show a high degree of overlap, and effective differentiation between these two conditions was not possible.

16.3 Infertility Is Both a Cause and Consequence of Sexual Dysfunction

Sexual dysfunction in an infertility setting represents an unusual yet complex problem. Sexual dysfunctions that lead to infertility in men include erectile disorder and ejaculatory dysfunction. In women, genitopelvic pain/penetration disorder results in nonconsummation of the marriage and prospectively results in infertility. A sexual dysfunction in an infertility setting can have organic or psychogenic cause, although a mixed aetiology is not uncommon. It is important to understand that all organically induced dysfunction will have some degree of psychogenic overlap. A diagnosis of infertility itself may result in some degree of dysfunction. Over 40 % of female patients diagnosed with infertility report lower desire and/or arousal and also report a reduction in the frequency of intercourse (Millheiser et al. 2010). Among males, in a cross-sectional survey conducted among 357 men from 8 academic fertility units, where an independent diagnosis of male factor infertility was made, the diagnosis resulted in highly significant ($p<0.004$) impact on sex life satisfaction and personal quality-of-life scores. The scores remained significant even after controlling for partner age, education status, race, religion, current employment status and duration of infertility (Smith et al. 2009). For most couples, a diagnosis of infertility exerts tremendous psychological, social, physical and financial burden. In a larger study involving over 843 couples, a greater degree of emotional distress and marital discordance was reported by the couples when a male factor infertility was exclusively diagnosed (Connolly et al. 1987). In another cross-sectional study, among

Table 16.3 72 of 544 patients, between February 2014 and January 2015, presented with sexual dysfunction at our clinic

Sexual dysfunction	No of patients
Erectile dysfunction (ED) only	27
Anejaculation with ED	2
Premature ejaculation (PE) with ED	2
Decreased libido with ED	9
Infertility with ED	6
Dyspareunia	2
Sexual Concern	6
Ejaculatory disorders	18
Total	*72*

200 infertile couples, over 41.5 % of couples reported a reduction in sexual desire, while over 52.5 % of couples reported a reduction in sexual satisfaction after a diagnosis of infertility was made (Ramezanzadeh et al. 2006). More importantly the duration of infertility varied inversely to the degree of sexual satisfaction and this relationship reached statistical significance ($p<0.05$).

In our clinic, the Department of Andrology and Reproductive Medicine, Chettinad Super Specialty Hospital, of the 544 male partners of couples who presented for an infertility evaluation between February 2014 and January 2015, 13 % of the men suffered from some form of sexual dysfunction (Table 16.3).

The management of infertility creates pressure and may cause or exacerbate an existing dysfunction. As a part of infertility management, the male partner may be forced to have sexual intercourse at a specific time of the month, around the time of ovulation. The stress to perform, on the day of ovulation, may thus result in a sexual dysfunction. The female partner may also lose interest in intercourse outside the fertile period. A situational dysfunction may result when the patient has difficulty in performing with a specific partner or in a particular situation or a definable circumstance. One example is the act of masturbation; normally a routine and/or pleasurable exercise may become stressful and/or embarrassing when the patient has to collect the entire sample in a wide-mouthed container, especially in a hospital setting.

From a clinical viewpoint, it should be remembered that one sexual dysfunction can frequently mask or exacerbate another dysfunction. One example of relevance would be the finding of a male patient stating that he loses his erection during attempted penetration and the female partner stating she has pain during penetration. One must not be hasty in making a diagnosis of erectile dysfunction in the male and/or vaginismus in the female. A thorough workup and charting of the sexual response cycle individually for each partner coupled with an in-depth history may simply point out that there was inadequate time allocated by the couple for foreplay which led to inadequate lubrication in the female consequently resulting in difficulties in penetration for the male and eventually erectile dysfunction over a period of time. A session of sex education describing the male and female sexual anatomy coupled with an explanation of the human sexual response cycle for these couples would ameliorate the problem.

16.4 Medical Conditions Affecting Sexual Function

Numerous medical conditions can affect sexual function either in a direct or an indirect manner (Ramezanzadeh et al. 2006; Gratzke et al. 2010; Phillips 1998). An in-depth history should comprehensively assess all medical/surgical conditions outlined in Table 16.4. An increased incidence of sexual dysfunction is reported in both men and women with poor physical and/or mental health (Weiner and Rosen 1997; Thranov and Klee 1994; Laumann et al. 1999). Cardiovascular status is an important parameter to be assessed during evaluation of sexual dysfunction in both men and women; patients should be stratified into low risk or high risk categories depending on the cardiac history before entailing on specific therapy for the sexual dysfunction (Miner et al. 2012; DeBusk et al. 2000). Specific medical causes of female sexual dysfunction are outlined in Table 16.5.

The presence of chronic illness can interfere with sexual function; the degree of impairment however depends on when the illness was diagnosed and whether the relationship started before or after a particular diagnosis was made. For an in-depth understanding as to how various chronic illness affects sexual function, please refer to Basson et al. (2010).

Numerous drugs and medications can affect the different phases of the sexual response cycle. These pharmacological agents work through a variety of mechanisms (Horowitz and Goble 1979). Adrenergic antagonists alter epinephrine

Table 16.4 Various medical/surgical conditions that can cause and/or exacerbate sexual dysfunction

Body system	Specific condition associated with sexual dysfunction
Cardiovascular disorders	Atherosclerosis, cardiac failure, aortic aneurysm repair, Leriche's syndrome
Endocrine disorders	Diabetes mellitus, metabolic syndrome, obesity, dyslipidemia, hyperprolactinemia, pituitary adenomas, craniopharyngioma, hypo- and hyperthyroidism, Cushing's syndrome
Genetic causes	Klinefelter's syndrome and bilateral anorchia
Haematological disorders	Anaemia, sickle cell disease and leukaemia
Hepatic disorders	Cirrhosis of the Liver
Infectious causes	Urethritis, vesiculitis, epididymo-orchitis, prostatitis, cystitis, gonorrhoea
Neurological causes	Parkinson's disease, amyotrophic lateral sclerosis, multiple sclerosis, spinal cord injuries, head Injuries, stroke and CNS tumours
Nutritional	Malnutrition, morbid obesity
Surgical	Prostatectomy both perineal and biopsy type, transurethral resection of prostate (TURP), retroperitoneal lymph node dissection (RPLND), lumbar sympathectomy
Andrological/urological disorders	Priapism, urethral strictures, Peyronie's disease, lower urinary tract symptoms (LUTS)
Others	Chemotherapy and radiotherapy, any systemic long-term chronic illness

Table 16.5 Specific causes of female sexual dysfunction

Specific causes of female sexual dysfunction
Genitopelvic pain syndrome, recurrent cystitis, vulvar dystrophy, vulvar vestibulitis, bartholinitis, genital herpes, genital myofascial pain syndrome, pelvic inflammatory disease, episiotomy scars and strictures, endometriosis, hyperprolactinemia, obesity
Chemotherapy and/or radiotherapy, neurogenic disease, breast cancer
Surgeries like hysterectomies, rectal cancer and surgery

Table 16.6 Common drug classes associated with sexual dysfunction

Drug induced dysfunction	
Psychoactive medications	Antipsychotics
	Barbiturates
	Benzodiazepines
	Selective serotonin reuptake inhibitors
	Tricyclic antidepressants
Cardiovascular and antihypertensive medications	Statins
	Antilipid medications
	Beta blockers
	Calcium channel blockers
	Clonidine
	Digoxin
	Spironolactone
	H2 Receptor antagonist
	Proton pump inhibitors
Hormonal preparations	Danazol
	GnRH agonists
	Oral contraceptives

release by blocking adrenergic receptors; examples include reserpine, methyldopa and prazosin. Sexual dysfunction is thus produced by alterations in the emissary or ejaculatory phase. Central nervous system sedating agents like alcohol, barbiturates, antihypertensive and anticonvulsants affect the person's libido and arousal by increasing brain serotonin levels and decreasing dopamine levels (Buffum 1982). Some medications can also cause dysfunction by increasing prolactin levels. An increase in prolactin reduces the testicular response to luteinizing hormone (LH) and results in reduced testosterone production (Segraves et al. 1985). Examples of such medications include cimetidine, phenothiazines and thioxanthenes. Drugs with atropine-like effects affect sexual arousal by their para-sympatholytic action; examples include antiemetics, antipsychotics and antihistamines. An outline of drug categories that affect sexual function is given in Table 16.6. An appropriate adjustment of medication dose or change in the medication itself may sometimes help in alleviating sexual dysfunction. The effect of medication on sexual function will depend on the patient's age, body type and duration of administration.

16.5 Psychosexual Factors Affecting Sexual Function

Sexual dysfunction is rarely caused by a single problem. Usually every sexual dysfunction will have some degree of a psychological involvement which requires evaluation. Depression and anxiety are common causes of sexual dysfunction, although they can also be a consequence of the sexual impairment (Epstein 1983). Other reported findings from empirical studies include diminished self-esteem, guilt and hostility. It is important to realize and understand that there is no clear-cut relationship between sex and marital problems (McCarthy and Fucito 2005). A couple may have a strained marital relationship yet normal sexual function; the vice versa is also true. Nevertheless, the most common factor in a relationship leading to dysfunction is marital dissatisfaction (Metz and McCarthy 2007). Marital dissatisfaction can arise due to unresolved relationship issues, unrealistic expectations from the marriage, problems with the family system and divergent sex values and/or preferences (Habke et al. 1999; Metz et al. 1997).

Other psychosexual factors causing sexual dysfunction include a previous failed sexual encounter, intellectual denial of perceiving sexual pleasure, religious beliefs and childhood and prior sexual trauma (Kaplan 1983). Interestingly, sexual paraphilias (voyeurism, transvestism) can also lead to sexual dysfunction and manifest themselves as erectile dysfunction; these disorders also seem more common than expected as per the task force report from the American Psychiatric Association 1999. In some cases, a sexual dysfunction can arise due to deficient knowledge about the normal sexual physiology.

16.6 Managing Sexual Dysfunction in a Primary Care Setting

The basic management strategy for sexual dysfunction starts with an easily remembered acronym termed as PLISSIT:

P stands for permission giving and includes taking a sexual history, being empathic to the patient and offering sexual information.

LI represents limited information, where the patient is given a limited knowledge about sexual function to alleviate any sexual ignorance if any.

SS stands for specific suggestion, where the practitioner can address and treat organic factors causing the specific sexual problem and also offer various treatment options for the specific dysfunction.

IT denotes intensive therapy; here the practitioner offers expert marital or psychotherapy after assessing the interpersonal conflicts. A referral at this stage can also be done (Taylor and Davis 2006).

A general medical management of all organically induced dysfunctions should be done. For patients presenting with diabetes and erectile dysfunction, meticulous control of blood sugars and lifestyle modification are strictly recommended. Erectile dysfunction is seen with a prevalence ranging from 45 to 70 % in men with coexistent type 2 diabetes. Advancing age, degree of glycemic control, the duration of diabetes, coexistent hypertension, dyslipidemia and sedentary lifestyle along with concomitant smoking and/or alcohol consumption is seen to be significantly associated with the severity of erectile dysfunction as suggested from large-scale studies (Malavige and Levy 2009). The onset of erectile dysfunction in diabetes is invariably secondary. An amalgamated therapeutic strategy involving lifestyle and dietary modification and stoppage of alcohol and/or smoking, along with specific sex therapy for the diagnosed dysfunction, may benefit the patient.

The basic ideology of any sex therapy is to emphasize to the patient his *right to sexual health* and that sexuality is a *normal physiological and psychological process*. The aim here is to train the patient to relax completely, laying the foundation for subsequent sexual excitement. The patient is taught to relax and *sensate focus* on his own bodily sensations and overcome the physiological impediments to a natural sexual response. Most sexual dysfunctions have also been managed by cognitive behavioural therapy, hypnosis and guided imagery. Hypnosis, where a technique of *guided imagery of successful performance* is given to the patient, has been tried for the treatment of non-organic erectile dysfunction, but much larger studies are required to verify the observed benefits (Aydin et al. 1996).

Recommended medical management of erectile dysfunction is with the utilization of phosphodiesterase inhibitors (PDE-5i's). PDE-5i's like sildenafil, tadalafil and vardenafil are recommended as first-line drugs for the management of both organic/psychogenic and mixed aetiology erectile dysfunction. A number of multicenter double-blind placebo controlled RCTs have proven the benefit of these agents in improving the erectile function significantly from baseline after 4 weeks of therapy (Goldstein et al. 2003). A cardiovascular history and risk stratification should be done before starting PDE-5i therapy. An absolute contraindication to PDE-5i therapy is when the patient is on nitrate therapy and if he has a history of unstable angina or an attack of myocardial infarction in the preceding 6 months. The side effect profile of PDE-5i is proven to be minimal, and therapy can be safely advocated for a period of 6 months (Morales et al. 1998).

Premature ejaculation is a common dysfunction seen in the clinic and is defined *as a male sexual dysfunction characterized by ejaculation which always or nearly always occurs before or within about one minute of vaginal penetration, and the inability to delay ejaculation on all or nearly all vaginal penetrations, and negative personal consequences, such as distress, bother, frustration and/or the avoidance of sexual intimacy* (McMahon et al. 2008). This definition is however not evidence based, and a global consensus on definition of PE is still lacking. Selective serotonin reuptake inhibitors have been used in the off-label management of PE (Khan and Pandiyan 2015). But concern has been raised about their safety profile. Other therapeutic modalities include behavioural techniques such as the start-stop technique proposed by Seman and squeeze-pinch technique of Masters (Grenier and Byers 1997). In this technique, during sexual autostimulation, as the man approaches orgasm, he squeezes firmly under the corona of the glans penis thereby inhibiting the ejaculatory reflex. A variation of this method utilizes the Kegel's technique, where the man is trained to relax his pubococcygeus muscle to further inhibit ejaculation. The combination of these techniques may work better than when utilizing a single technique alone (Elia and Bergman 1993). Kegel's exercise has also been recommended for the management of psychogenic erectile disorder in men apart from PE.

Kegel's exercises in women help in improving the perivaginal muscle tone, as there is a certain degree of correlation between the muscle tone and sexual arousal felt. Kegel's exercises if done regularly can improve the tone of the pubococcygeus muscle and when combined with sex education/cognitive behavioural therapy and/or systematic desensitization may help alleviate disorders of orgasm in women. These empirical treatments are better than placebo, and currently there are no pharmacological agents that can be used for the management of female disorders of orgasm (Meston et al. 2004). Flibanserin, an antidepressant, has recently been approved by the FDA to treat hypoactive sexual desire disorders in postmenopausal women, amidst much controversy (Simon et al. 2014).

Some general treatment measures which could be followed for the management of female sexual dysfunction encourage the utilization of explicit sexual material like erotic videos, break the routine and fix up a *date* for 'sexual activity', sensate focus exercises, encourage noncoital behaviour, application of topical lidocaine and warm baths before intercourse, biofeedback and lastly adoption of a change in sex position, i.e. like the 'women on top' (Striar and Bartlik 1999). Estrogens have been used to improve sexual desire, although benefits are not seen uniformly across all patients. The exact relation between sexual function and hormonal levels remains yet to be established (Laan and van Lunsen 1997). There is currently insufficient evidence to suggest the use of testosterone to treat disorders of desire or arousal in females, an added concern in testosterone therapies is the development of virilising effects in women like hirsutism and acne.

Disorders of arousal usually develop secondary to inadequate stimulation at least in older women. Management strategies involve the use of commercially available lubricants along with sex education/cognitive behavioural therapy. Genitopelvic pain disorders in the female can be categorized depending on the nature of pain whether superficial or deep. Superficial pain is related to urogenital atrophy and/or a lack of arousal and is associated with penetration, whereas deep pain is related to pelvic pathology. Recommended treatment is by utilizing a technique of progressive vaginal muscle relaxation and utilization of commercially available vaginal dilators (Phillips 2000). Once a sufficient degree of dilatation is achieved, the partner may attempt penile penetration.

Conclusion

Sexual dysfunction in an infertility clinic represents a common yet complex problem. The key to successful management is by eliciting a proper sexual history, investigating with appropriate laboratory tests and utilizing standardized treatment guidelines recommended for the suspected dysfunction. Proper management of sexual dysfunction requires a multidisciplinary team-based approach. An important point to understand is that the very diagnosis of infertility itself can result in dysfunction in either the male and/or the female partner. The couple must be counselled on the fact that infertility and sexual dysfunction are two distinct issues that have to be managed separately. Patients should be advised and reassured that they have a right to enjoy and relish their sexual health. Patient referral to an expert is warranted in complicated cases, when preliminary management strategies fail.

References

Abramson PR, Pinkerton SD. With pleasure: thoughts on the nature of human sexuality. New York: Oxford University Press; 2002.

American Psychiatric Association. Task force on sexually dangerous offenders. Dangerous sex offenders: a task force report of the American Psychiatric Association. Washington, D.C: American Psychiatric Pub; 1999.

American Psychiatric Association. Diagnostic and statistical manual of mental disorders (DSM-5®). Washington, DC: American Psychiatric Publication; 2013.

Aydin S, Odabas Ö, Ercan M, Kara H, Agargün MY. Efficacy of testosterone, trazodone and hypnotic suggestion in the treatment of non-organic male sexual dysfunction. Br J Urol. 1996;77(2):256–60.

Basson R, Rees P, Wang R, Montejo AL, Incrocci L. Sexual function in chronic illness. J Sex Med. 2010;7(1pt2):374–88.

Buffum J. Pharmacosexology: the effects of drugs on sexual function–a review. J Psychoactive Drugs. 1982;14(1–2):5–44.

Connolly KJ, Edelmann RJ, Cooke ID. Distress and marital problems associated with infertility. J Reprod Infant Psychol. 1987;5(1):49–57.

DeBusk R, Drory Y, Goldstein I, Jackson G, Kaul S, Kimmel SE, Kostis JB, Kloner RA, Lakin M, Meston CM, Mittleman M. Management of sexual dysfunction in patients with cardiovascular disease: recommendations of the Princeton Consensus Panel. Am J Cardiol. 2000;86(2):62–8.

Dunn ME, Trost JE. Male multiple orgasms: a descriptive study. Arch Sex Behav. 1989;18:377–87.

Elia G, Bergman A. Pelvic muscle exercises: when do they work? Obstetrics Gynecol. 1993;81(2):283–6.

Epstein N. Cognitive therapy with couples. Springer, Pennsylvania; 1983.

Frank E, Anderson C, Rubinstein D. Frequency of sexual dysfunction in normal couples. N Engl J Med. 1978;299(3):111–5.

Goldstein I, Young JM, Fischer J, Bangerter K, Segerson T, Taylor T. Vardenafil, a new phosphodiesterase type 5 inhibitor, in the treatment of erectile dysfunction in men with diabetes a multicenter double-blind placebo-controlled fixed-dose study. Diabetes Care. 2003;26(3):777–83.

Gratzke C, et al. Anatomy, physiology, and patho-physiology of erectile dysfunction. J Sex Med. 2010;7(1 Pt 2):445–75.

Grenier G, Byers ES. The relationships among ejaculatory control, ejaculatory latency, and attempts to prolong heterosexual intercourse. Arch Sex Behav. 1997;26(1):27–47.

Habke AM, Hewitt PL, Flett GL. Perfectionism and sexual satisfaction in intimate relationships. J Psychopathol Beha Asses. 1999;21(4):307–22.

Halvorsen JG, Metz ME. Sexual dysfunction, part II: diagnosis, management, and prognosis. J Am Board Fam Pract. 1992;5(2):177–92.

Horowitz JD, Goble AJ. Drugs and impaired male sexual function. Drugs. 1979;18(3):206–17.

Kaplan HS. The evaluation of sexual disorders: psychological and medical aspects. New York: Psychology Press; 1983.

Kaplan HS. The new sex therapy. Springer, New York; 1980.

Khan SD, Pandiyan N. Ejaculatory dysfunction—a mini review. Adv SexMed. 2015;5(02):39.

Laan E, van Lunsen RH. Hormones and sexuality in postmenopausal women: a psychophysiological study. J Psychosom Obstet Gynecol. 1997;18:126–33.

Laumann EO, et al. The epidemiology of erectile dysfunction: results from the national health and social life survey. Int J Impot Res. 1999;11 Suppl 1:S60–4.
Malavige LS, Levy JC. Erectile dysfunction in diabetes mellitus. J Sex Med. 2009;6(5):1232–47.
Masters WH, Masters VJ. Human sexual response. New York: Bantam Books; 1986.
McCarthy BW, Fucito LM. Integrating medication, realistic expectations, and therapeutic interventions in the treatment of male sexual dysfunction. J Sex Marital Ther. 2005;31(4):319–28.
McMahon CG, Althof SE, Waldinger MD, Porst H, Dean J, Sharlip ID, Adaikan PG, Becher E, Broderick GA, Buvat J, Dabees K. REPORT: an evidence-based definition of lifelong premature ejaculation: report of the International Society for Sexual Medicine (ISSM) Ad Hoc committee for the definition of premature ejaculation. J Sex Med. 2008;5(7):1590–606.
Meston CM, Buss DM. Why humans have sex. Arch Sex Beha. 2007;36(4):477–507.
Meston CM, Hull E, Levin RJ, Sipski M. Disorders of orgasm in women. J Sex Med. 2004;1(1):66–8.
Metz ME, McCarthy BW. The "Good-Enough Sex" model for couple sexual satisfaction. Sex Relation Therapy. 2007;22(3):351–62.
Metz ME, Pryor JL, Nesvacil LJ, Abuzzahab Sr F, Koznar J. Premature ejaculation: a psychophysiological review. J Sex Marital Ther. 1997;23(1):3–23.
Millheiser LS, Helmer AE, Quintero RB, Westphal LM, Milki AA, Lathi RB. Is infertility a risk factor for female sexual dysfunction? A case–control study. Fertil Steril. 2010;94(6):2022–5.
Miner M, et al. Cardiometabolic risk and female sexual health: the Princeton III summary. J Sex Med. 2012;9(3):641–51.
Morales A, Gingell C, Collins M, Wicker PA, Osterloh IH, Montorsi F, Wagner G. Clinical safety of oral sildenafil citrate (ViagraTM) in the treatment of erectile dysfunction. Int J Impot Res. 1998;10(2):69–74.
Padma-Nathan H, Steers WD, Wicker PA. Efficacy and safety of oral sildenafil in the treatment of erectile dysfunction: a double-blind, placebo-controlled study of 329 patients. Sildenafil Study Group. Int J Clin Pract. 1998;52(6):375–9.
Phillips NA. The clinical evaluation of dyspareunia. Int J Impot Res. 1998;10 Suppl 2:S117–20.
Phillips NA. Female sexual dysfunction: evaluation and treatment. Am Fam Physician. 2000;62(1):127–48.
Ramezanzadeh F, Aghssa MM, Jafarabadi M, Zayeri F. Alterations of sexual desire and satisfaction in male partners of infertile couples. Fertil Steril. 2006;85(1):139–43.
Read S, King M, Watson J. Sexual dysfunction in primary medical care: prevalence, characteristics and detection by the general practitioner. J Public Health. 1997;19(4):387–91.
Rosen R, Altwein J, Boyle P, Kirby RS, Lukacs B, Meuleman E, O'Leary MP, Puppo P, Robertson C, Giuliano F. Lower urinary tract symptoms and male sexual dysfunction: the multinational survey of the aging male (MSAM-7). Eur Urol. 2003;44(6):637–49.
Segraves RT, Madsen R, Carter CS, Davis JM. Erectile dysfunction associated with pharmacological agents. In: Diagnosis and treatment of erectile disturbances. Springer, New york; 1985. p. 23–63.
Simon JA, Kingsberg SA, Shumel B, Hanes V, Garcia Jr M, Sand M. Efficacy and safety of flibanserin in postmenopausal women with hypoactive sexual desire disorder: results of the SNOWDROP trial. Menopause. 2014;21:633–40.
Smith JF, Walsh TJ, Shindel AW, Turek PJ, Wing H, Pasch L, Katz PP. Sexual, marital, and social impact of a man's perceived infertility diagnosis. J Sex Med. 2009;6(9):2505–15.
Striar S, Bartlik B. Stimulation of the libido: the use of erotica in sex therapy. Psychiatric Anna. 1999;29(1):60–2.
Taylor B, Davis S. Using the extended PLISSIT model to address sexual healthcare needs. Nurs Stand. 2006;21(11):35–40.
Thranov I, Klee M. Sexuality among gynaecologic cancer patients—a cross-sectional study. Gynecol Oncol. 1994;52:14–9.
Weiner DN, Rosen RC. Medications and their impact. In: Sipski ML, Alexander CJ, editors. Sexual function in people with disability and chronic illness: a health professional's guide. Gaithersburg: Aspen; 1997.

Index

K. Gunasekaran, N. Pandiyan (eds.), *Male Infertility*,
DOI 10.1007/978-81-322-3604-7